The Older Cancer Patient

A Guide for Nurses and Related Professionals

Janine Overcash, PhD, ARNP, is an Assistant Professor of Nursing at the University of South Florida, College of Nursing in Tampa, Florida. Dr. Overcash received her PhD in Anthropology from the University of the South and did her graduate research on breast cancer of the older woman at the H. Lee Moffitt Cancer Center and Research Institute in Tampa, Florida.

Dr. Overcash has published many articles on the assessment of the older cancer patient. She is currently engaged in research to examine the ways of applying the comprehensive geriatric assessment to cancer patients in the outpatient setting. Dr. Overcash has given many lectures nationally and internationally concerning the needs of the older cancer patient.

Lodovico Balducci, MD, is Professor of Medicine & Oncology, University of South Florida College of Medicine, and Program Leader of the Senior Adult Oncology Program at the H. Lee Moffitt Cancer Center & Research Institute in Tampa, Florida. Dr. Balducci received his medical degree from Catholic University, Rome, Italy, and his residency training and fellowship at the University of Mississippi Medical Center, Jackson, Mississippi.

Dr. Balducci has edited the only two existing textbooks on geriatric oncology. He is currently the Program Leader of the only existing geriatric oncology program in the country and the world. Dr. Balducci has published over 130 articles in various medical journals on the subject of geriatric oncology, and five monographs on geriatric oncology. Dr. Balducci's clinical research activities include cancer and aging, management of the frail elderly, assessment of quality of life in the older cancer patient, prognostic assessment of the older cancer patient, and interactions of comorbidity and function in the older cancer patient. Dr. Balducci is a member of ASCO's Public Issues Committee and Task Force on Cancer and Aging.

Dr. Balducci is board certified in Geriatric Medicine and Medical Oncology/Hematology. He is a member of the American Geriatrics Society, the American Society of Clinical Oncology, American Association for Cancer Research, American Society of Hematology, American Society of Breast Disease, and a fellow of the American College of Physicians. Dr. Balducci has lectured throughout the USA, Europe, Asia, Australia, and South America.

The Older Cancer Patient

A Guide for Nurses and Related Professionals

Janine Overcash, PhD, ARNP
Lodovico Balducci, MD

Editors

 Springer Publishing Company

FREY
RC
281
.A34
O435
2003

Springer Publishing Company, Inc.
536 Broadway
New York, NY 10012-3955

Acquisitions Editor: Ruth Chasek
Production Editor: Jeanne Libby
Cover design by Joanne Honigman

03 04 05 06 07 / 5 4 3 2 1

Library of Congress Cataloging-in-Publication Data

The older cancer patient : a guide for nurses and related professionals /
Janine Overcash, Lodovico Balducci, editors
    p. cm.
    Includes bibliographical references and index.
    ISBN 0-8261-1805-4
    1. Geriatric oncology. 2. Cancer—Nursing. I. Overcash, Janine.
II. Balducci, Lodovico.
    [DNLM: 1. Neoplasms—therapy—Aged. 2. Neoplasms—
diagnosis—Aged. 3. Quality of Life—Aged. 4. Social Support—
Aged QZ 266 O44 2003]
    RC281.A34.O435 2003
    618.97'6994—dc21

                  2003042360

Printed in the United States of America by Maple-Vail Book Manufacturing Group.

Contents

Contributors

John Barrett
Department of Psychology
Xavier University
Cincinnati, Ohio

Scott D. Barnett
Director of Epidemiology and
    Biostatistics
Inova Heart Center
Falls Church, Virginia

Ira Byock
Research Professor of Philosophy
Director of the Palliative Care
    Service
University of Montana
Missoula, Montana

Linda Casey
James A. Haley Veterans Hospital
University of South Florida
Tampa, Florida

Hongbin Chen
Research Associate in the Senior
    Adult Oncology Program
Moffitt Cancer Center and
    Research Institute
University of South Florida
Tampa, Florida

Yvonne Corbeil
Director of Program Development
Palliative Care Services
University of Montana
Missoula, Montana

Kathy Effingham
Primary Care Nurse
Senior Adult Oncology Program
Moffitt Cancer Center and
    Research Institute
University of South Florida
Tampa, Florida

Martine Extermann
Senior Adult Oncology Program
Moffitt Cancer Center and
    Research Institute
University of South Florida
Tampa, Florida

Adam Golden
Department of Internal Medicine
Orlando Regional Healthcare
Orlando, Florida

William Haley
Chair of the Department of
    Gerontology
University of South Florida
Tampa, Florida

Janice T. Hoff
Nurse Practitioner
West Florida Hospital Senior
  Health Services
Pensacola, Florida

Sandra Holley
Nurse Scientist
Post-doctoral Research Fellow
VISN 8 Patient Safety Center of
  Inquiry
Tampa, Florida

Mary Ann Marsh
Primary Care Nurse
Senior Adult Oncology Program
Moffitt Cancer Center and
  Research Institute
University of South Florida
Tampa, Florida

Julie Meyer
Nurse Practitioner
Coordinator of the Senior Adult
  Oncology Program
Moffitt Cancer Center and
  Research Institute
University of South Florida
Tampa, Florida

Neil Nesbaum
Geriatrics/Long Term Care
  Service Line Director
Veterans Affairs Capital Health
  Care Network
Fort Howard, Maryland

Patricia Ryan
Clinical Program Director
VISN 8 e-Care Coordination
  Service
VA Medical Center, Bay Pines,
  Florida

Michael A. Silverman
VA Medical Center
Clinical Professor of Medicine
West Virginia School of
  Osteopathic Medicine
Martinsburg, West Virginia

Leah Sisler
Department of Nursing
University of South Florida
Tampa, Florida

Katherine K. Stanley
Nurse Practitioner
West Florida Hospital Senior
  Health Services
Milton, Florida

Babu Zachariah
James A. Haley Veterans
  Hospital
University of South Florida
Tampa, Florida

Introduction

The aging of the population involves a number of medical and ethical consequences. These include management of patients with multiple conditions, and of vulnerable, demented, socially isolated, and frail patients. The diverse face of aging calls for a multidisciplinary, yet individualized approach to the older person that somehow transcends the traditional nursing models. A disease process is an aspect of a multidimensional picture in which medical, functional, emotional, cognitive, and social issues are interwoven. No single provider has the competence and the expertise to address these different issues simultaneously. He or she treating the disease needs to interpret findings in the social, nutritional, and pharmacological areas with the help of specialists in these fields. This is where the need for a multidisciplinary treatment team becomes apparent. In addition, the treatment plans need to be coordinated by a person capable of implementing a complex and multidisciplinary intervention. Hence, the emergence of the nurse as a central figure in the multidisciplinary team, who is involved in assessment, treatment, and evaluation of the senior patient. Geriatrics has certainly highlighted the central role of nursing in the management of the patient. In this book we apply the principles of care of the elderly to the special problem of the older person with cancer.

Cancer is an ideal model to study elderly management for the following reasons:

- Cancer is a disease of aging: 60% of all neoplasms in the USA occur in the 12% of the population aged 65 and over;
- Cancer is still the second most common cause of death for older individuals, and is expected to become the first, due to the decline in cardiovascular death;

- Cancer is generally a chronic disease, involving a prolonged and multifaceted relationship with the provider;
- The management of cancer is influenced by other diseases, poor function, malnutrition, cognitive impairment, depression, social isolation: virtually all older cancer patients do benefit from a multidisciplinary intervention;
- Cancer affects mostly a population of so-called vulnerable elderly which is a population most likely to experience a loss of functional dependence and a decline in general health as a result of cancer and its treatment. Arguably, this is the population that benefits most from astute case management.

This book was conceived as a reference primarily for nurses and advanced practice nurses managing older patients with cancer. In addition to the practical principles relating to the prevention and the treatment of cancer in older patients, and the implementation of a multidisciplinary team, nurses and other health care providers will find an outline of urgent research issues that pertain to the care of the elderly in this book. As management of the older person is largely uncharted water, well-planned research in geriatrics is essential to effective care.

The goal of this book is threefold. First, we want to present an overview of cancer in the elderly. In particular we want to underscore three points:

1. that cancer in the older person is more often than not preventable and treatable;
2. that a multidisciplinary team is necessary for the optimal management of the older person;
3. that the role of the nurse as case-manager needs to be contained with the role of patient advocate.

To make these points we review the epidemiology of cancer and aging, the benefits of cancer prevention and cancer treatment in the older person, the role of the multidisciplinary team, and the barriers to effective prevention and treatment. To assist practitioners in complex medical decisions, we provide a thorough description of clinical trials involving older cancer patients, a description of current guidelines for ameliorating the toxicity of chemotherapy in older individuals, a description of geriatric assessment and its value under specific circumstances, and practical application of quality-of-life assessment and decision-analysis. In addition we highlight the importance of cultural competence and end-of-life care issues.

Second, we wish to open a forum for practitioners of different specialties regarding the management of cancer in the older person. In a society that is rapidly evolving, the current approach to medicine is becoming obsolete. An ongoing discussion of new findings, and an ongoing exchange of experiences is the only way to translate into clinical practice new research findings, and at the same time to maintain health care that is congruent with the population it is supposed to serve. Here the time-honored nursing role of mediator between the scientific and the human aspects of medicine becomes important. The description of clinical approaches to the older patient is purposefully provocative to fuel the debate and to entreat the attention of the reader.

Last, but not least, this book is the description of the personal adventure of a nurse and a physician who planned single-handedly almost nine years ago, a multidisciplinary program devoted to the treatment of the older cancer patient, within a major cancer center. At that time our approach was unique and highly controversial. The success of our collaboration is witnessed by the fact that our model is now reproduced around the country and around the world, and by the fact that the American Society of Clinical Oncology has now established a special curriculum for the management of older persons with cancer and has instituted 15 experimental fellowships in Geriatric Oncology. We hope we are not the best, because we wish to see a progressive improvement in this important field, but we certainly have been the first. We feel it is only fair to share with our readers our sense of accomplishment that includes a deeply felt and lasting friendship.

We wish to thank the persons who have been the main participants in our endeavor: Anita Klamo, the program secretary, has been since the very beginning the soul of the program. Kathy Effingham, RN, Carolyn Kline, RN, and Paulette Daniels, RN, and her predecessor Margaret Bina, RN, have mostly inspired this book thanks to the compassionate care they have provided. Julie Meyer, the ARPN who recently joined the program has become an example of care coordinator; Martine Extermann, MD, PhD, who has joined us from Switzerland, has become the director of the program for innovative research; Margaret McGinnis, MSW has provided invaluable assistance both to our patients and to our research plans; Theresa Thomasewski, RD has provided a continuous, reliable, and highly appreciated dietary assessment of the older persons with cancer; and Mary Beth Corcoran, the program pharmacist, has fought harder than anybody the plague of polypharmacy. And, most of all, we'd like to thank the thousands of patients who have walked through our program and to whom this book is dedicated.

JANINE OVERCASH, PhD, ARNP
LODOVICO BALDUCCI, MD

Overview

Kathy's Diagnosis

Kathy Clark finished her jog, as she has done for the last 30 years in the mornings. The mornings in California were beautiful and Kathy loved rising early and getting her day started. Kathy was 72 but could pass for someone twenty years younger. Kathy had always thought the key to youth was keeping busy, something she practiced faithfully, especially since her divorce was about to be final. Kathy loved dining out, late night card games, beach outings, and church activities, all of which kept her social calendar packed. Kathy was determined not to slow down and become that 72-year-old, old lady.

A familiar car pulled into the driveway. It was Mary, Kathy's youngest daughter, who was in her sixth month of pregnancy and looked beautiful. Kathy was initially worried about Mary being pregnant, because Mary is single and an independent career woman with a great job in the record industry. Kathy is now very excited about the birth of her grandchild, her first grandchild. Out from the red car bounded Mary, suntanned, full of youth, and not physically limited by pregnancy in the least. Kathy always thought her daughter looked very young. "Mary will be 38 next year," thought Kathy as Mary's thick black heels clicked on the driveway as she hurried to give her mother a hug.

"I stopped by before work so I could be the first to congratulate you on such a momentous day," exclaimed Mary as she released her mother from a vigorous hug.

"Thanks, but I haven't heard anything yet this morning. The attorney is probably not in the office yet, " replied Kathy flatly. "Just think, after three years of hell everything will be final today. You will get closure on this whole ordeal," said Mary as she took off her sunglasses, turning her face to the rising morning sun.

"Three years of hell? Try 41 years of hell. Your Dad was never easy to live with. When I get the divorce papers, then I'll have my cloooossure, as you call it," responded Kathy.

"So mom, would you like to get something to eat after I get home tonight? I shouldn't be too late and we could go to Bert's and get a burger."

"No, I'm going to play cards with the girls tonight, but I can go tomorrow," replied Kathy, thinking about how much she enjoyed her card games with Sarah, Kim, and Carol. "OK, well, I'll call later," muttered Mary, looking a little hurt as she jumped back into her car and started the engine.

Mary spun down the drive. Kathy watched after her, already beginning to regret her decision. She thought as she turned to open the front door, "I've spent my life worrying, protecting, and loving my family. Today I start to live for myself."

The phone was ringing as Kathy walked across the cool living room.

"Hello," answered Kathy while looking at her calendar, realizing she had made dinner plans for tomorrow night with girls from the literary club.

"Hello, Mrs. Clark?" said a vaguely familiar voice.

"Yes," responded Kathy, thinking that she would have to break her plans with the girls tomorrow and go out with Mary.

"This is Catherine Phillips, the nurse from Dr. Tate's office. A small abnormality was found on your mammogram yesterday, and we would like you to come in so we can rule out any problems."

"OK, what kind of problems? asked Kathy, knowing full well the kind of problems to which the young nurse was referring. Kathy had many friends that had been diagnosed with various forms of cancer. She had frequently fantasized how she would handle such an insult to her health.

"Well, Mrs. Clark, whenever an abnormality is discovered on a mammogram, further testing must be performed to detect breast cancer. Most likely the spot is nothing, but we would like you to come in and have us check it out. Can you come in today?" asked Ms. Phillips.

"Sure," replied Kathy involuntarily. "Let's get this over with so I don't worry about this for nights on end."

"We have an opening at 2:00?"

"That would be fine." Kathy put down the phone and fed the cats. She began telling herself, that worrying was not going to help. "I just survived an awful divorce. I guess I can survive anything." Kathy had always maintained her calm in a crisis. Historically, she had silently dealt with previous hardships and crises as times or events to move through, not to be belabored with heightened anxiety or emotion.

Dr. Tate's office was characteristically busy. Kathy could not find a seat, so she leaned against the wall in a dimly lit corner with the latest edition of Glamour. *After two hours of waiting, an attendant finally led her into an extremely cold examination room. She seemed indifferent to the reason for Kathy's visit. A flimsy green hospital gown awaited Kathy on the examination table. As the attendant was leaving the room, she muttered, "The doctor will be right in." Approximately 10 minutes later, the handsome Dr. Tate burst through the exam room door.*

"Good afternoon, Mrs. Clark, I'm glad you're here. Looks like the mammogram showed a small abnormality on your left breast. I just wanted to get a biopsy today to rule out any problems. We should have the results later today or early tomorrow," said Dr. Tate in a calm and even manner.

"Just my luck," thought Kathy, "as soon as I get free from my husband, I come down with cancer."

Kathy left the doctor's office feeling down. "The doctor said that it most likely was nothing, but the way my luck has been running, I wouldn't be surprised if it were something." Kathy turned off the interstate and proceeded down the beautiful tree-lined streets of her neighborhood. "Well, I'm not going to let this worry me." "There's nothing I can do about it now." Suddenly, she remembered that she was planning to meet the girls for cards. Carol lives about 20 minutes from Kathy. Kathy has known Carol for over forty years, seeing her regularly for shopping, card games, and movies. Mary and Margaret, Carol's daughter, went to school together. Kim and Sarah have also been longtime friends, but Kathy has never had the connection with them she has with Carol. Kathy began imagining how her friends might react if she told them of her possible cancer diagnosis. Her mind played many scenes, none of which Kathy remotely liked. If this thing did indeed turn up cancerous, she did not want people to feel sorry for her, react fatalistically, or even treat her the least bit differently. Her decision was made as she opened the door to Carol's home; she would not tell her friends.

The next morning Kathy was awakened by the phone. It was the call she had been awaiting earnestly for three years.

"Hello, Mrs. Clark?" asked a woman's voice

"Yes," answered Kathy, as her voice was slow to respond in the morning.

"This is Sheila from Ms. Lambert's office. It looks like all the paper-work is done. We received Mr. Jone's signatures late yesterday, so it looks like everything is final. Your divorce is finally over."

"Thank you," replied Kathy, "You've made my day!"

Kathy bounced from bed and opened the blinds. The pale morning sun entered the room. Kathy threw on her robe and made her way to the kitchen. As she was filling the coffeepot, her thoughts began to focus on her garden and how she was going to plant more lavender around the little pond. "That will be a good project for today."
Kathy spent the entire day planting and replanting lavender, day lily, and several types of field daisies. At about 3:00 the phone rang.

"Kathy, the biopsy is back and it looks like there is some cancer. I want to refer you to a surgeon at the university," says Dr. Tate in a very clinical tone.

"Yes," replied Kathy, barely able to speak.

"Someone from his office will most likely call you today," said Dr. Tate as the sound of shuffling papers made its way through the phone.

"Yes," said Kathy in disbelief.

As Kathy put down the phone, she began to feel numb. "How could such a thing happen to me? Haven't I been through enough? After 41 years of a bad marriage, I'm now rewarded with a cancer diagnosis on the day my divorce is final. Great!" thought Kathy as she sat at the kitchen table to collect her thoughts. "Well, if this is what I'm dealt, then I have to deal with it." Kathy got up and headed for the shower. She was scheduled to meet her daughter for dinner. As she pulled off her shirt, Kathy stared at her breasts. She had always had a beautiful body, healthy, very athletic. How could she have cancer? Kathy finished her shower and selected her outfit. As she dressed, she considered the possibility of losing her breast. What would my body look like? How would I look in clothes? Does this mean I have to take chemotherapy and lose my hair? I just had a mammogram last year. This thing could not be very big.

The door opened and Mary appeared looking as beautiful as ever, her abdomen filling her maternity blouse. "Guess what, mom?" Mary asked, smiling broadly. "I got my promotion and they're transferring me to Florida! It will only be for a little while, but I'm very excited. Did you hear anything from the attorney?

"Yes, everything is final. Finally," replied Kathy.

"Well, you don't sound too happy."

"I am. I'm just tired," said Kathy as she picked up her keys and led the way out the door.

As they reached the restaurant, Mary chatted about her job and her upcoming move.

"Oh, mom, things are beginning to look up for us. You are a free woman, and I am moving on with my career! Let's order something sinful, with lots of chocolate!"

Dinner proceeded, with Mary continuously chirping about various issues, mostly concerning her work and her friends. Dessert came and Mary noticed that her mother had been uncharacteristically quiet and didn't even eat much of her dinner.

"Mom, what's wrong? You've been quiet all night."

"Mary, I had a breast biopsy yesterday, and the doctor has found cancer," said Kathy in a very calm, matter-of-fact voice.

"Oh, my God! What does this mean?" said Mary as tears began filling her eyes.

"I'm not sure, I have to go to the doctor tomorrow. Some surgeon Dr. Tate suggested."

"Well, mom, I would like to be there," squeaked Mary, her voice hindered by emotion.

"No, Mary, don't get too upset yet. Let's see what we're dealing with." Kathy concluded the dinner much like a business woman ending a meeting.

CHAPTER ONE

Epidemiology and Pathology of Cancer and Aging

Janine Overcash and Lodovico Balducci

T his chapter reviews the epidemiology of cancer in the elderly. Epidemiology represents an opportunity to pursue the following:

- To illustrate the extent and scope of the problem;
- To explain that reduction in cancer-related morbidity and mortality in the older person is paramount to cancer control;
- To explore the biological mechanisms linking age and cancer, and the possibility of preventative interventions;
- To describe a profile of the older person with cancer. This profile will demonstrate that the benefits of cancer prevention and cancer treatment generally overwhelm the risks, even in the aged.

THE CHANGING DEMOGRAPHIC LANDSCAPE

The average life expectancy in the United States has been progressively increasing (Table 1.1), while at the same time the birth rate has declined (National Center for Health Statistics, 1991). The combination of these events has led to a phenomenon known by demographers as "squaring of the pyramid" (Figure 1.1) (Yancik & Ries, 1998). At the beginning of the century, a graphic description of the population of the USA (and of the other Western countries) appeared as a pyramid, with a large base of persons under 20 and a small top of persons over 65. In 1990, the picture looked more like a trapezoid,

TABLE 1.1 Estimated life expectancy at birth in years, by race and sex: Death-registration States, 1900–28, and United States, 1929–99*

Area and year[1]	All races			White			Black[4]		
	Both sexes	Male	Female	Both sexes	Male	Female	Both sexes	Male	Female
United States[1]									
1999	76.7	73.9	79.4	77.3	74.6	79.9	71.4	67.8	74.7
1998	76.7	73.8	79.5	77.3	74.5	80.0	71.3	67.6	74.8
1997	76.5	73.6	79.4	77.2	74.3	79.9	71.1	67.2	74.7
1996	76.1	73.1	79.1	76.8	73.9	79.7	70.2	66.1	74.2
1995	75.8	72.5	78.9	76.5	73.4	79.6	69.6	65.2	73.9
1994	75.7	72.4	79.0	76.5	73.3	79.6	69.5	64.9	73.9
1993	75.5	72.2	78.8	76.3	73.1	79.5	69.2	64.6	73.7
1992	75.8	72.3	79.1	76.5	73.2	79.8	69.6	65.0	73.9
1991	75.5	72.0	78.9	76.3	72.9	79.6	69.3	64.6	73.8
1990	75.4	71.8	78.8	76.1	72.7	79.4	69.1	64.5	73.6
1989	75.1	71.7	78.5	75.9	72.5	79.2	68.8	64.3	73.3
1988	74.9	71.4	78.3	75.6	72.2	78.9	68.9	64.4	73.2
1987	74.9	71.4	78.3	75.6	72.1	78.9	69.1	64.7	73.4
1986	74.7	71.2	78.2	75.4	71.9	78.8	69.1	64.8	73.4
1985	74.7	71.1	78.2	75.3	71.8	78.7	69.3	65.0	73.4
1984	74.7	71.1	78.2	75.3	71.8	78.7	69.5	65.3	73.6
1983	74.6	71.0	78.1	75.2	71.6	78.7	69.4	65.2	73.5
1982	74.5	70.8	78.1	75.1	71.5	78.7	69.4	65.1	73.6
1981	74.1	70.4	77.8	74.8	71.1	78.4	68.9	64.5	73.2
1980	73.7	70.0	77.4	74.4	70.7	78.1	68.1	63.8	72.5
1979	73.9	70.0	77.8	74.6	70.8	78.4	68.5	64.0	72.9
1978	73.5	69.6	77.3	74.1	70.4	78.0	68.1	63.7	72.4

TABLE 1.1 *(continued)*

Area and year	All races			White			Black[4]		
	Both sexes	Male	Female	Both sexes	Male	Female	Both sexes	Male	Female
United States *(continued)*									
1977	73.3	69.5	77.2	74.0	70.2	77.9	67.7	63.4	72.0
1976	72.9	69.1	76.8	73.6	69.9	77.5	67.2	62.9	71.6
1975	72.6	68.8	76.6	73.4	69.5	77.3	66.8	62.4	71.3
1974	72.0	68.2	75.9	72.8	69.0	76.7	66.0	61.7	70.3
1973	71.4	67.6	75.3	72.2	68.5	76.1	65.0	60.9	69.3
1972	71.2	67.4	75.1	72.0	68.3	75.9	64.7	60.4	69.1
1971	71.1	67.4	75.0	72.0	68.3	75.8	64.6	60.5	68.9
1970	70.8	67.1	74.7	71.7	68.0	75.6	64.1	60.0	68.3
1969	70.5	66.8	74.4	71.4	67.7	75.3	64.5	60.6	68.6
1968	70.2	66.6	74.1	71.1	67.5	75.0	64.1	60.4	67.9
1967	70.5	67.0	74.3	71.4	67.8	75.2	64.9	61.4	68.5
1966	70.2	66.7	73.9	71.1	67.5	74.8	64.2	60.9	67.6
1965	70.2	66.8	73.8	71.1	67.6	74.8	64.3	61.2	67.6
1964	70.2	66.8	73.7	71.0	67.7	74.7	64.2	61.3	67.3
1963[3]	69.9	66.6	73.4	70.8	67.4	74.4	63.7	61.0	66.6
1962[3]	70.1	66.9	73.5	70.9	67.7	74.5	64.2	61.6	66.9
1961	70.2	67.1	73.6	71.0	67.8	74.6	64.5	62.0	67.1
1960	69.7	66.6	73.1	70.6	67.4	74.1	63.6	61.1	66.3
1959	69.9	66.8	73.2	70.7	67.5	74.2	63.9	61.3	66.5
1958	69.6	66.6	72.9	70.5	67.4	73.9	63.4	61.0	65.8
1957	69.5	66.4	72.7	70.3	67.2	73.7	63.0	60.7	65.5
1956	69.7	66.7	72.9	70.5	67.5	73.9	63.6	61.3	66.1
1955	69.6	66.7	72.8	70.5	67.4	73.7	63.7	61.4	66.1

TABLE 1.1 (continued)

Area and year	All races Both sexes	All races Male	All races Female	White Both sexes	White Male	White Female	Black[4] Both sexes	Black[4] Male	Black[4] Female
United States (continued)									
1954	69.6	66.7	72.8	70.5	67.5	73.7	63.4	61.1	65.9
1953	68.8	66.0	72.0	69.7	66.8	73.0	62.0	59.7	64.5
1952	68.6	65.8	71.6	69.5	66.6	72.6	61.4	59.1	63.8
1951	68.4	65.6	71.4	69.3	66.5	72.4	61.2	59.2	63.4
1950	68.2	65.6	71.1	69.1	66.5	72.2	60.8	59.1	62.9
1949	68.0	65.2	70.7	68.8	66.2	71.9	60.6	58.9	62.7
1948	67.2	64.6	69.9	68.0	65.5	71.0	60.0	58.1	62.5
1947	66.8	64.4	69.7	67.6	65.2	70.5	59.7	57.9	61.9
1946	66.7	64.4	69.4	67.5	65.1	70.3	59.1	57.5	61.0
1945	65.9	63.6	67.9	66.8	64.4	69.5	57.7	56.1	59.6
1944	65.2	63.6	66.8	66.2	64.5	68.4	56.6	55.8	57.7
1943	63.3	62.4	64.4	64.2	63.2	65.7	55.6	55.4	56.1
1942	66.2	64.7	67.9	67.3	65.9	69.4	56.6	55.4	58.2
1941	64.8	63.1	66.8	66.2	64.4	68.5	53.8	52.5	55.3
1940	62.9	60.8	65.2	64.2	62.1	66.6	53.1	51.5	54.9
1939	63.7	62.1	65.4	64.9	63.3	66.6	54.5	53.2	56.0
1938	63.5	61.9	65.3	65.0	63.2	66.8	52.9	51.7	54.3
1937	60.0	58.0	62.4	61.4	59.3	63.8	50.3	48.3	52.5
1936	58.5	56.6	60.6	59.8	58.0	61.9	49.0	47.0	51.4
1935	61.7	59.9	63.9	62.9	61.0	65.0	53.1	51.3	55.2
1934	61.1	59.3	63.3	62.4	60.5	64.6	51.8	50.2	53.7
1933	63.3	61.7	65.1	64.3	62.7	66.3	54.7	53.5	56.0
1932	62.1	61.0	63.5	63.2	62.0	64.5	53.7	52.8	54.6

TABLE 1.1 (*continued*)

Area and year	All races			White			Black[4]		
	Both sexes	Male	Female	Both sexes	Male	Female	Both sexes	Male	Female
United States (*continued*)									
1931	61.1	59.4	63.1	62.6	60.8	64.7	50.4	49.5	51.5
1930	59.7	58.1	61.6	61.4	59.7	63.5	48.1	47.3	49.2
1929	57.1	55.8	58.7	58.6	57.2	60.3	46.7	45.7	47.8
Death-registration States									
1928	56.8	55.6	58.3	58.4	57.0	60.0	46.3	45.6	47.0
1927	60.4	59.0	62.1	62.0	60.5	63.9	48.2	47.6	48.9
1926	56.7	55.5	58.0	58.2	57.0	59.6	44.6	43.7	45.6
1925	59.0	57.6	60.6	60.7	59.3	62.4	45.7	44.9	46.7
1924	59.7	58.1	61.5	61.4	59.8	63.4	46.6	45.5	47.8
1923	57.2	56.1	58.5	58.3	57.1	59.6	48.3	47.7	48.9
1922	59.6	58.4	61.0	60.4	59.1	61.9	52.4	51.8	53.0
1921	60.8	60.0	61.8	61.8	60.8	62.9	51.5	51.6	51.3
1920	54.1	53.6	54.6	54.9	54.4	55.6	45.3	45.5	45.2
1919	54.7	53.5	56.0	55.8	54.5	57.4	44.5	44.5	44.4
1918	39.1	36.6	42.2	39.8	37.1	43.2	31.1	29.9	32.5
1917	50.9	48.4	54.0	52.0	49.3	55.3	38.8	37.0	40.8
1916	51.7	49.6	54.3	52.5	50.2	55.2	41.3	39.6	43.1
1915	54.5	52.5	56.8	55.1	53.1	57.5	38.9	37.5	40.5
1914	54.2	52.0	56.8	54.9	52.7	57.5	38.9	37.1	40.8
1913	52.5	50.3	55.0	53.0	50.8	55.7	38.4	36.7	40.3
1912	53.5	51.5	55.9	53.9	51.9	56.2	37.9	35.9	40.0
1911	52.6	50.9	54.4	53.0	51.3	54.9	36.4	34.6	38.2
1910	50.0	48.4	51.8	50.3	48.6	52.0	35.6	33.8	37.5

13

TABLE 1.1 (*continued*)

Area and year	All races Both sexes	All races Male	All races Female	White Both sexes	White Male	White Female	Black[4] Both sexes	Black[4] Male	Black[4] Female
United States (*continued*)									
1909	52.1	50.5	53.8	52.5	50.9	54.2	35.7	34.2	37.3
1908	51.1	49.5	52.8	51.5	49.9	53.3	34.9	33.8	36.0
1907	47.6	45.6	49.9	48.1	46.0	50.4	32.5	31.1	34.0
1906	48.7	46.9	50.8	49.3	47.3	51.4	32.9	31.8	33.9
1905	48.7	47.3	50.2	49.1	47.6	50.6	31.3	29.6	33.1
1904	47.6	46.2	49.1	48.0	46.6	49.5	30.8	29.1	32.7
1903	50.5	49.1	52.0	50.9	49.5	52.5	33.1	31.7	34.6
1902	51.5	49.8	53.4	51.9	50.2	53.8	34.6	32.9	36.4
1901	49.1	47.6	50.6	49.4	48.0	51.0	33.7	32.2	35.3
1900	47.3	46.3	48.3	47.6	46.6	48.7	33.0	32.5	33.5

[For selected years, life table values shown are estimates; see Technical notes. Beginning 1970 excludes deaths of nonresidents of the United States; see Technical notes]

[1]Alaska included in 1959 and Hawaii in 1960.

[2]Deaths based on a 50–percent sample.

[3]Figures by race exclude data for residents of New Jersey; see Technical notes.

[4]Prior to 1970, data for the black population are not available. Data shown for 190G-69 are for the nonwhite population. See Technical notes.

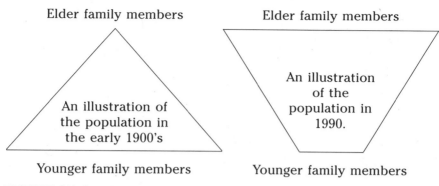

FIGURE 1.1 Squaring of the aging pyramid.

with a larger top and a smaller base. If this trend continues, one may expect that one third of the US population will be aged 65 and over by the year 2000 (Yancik & Ries, 2000). Of special concern to health care operators is the fact that the population increasing more rapidly is aged 85 and older, the so-called "oldest old" (Kennedy, 1993), arguably the population most in need of health and supportive care.

The expansion of the older population has led to new clinical problems related to a concentration of chronic diseases among the elderly. The focus of this chapter is cancer, but the problems related to cancer are common to other conditions as well and concern the following:

- Causes of the association of chronic diseases and aging;
- Biology of chronic disease in the older person, especially for what concerns the influence of multiple comorbidities (Fried, Storer, King, & Lodder, 1991; Hammermann et al., 1999; Yancik, et al. 2001);
- Management-related problems related to both prevention and treatment. In particular, in cancer prevention and cancer treatment, the benefits of the intervention may be fewer, due to decreased life expectancy, and the risks higher, due to a reduction in functional reserve (Balducci & Extermann, 2001).

Goals of prevention and treatment often reflect a popular outcome alternative to prolongation of survival, which is compression of morbidity (Crimmins & Saito, 2001). This construct stems from two considerations. First, human life span (that is, the time each person is programmed to live, irrespective of external factors, such as diseases, accidents, or wars), is limited. Second, after age 40, disease and disability precede death for an average of 30 and 20 years, respectively

TABLE 1.2 Probability of Developing Invasive Cancers Over Selected Age Intervals, by Sex, US, 1995–1997*

	Gender	Birth to 39 (%)	40 to 59 (%)	60 to 79 (%)	Birth to Death (%)
All sites†	Male	1.56 (1 in 64)	8.25 (1 in 12)	33.13 (1 in 3)	43.48 (1 in 2)
	Female	1.97 (1 in 51)	9.37 (1 in 11)	22.39 (1 in 4)	38.34 (1 in 3)
Bladder‡	Male	0.03 (1 in 3,437)	0.44 (1 in 226)	2.39 (1 in 42)	3.40 (1 in 29)
	Female	Less than 1 in 10,000	0.14 (1 in 699)	0.68 (1 in 146)	1.18 (1 in 85)
Breast	Female	0.44 (1 in 225)	4.15 (1 in 24)	7.0-2 (1 in 14)	12.83 (1 in 8)
Colon &	Male	0.07 (1 in 1,531)	0.87 (1 in 115)	4.00 (1 in 25)	5.78 (1 in 17)
Rectum	Female	0.05 (1 in 1,855)	0.69 (1 in 146)	3.04 (1 in 33)	5.55 1 in 18)
Leukemia	Male	0.15 (1 in 654)	0.21 (1 in 467)	0.84 (1 in 119)	1.42 (1 in 70)
	Female	0.11 (1 in 900)	0.15 (1 in 671)	0.50 (1 in 199)	1.05 (1 in 95)
Lung &	Male	0.04 (1 in 2,499)	1.24 (1 in 80)	6.29 (1 in 16)	8.09 (1 in 12)
Bronchus	Female	0.03 (1 in 2,997)	0.92 (1 in 108)	4.04 (1 in 25)	5.78 (1 in 17)
Melanoma	Male	0.13 (1 in 744)	0.53 (1 in 190)	0.94 (1 in 106)	1.68 (1 in 60)
of the Skin	Female	0.22 (1in 453)	0.40 (1 in 249)	0.48 (1 in 207)	1.25 (1 in 80)
Non-Hodgkin's	Male	0.19 (1 in 513)	0.50 (1 in 198)	1.21 (1 in 83)	2.11 (1 in 47)
Lymphoma	Female	0.08 (1 in 1,296)	0.32 (1 in 312)	0.97 (1 in 103)	1.74 (1 in 57)
Prostate	Male	less than 1 in 10,000	2.06 (1 in 49)	13.42 (1 in 7)	15.89 (1 in 6)
Uterine Cervix	Female	0.17 (1 in 576)	0.30 (1 in 332)	0.26 (1 in 387)	0.78 (1 in 129)
Uterine Corpus	Female	0.05 (1 in 2,142)	0.74 (1 in 136)	1.67 (1 in 60)	2.73 (1 in 37)

*For those free of cancer at beginning of age interval. Based on cancer cases diagnosed during 1995–1997. The "1 in" statistic and the inverse of the percentage may not be equivalent due to rounding. †Excludes basal and squamous cell skin cancers and in situ carcinomas except urinary bladder. ‡Includes invasive and in situ cancer cases.

Source: DEVCAN Software, Version 4.0, Surveillance, Epidemiology, and End Results Program, 1973–1997, Division of Cancer Control and Population Sciences, National Cancer Institute, 2000. American Cancer Society, Surveillance Research, 2001

(Table 1.2). Hence, the most reasonable goal of health interventions in the older person may be reducing the time gap between disease, disability, and death. In other words, one can say that preservation of function and quality of life may be a more realistic goal than cure of the disease in the older person.

ASSOCIATION OF CANCER AND AGE: MECHANISMS AND CLINICAL IMPLICATIONS

The incidence of most common cancer increases with age (Table 1.2); currently approximately 50% of all malignancies occur in persons aged 65 and older; by the year 2030, this proportion may rise to 60% due to the expansion of the older population (Yancik & Ries, 2000). Together with the incidence of cancer, (ACS,2001) the prevalence of cancer may also increase with age (Verdecchia et al., 2001). A number of factors may contribute to the increased prevalence of cancer. In addition to the increased incidence, probably the fact that common cancers, such as breast and lung cancer, generally have a more indolent course in older individuals, and the survival of these individuals with metastatic cancer may be longer, explains the increased prevalence (Crimmins & Saito, 2001). Also, prostate cancer, which affects mostly older men, is associated with many years of survival and accounts for the higher prevalence of cancer among the elderly.

Cancer is currently a common cause of death in individuals over 65, second only to cardiovascular diseases (Anisimov, 1998). Of interest, death rate from cardiovascular diseases is declining among the elderly, however, probably as a consequence of smoking cessation, improved diet, and more frequent exercise, whereas death rate from cancer has remained constant or has slightly increased, however hypertension remains the leading cause of death (Figure 1.2) (Lavecchia, 2001). It is reasonable to expect that cancer may become the first cause of death during the next two decades.

The association of cancer and aging may be explained by three non-mutually exclusive mechanisms. Carcinogenesis, the process leading to the formation of clinical cancer from a normal cell, is time consuming. Though it is impossible to calculate precisely the carcinogenic time of human cancer, it is reasonable to think that in some cases it may approach 20 or more years (Fernandez-Pol & Douglas, 2001; Minton & Shaw, 1998). It is not surprising then to find the highest concentration of cancer in older individuals.

Carcinogenesis involves a number of serial steps that must occur in a precise order to produce cancer (Fernandez-Pol & Douglas, 2001). Each step is effected by different substances. The initial carcinogenic

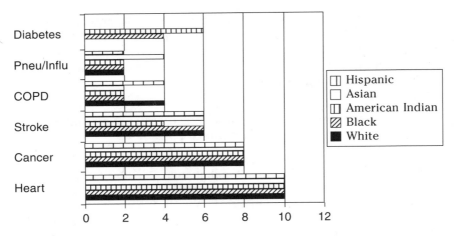

FIGURE 1.2

Sahyoun, N.R., Lentzner, H., Hoyert, D., & Robinson, K. N. (2001). Trends in causes of death among the elderly. *Aging Trends, 1*. Hyattsville, MD: National Center for health Statistics, 2001.

steps involve the activation of oncogenes or the suppression in the activity of anti-proliferative genes (antioncogenes), which are acted upon by substances called "early-stage carcinogens" and are considered irreversible. The subsequent steps may involve the release of substances that stimulate tumor growth, are effected by "late-stage carcinogens" and may be reversible. Chemoprevention of cancer acts primarily by reversing the late carcinogenic steps (Balducci & Beghe, 2000; Hong, Spiz & Lippman, 2000; Minton & Shaw, 1998). Preponderant evidence suggests that aging cells may be in an advanced carcinogenic status and thus more susceptible to late stage carcinogens. In cell cultures, some molecular changes of aging, including formation of DNA adducts, DNA hypomethylation, point mutations, and DNA translocation, mimic the changes of early carcinogenic steps. In addition, the tissues of older animals, including the cutaneous, the lymphatic, the hepatic, and the nervous tissues, are more likely to develop cancer when exposed to late-stage carcinogens than are those of younger animals (Anisimov, 2001; Anisimov et al., 2001).

Several lines of circumstantial evidence suggest that the tissues of aging humans may also be primed to the effects of late-stage carcinogens. The incidence of non-melanomatous skin cancer and of prostate cancer (Balducci et al., 1997) increases logarithmically with age, which suggests increased susceptibility of older persons to these types of cancer. The incidence of non-Hodgkin's lymphoma increased 80% in people over 60 between 1970 and 1990 (Monfardini & Carbone, 1998) and that of malignant brain tumors has increased 700%, or sevenfold, in persons aged 70 and older (Flowers, 1998). This increment, which concerns older individuals exclusively, suggests that these individuals may be more susceptible to new environmental carcinogens. Perhaps the most convincing demonstration of this enhanced susceptibility comes from an unfortunate natural experiment that occurred in the early 1970s in the Eastern Italian town of Trieste, when a leak of dioxin affected the whole town. Fifteen years later it was found that the risk of lung cancer from dioxin was more than twice as high for persons who were over 70 at the time of exposure than for those who were under 50 (Barbone et al., 1995).

The aging biological environment may also favor carcinogenesis. Paradoxically, proliferative senescence may be one of these factors (Campisi, 1997). This finding is counterintuitive, because proliferative senescence implies the loss of a cell's ability to replicate itself. However, the senescent cells may lose in the meantime the ability to undergo programmed cell death (apoptosis), and consequently their population may continue to grow even if the proliferative rate is decreased. This is one of the mechanisms of indolent small lymphocytic follicular lymphoma, whose cells over-express an abnormal form of Bcl2, which prevents apoptosis (Cotter, Waters & Cunningham, 1999; Warner, 1997). In addition, the senescent cells may favor the growth and spreading of tumors in surrounding tissues. Proliferative senescence is associated with increased production of heregulin, a powerful tumor growth factor, and of metalloproteinases, which dissolve the basal membranes of tissues (Campisi, 1997). Immune-senescence implies a progressive loss in cell-mediated immunity (Burns & Goodwin, 1998), an important natural bulwark against tumor growth.

The increased susceptibility of older persons to environmental carcinogens has important clinical consequences. First, it overturns a widely held tenet that primary prevention of cancer is futile in older individuals, because all carcinogenic changes have already occurred. It suggests instead that removal of environmental carcinogens, such as smoking cessation, may be mostly beneficial to older individuals. Second, it suggests that older individuals may be prime candidates for chemoprevention, which prevents and reverses late carcinogenic steps (Hong, Spits, & Lippman, 2000).

THE PROFILE OF THE OLDER PERSON WITH CANCER

The critical question in geriatric oncology is whether older individuals die with cancer or of cancer. The answer determines whether cancer prevention and cancer treatment in older individuals are worthwhile goals. Diab et al. (2000) compared the survival of breast cancer patients and that of women without breast cancer of the same age, using the SEER (Surveillance, Epidemiology and End Results) database. It was found that breast cancer was associated with lower life expectancy in women aged 50 to 65, but did not affect the survival of those aged 70 to 75. For those over 80, survival tended to increase. The most likely explanation of these findings is that the general health of older women with breast cancer is better than that of the whole population of women approximately the same age. This study confirms previous observations by other authors, in that Repetto et al. (1998) found that the incidence of comorbidity and functional dependence was lower among patients aged 65 and older with cancer than among age-matched controls of the same age. Ferrucci (1998) compared the functional status and comorbidity of all cancer patients aged 65 and older and persons of the same age in the small Italian town of Cusumano, and found that cancer patients had an overall better health condition (Ferrucci, L; Personal Communication, Fourth International Conference of Geriatric Oncology, Sheraton Hoelt, Rome, Italy, October 1998). Stanta et al. (1997) found that the prevalence of comorbidity at autopsy was lower among cancer patients aged 70 to 95 than among aged-matched controls without cancer. On this basis, it is reasonable to assume that cancer is the cause of death for a large portion, perhaps the majority of older cancer patients, and cancer control is highly worthwhile for these individuals (Stanta et al., 1997).

The fact that cancer should develop preferentially in healthy and independent older individuals is not clear, but reasonable speculations may be made based on recent insights in the biology of aging. Aging is associated with a progressive accumulation in the circulation of catabolic cytokines, including interleukin-6 and tumor necrosis factor (Balducci & Extermann 2001). Seemingly, these cytokines, which are a chemical hallmark of frail elderly, may oppose tumor growth. Even the dysfunction of the immune system due to aging may act as a two-edged sword, and in some cases, it may inhibit tumor growth (Hurz et al., 1990). A number of other environmental changes characteristic of frail elderly include reduced production of growth hormone and consequently of insulin-like growth factor 1 (IGF-1), one of the most powerful tumor growth factors (Rosen, 2000) .

CONCLUSIONS

Clearly, cancer will become mostly a disease of older individuals, if the current demographic trend continues. The association of cancer and aging may be accounted for by the length of time of carcinogenesis, by molecular changes of aging that prime the older tissue to the effects of late-stage carcinogens, and by a number of age-related environmental changes that favor cancer growth. Those factors that make older individuals more susceptible to cancer may partly be reversed by elimination of environmental carcinogens and by chemoprevention. Cancer is mostly a disease of healthy and functional elderly, whose survival may be shortened and whose quality of life may be deranged by cancer. Cancer prevention and cancer treatment appear highly worthwhile in older individuals.

REFERENCES

Anderson, R. N. (1998). *United States abridged life tables, 1996. National vital statistics reports, 47*(13), Hyattsville, Maryland: National Center for Health Statistics.

Anisimov, V. N. (1998). Age as a risk factor in multistage carcinogenesis. In Balducci, L., Lyman, G. H., Ershler, W. B. (Eds.), *Comprehensive geriatric oncology,* Harwood Academic Publishers, Amsterdam, 157–178.

Anisimov, V. N., Zavarzina, N. Y., Zabezhinski, M. A., Popovich, I. G., Zimina, O. A., Shtylick, A. V., Arutjunyan, A. V., Oparina, T. I., Prokopenkp, V. M., Mikhalski, A. I., & Yashin, A. I. (2001). Melantonin increases both life span and tumor incidence in female CBA mice. *The Journals of Gerontology. Series A, Biological Sciences and Medical Sciences, 56*(7), B311–323.

Balducci, L., & Beghe, C. (2000). The application of the principles of geriatrics to the management of the older person with cancer (2000). *Critical Reviews in Oncology/Hematology, 35*(3), 147–154.

Balducci, L., & Extermann, M. (2001). A practical approach to the older patient with cancer. *Current Problems in Oncology, 37,* 137–145.

Balducci, L., Pow-Sang, J., & Friedland, J. (1997). Prostate cancer. *Clinical Geriatric Medicine, 13,* 182–206.

Barbone, F., Bovenzi, M., & Cavallieri, F. (1995). Air pollution and lung cancer in Trieste, Italy. *American Journal of Epidemiology, 141,* 1161–1169.

Burns, E. A., & Goodwin, J. S. (1998). Immunological changes of aging. In: L. Balducci, G. H. Lyman, & W. B. Ershler (Eds.), *Comprehensive geriatric oncology* (pp. 213–222). London: Harwood Academic Publishers.

Campisi, J. (1997). Aging and cancer: the double-edged sword of replicative senescence. *Journal of the American Geriatric Society, 45*(4):482–488.

Cotter, F. E., Waters, J., & Cunningham, D. (1999). Human Bcl-2 antisenescence therapy for lymphomas. *Biochemistry Biophysics Acta, 1489,* 97–106.

Crimmins, E. M., & Saito, Y. (2001). Trends in healthy life expectancy in the United States, 1970–1990: Gender, racial, and educational differences. *Social Sciences & Medicine, 52*(11), 1629–1641.

Diab, S. G., Elledge, R. M., & Clark, G. M. (2000). Tumor characteristics and clinical outcome of elderly women with breast cancer. *Journal of the National Cancer Institute, 92,* 550–556.

Fernandez-Pol, A., & Douglas, M. G. (2000). Molecular interactions of cancer and aging. *Hematology Oncology Clinics of North America, 14,* 25–45

Flowers, A. (1998). Brain tumors. In L. Balducci, G. H. Lyman, & W. B. Ershler (Eds.), *Comprehensive geriatric oncology* (pp. 703–720). London: Harwood Academic Publishers.

Fried, L. P., Storer, D. J., King, D. E., & Lodder, F. (1991). Diagnosis of illness presentation in the elderly. *Journal of the American Geriatrics Society, 39*(2):117–123.

Glass, A. G., & Hoover, R. H. (1989). The emerging epidemic of melanoma and squamous cell cancer. *Journal of the American Medical Association, 262,* 2097–2100.

Hamermann, D., Berman, J. W., & Albers, G. W. (1999). Emerging evidence for inflammation in conditions frequently affecting older adults: report of a symposium. *Journal of the American Geriatrics Society, 47,* 995–999

Hong, W. K., Spita, M. R., & Lippman, S. M. (2000). Cancer chemoprevention in the 21st century: genetics, risk modeling, and molecular targets. *Journal of Clinical Oncology, 18*(21 suppl), 9S–18S.

Kennedy, B. J. (1993). Specific considerations for the older patient with cancer. In P. Calabresi & P. S. Schein (Eds.), *Medical Oncology* (pp. 1219–1223). New York: McGraw-Hill, Inc.

Kurz, J. M., Jacquemier, J., & Amalric, R. (1990). Why are local recurrences after breast-conserving therapy more frequent in younger persons. *Journal of Clinical Oncology, 10,* 141–152.

La Vecchia, C., Lucchini, F., Negri, E., & Levi, F. (2001). Cancer mortality in the elderly, 1960–1998: a worldwide approach. *Oncology Spectrum, 12,* 356–394.

Minton, S., & Shaw, G. (1998). Chemoprevention of cancer in the elderly. In L. Balducci, G. H. Lyman, W. B. Ershler (Eds.), *Comprehensive geriatric oncology* (pp. 307–324). London: Harwood Academic Publishers.

Monfardini, S., & Carbone, A. (1998). Non-Hodgkin's lymphomas. In L. Balducci, G. H. Lyman, W. B. Ershler (Eds.), *Comprehensive geriatric oncology* (pp. 577–595). London: Harwood Academic Publishers.

National Center for Health Statistics: Vital statistics of the United States 1989. Mortality. Part B Hyattsville MD, National Center for Health Statistics, 1991.

Newschaffer, C. J., Bush, T. L., & Penberthy, L. E. (1998). Does comorbid disease interact with cancer? An epidemiological analysis of mortality in a cohort of elderly breast cancer patients. *Journal of Gerontology, 53A,* M372–378.

Pasternak, G., & Wunderlich, V. (1995). The thirteenth meeting of the European Association for Cancer Research. *Journal of Molecular Medicine, 73*(3), 153–155.

Repetto, L., Granetto, C., Venturino, A., Rosso, R., Gianni, W., & Santi, L. (1998). Prognostic evaluation of the older cancer patient. In L. Balducci, G. H. Lyman, & W. B. Ershler (Eds.), *Comprehensive geriatric oncology* (pp. 281–286). London: Harwood Academic Publishers.

Rosen, C. J. (2000). Growth hormone and aging. *Endocrine, 12,* 197–201

Stanta, G., Campagner, L., Cavallieri, F., & Giarelli, L. (1997). Cancer of the oldest old: What we have learned from autopsy studies. *Clinical Geriatric Medicine, 13,* 55–68.

Verdecchia, A., Mariotto, A., Capocaccia, R., Gatta, G., Micheli, A., Sant, M., & Berrion, F. (2001). Incidence and prevalence of all cancerous disease in Italy: trends and implications. *European Journal of Cancer, 37*(9), 1149–1157.

Warner, H. R. (1997). Aging and regulation of apoptosis. *Current Topics in Cellular Regulation, 35,* 107–121.

Yancik, R., & Ries, L. A. (1998). Magnitude of the problem-How we apply what we know? In L. Balducci, G. H. Lyman, W. B. Ershler (Eds.), *Comprehensive geriatric oncology* (pp. 95–103). London: Harwood Academic Publishers.

Yancik, R., & Ries, L. A. (2000). Aging and cancer in America: Demographic and epidemiological perspectives. *Hematology/Oncology Clinics of North America, 14,* 17–24.

Yancik, R., Wesley, M. N., Ries, L. A., Havlik, R. J., Edwards, B. K., & Yates, J. W. (2001). Effect of age and comorbidity in postmenopausal breast cancer patients aged 55 years and older. *Journal of the American Medical Association, 285*(7), 885–892.

CHAPTER TWO

Issues in the Care of the Older Cancer Patient: Delayed Diagnosis, Inadequate Treatment, and Information Gaps

Lodovico Balducci, Martine Extermann, and Janine Overcash

This chapter explores the quality of cancer care received by older individuals. The goal of this chapter is to highlight the opportunity for improvement of care in the older cancer patient in three areas: delayed diagnosis, treatment adequacy, and appropriate evaluation and to emphasize the pivotal role of the nurse in these endeavors.

We navigate uncharted waters. Whereas an abundance of guidelines directs the management of the frail patient at home or in long-term care facilities (Bates-Jensen, 2001; Lagergren, 1993; Maclean, 2001; Olivotto & Levine, 2001; Pearson et al.; Rhew, 2001; Schostak, 1991), guidelines for the management of specific diseases in older individuals living in the community are still needed. Only last year, the National Cancer Center Network (NCCN) issued a set of general guidelines for the management of cancer in the older person (Balducci & Yates, 2000).

The paucity of guidelines reflects the paucity of information on optimal management of cancer in the older person, and this in turn reflects the difficulty of including older individuals in clinical trials (Begg & Carbone, 1982; Hutchins, Unger, Crowley, Coltman, & Albain,

1999). This difficulty is mainly due to the elusive definition of aging (Balducci & Extermann, 2001). The population mostly at risk for inadequate or inappropriate management is the population mostly affected by cancer, who are those aged 70–90 (Yancik & Ries, 2000). This is the most diverse and hard to classify population. The majority of persons aged 70–90 experience a loss of functional reserve that is progressive with age and that varies from person to person: they are neither totally independent nor frail, rarely do they fulfill the exacting eligibility conditions of clinical trials, but at the same time they may benefit from some form of cancer treatment, when special provisions are made (Balducci & Extermann, 2001). These persons are most vulnerable to the opposite risks involved in the management of cancer and age: overtreatment and high risk of serious toxicity, and undertreatment and inadequate cancer control.

DELAYED DIAGNOSIS

Several reports showed that the presentation of common cancer in older individuals occurred at a more advanced stage than in the young, during the 1980s (Mor et al., 1988; Samet, Hunt, Lerchen & Goodwin, 1988). These studies were based on large tumor registries and showed that the percentage of patients with advanced stage breast, bladder, ovarian, endometrial, and cervical cancer, and lymphoma was higher after age 65. The possibility that cancer presents at a more advanced stage because it is more aggressive is unlikely. In the case of breast cancer it is clear that the disease becomes more indolent with aging (Balducci, Silliman, & Diaz, 2002). The percentage of hormone-receptor rich, well-differentiated, low-grade, slowly proliferating breast cancer increases with age (Nixon et al., 1994; Valentinis, Silvestrini, & Daidone, 1991). At the same time, a number of patient-related conditions, such as reduced concentration of circulating estrogen and insulin-like growth factor 1, reduced angiogenesis and immune-senescence, disfavor the growth of breast cancer in the elderly (Balducci et al., 2002; Kurtz et al., 1990; Nixon et al., 1994). Clinically, slow-growing bone and cutaneous metastases are more common in older than younger women, whereas visceral and cerebral metastases are more common in those younger (Holmes, 1994). The most likely explanation of more advanced disease is delayed diagnosis.Delayed diagnosis might have prevented surgical cure and have been responsible for worse outcome. Delayed diagnosis might also have led to increased utilization of emergency surgery, especially for the management of intestinal obstruction from cancer of the large bowel (Berger & Roslyn, 1997;

Kemeny & Peakman, 1998), which in older individuals is associated with increased risk of death and of perioperative complications. Likely causes of delayed diagnosis include:

- Decreased utilization of screening services;
- Failure to recognize timely the signs and symptoms of cancer;
- Reduced access to diagnostic and treatment facilities; and
- Cultural barriers, due to ageism and lack of information.

In the 1980s it was found that the utilization of screening services declined with age and only one in ten women aged 70 and older received mammographic screening for breast cancer (Fox, Roetzheim & Kington, 1997). The utilization of other screening services was even lower. In the last decade this trend has reversed and by 1990 more than 50% of Caucasian women living in urban areas had undergone at least one mammographic exam after age 70 (Fox et al., 1997; Mandelblatt, Wheat, Monane, Moshief & Hollenberg, 1992). Unfortunately, the use of mammography still lags behind for elderly women belonging to minority groups, especially blacks and Hispanics (Fox et al., 1997; Fox, Stein, Sockloskie & Ory, 2001; Zambrana, Breen, Fox & Gutierrez-Mohamed, 1999) and those living in rural areas (Fox et al., 2001). Underutilization of mammography appears the most likely explanation for the poorer outcome of breast cancer among African American and Hispanic women (Bain, Greenburg, & Whitekar, 1986; Rawl et al., 2000; Ramirez, Talavera, Villarreal et al., 2000). A number of patient-related and provider-related barriers prevent the screening of older women (Fox et al., 1997; Roetzheim, Fox & Leake, 1995) (Table 2.1). Most of these barriers are self-explanatory. Cultural barriers may include religious views such as those held by Muslim women who may not be allowed to attend a physician visit alone, Christian Scientists who may refuse any form of preventative intervention, or special sociopolitical circumstances (for example, Hispanic women might have been reluctant to be screened in California, for fear of being reported as illegal aliens). Screening for cancer may be a low priority in high-crime areas when compared to other higher risk factors that can result in mortality. Another important finding of these studies is the fact that physician recommendation was the single most important factor in determining attendance of a screening program (Fox, Siu & Stein, 1994) and that the stronger the certainty about the value of screening the women perceived behind the recommendation, the more likely they were to be screened. Clearly, this finding provides a unique opportunity of intervention to improve the screening rate of asymptomatic older persons. A number of programs currently try a capillary form of

TABLE 2.1 Age-related Barriers to Screening

Patient-Related
Lack of information
Ageism
Limited access to health-care facility
Limited income
Cultural barriers
Inadequate physician support

Provider-Related
Lack of information
Ageism
Low intervention priority

professional education, aimed specially at minority providers, to illustrate both the effectiveness of screening and the most effective communication techniques to convey the message to older individuals (Fox et al., 1999; Zambrana et al., 1999).

Failure to recognize early symptoms of cancer by older individuals is well documented (Balducci, 1994; Bausell, 1986; Fried, Storer, King & Lodder, 1991; Mor, Masterson-Allen, Goldberg, Guadagnoli, Wool et al., 1990; Samet et al, 1988). The most common mechanisms of this failure include:

- A common misconception that symptoms like pain, bleeding, constipation, hesitancy are a natural consequence of aging and do not deserve special attention;
- Masking of new symptoms of cancer from preexisting symptoms due to comorbid conditions (for example, worsening bone pain due to metastatic disease may be masked by preexisting arthritis or osteoporosis);
- Lack of appreciation of new symptoms, from cognitive disorders and drugs;
- Social situations that prevent timely pursuance of medical attention (for example, older person who is also the caregiver of a demented or debilitated spouse may try to delay as much as possible the discovery of a disease that may hinder his/her role).

Nurses are in an ideal position to approach these problems. For persons in assisted living facilities, the initial findings of cancer, which may present as a skin lesion, abnormal bleeding, masses, or even new pains, are often detected by the nurse or the nursing aide caring for the patients. For patients living at home, nurses working in a primary care office, home care agency, or employed as geriatric managers (Mackey, 2001; Mahon, 2000) are in a strategic position to recognize early symptoms and signs of cancer and free the patient of social impediments to timely care. Screening programs must be put in place that are accessible to all parts of the community.

Along with the importance of screening, it is essential to provide education as part of the process. Treacy and Mayer (2000) define cancer education as the "process of influencing behavior to elicit changes in the knowledge, attitudes, and skills required to maintain and improve health" (p. 48). Although it is common sense, it is important to provide pamphlets to people who smoke cigarettes, who do not regularly undergo screening examinations, or do not perform breast self-examinations, so the information can be considered at a later time. Health education material should be assessed for larger print and overall ease of readability. Glossy, small print brochures packed with information may be physically difficult for many seniors to read. External factors influence the educational process at any age, and a well-lighted environment, minimized interruptions, and timing of teaching is very important (Treacy & Mayer, 2000). Attempting to conduct teaching in the middle of a busy screening center or clinic is difficult both for the teacher and for the person gaining the information. If possible, a teaching room or area where materials can be displayed, videos played, and stimuli reduced may help increase the results of the cancer education component of the teaching.

Teaching right after screening may have revealed a potential malignancy may not be appropriate either. In this case it might be best to simply tell the person where to go for further examination and what to expect. The screening participant may be very anxious concerning the threat of a potential cancer and therefore it is not the time to go into the importance of screening and life-modifying behaviors. As nurse educators, it is important that you assess your students, whether they are students in the classroom, or people in the community. People who are thinking about other issues are less likely to retain new information.

Age-related restriction in social and economic resources may also hamper access to care. Aging is associated with a decline both in income (Ahacic, Parker, & Thorslund, 2000) and in mobility. At the same time, the proliferation of increasingly specialized care centers makes it more and more difficult for older individuals to receive all diagnostic tests in a single trip. Special care centers capable of providing the older person with a battery of diagnostic tests on the same day are highly desirable.

Ageism is a pervasive, albeit poorly defined prejudice that may adversely affect the quality of care of older individuals (Chafetz, 2001; Muss, 2001). Some of the most common misconceptions are that cancer is not curable in older individuals, or that the complications of treatment, especially chemotherapy, are worse than cancer in the older person. These misconceptions are frequently held by patients, physicians, and nurses, thus the need for education is great. Cancer is not a consequence of aging, and many older people are viable candidates for the same types of cancer treatment as younger people. These types of misconceptions are promoted due to lack of education, and the effects of this type of mindset can be detrimental to many families. Ageism infects patients, families, health care providers, and legislators, who may feel that older individuals utilize an excess of health resources and should be entitled at most to a dignified and comfortable death, as suggested by the former Colorado governor Mr. Ladd in a now-infamous conference, during which he stated, "Older persons have a duty to die."

In addition to gaining awareness of one's own aging and espousing the sacredness of each human life, ageism can be overcome by a process of public and professional education aimed to highlight the benefits of medical interventions in older persons with cancer. New advances in cancer treatments are prime motivations for why older people should undergo cancer treatment. An improved cure rate of breast cancer by 30% in the adjuvant setting has been shown with selective estrogen receptor modulators (SERMs), which are agents such as tamoxifen and raloxifene (Early Breast Cancer Trialists Collaborative Group, A, 1998; Holly, Valavaara, & Blanco, 2001). New forms of hormonal treatment, including aromatase inhibitors, are capable of inducing a 40% or higher response rate in patients with metastatic breast cancer, including visceral disease and tumors strongly expressing HER2Neu (Goss & Strasser, 2001). The cure rate of large cell lymphoma of 30–45% in persons over 70 (Monfardini & Carbone, 1998) is also another motivation for continued treatment of older persons. Regarding treatment modalities, the potential of new, targeted forms of systemic treatment in older individuals such as capecitabine (Balducci, Extermann, & Carreca, 2001), monoclonal antibodies (Seidman et al., 2001), and inhibitors of tumor-specific enzymes, such as thymidine phospokinase (Drucker, 2001) and farnesyl transferase, promise to minimize the complications of treatment. In terms of support measures, colony-stimulating factors (Balducci & Yates, 2000), erythropoietin (Balducci & Extermann, 2001), keratinocyte-growth factor (Spielberger, Stiff & Emmanouilides, 2001), and bisphosphonates (Lipton et al., 2000) are critical in preventing neutropenic infections, fatigue, bone pain, and fractures.

Of course the prevention and treatment of cancer in older individuals will further squeeze limited health care resources. The answer to this important problem, however, cannot involve denying life-saving treatment to a whole segment of the population because of its age. A more constructive solution is to target the population more likely to benefit. For example, Kerlikowske, Salzmann, Phillips, Cauley and Cummings (1999) have calculated that by limiting the use of screening mammography to women in the upper quintile of bone density, who are also those at higher risk of breast cancer, 90% of cancers would still be detected and the cost of screening would be reduced by half. Extermann, Balducci, and Lyman (2000) have established that adjuvant chemotherapy for breast cancer may be beneficial to women aged 70 only if their risk of dying of breast cancer is 13% or higher, and for women aged 80 only if the risk is 30% or higher (Extermann et al., 2000). This type of decision analysis provides the direction for the most productive investment of limited health care resources in the elderly.

TREATMENT ADEQUACY

Three lines of evidence suggest that older individuals may receive substandard cancer treatment:

In a number of retrospective studies, concerning mainly breast cancer, the percentage of patients undergoing complete staging, full lymph node dissection, and receiving postoperative radiation therapy and adjuvant systemic therapy declined with age (Bergman et al., 1992; Greenfield, Blanco, & Elashoff, 1987; Hillner et al., 1996). Similar observations were reported also with other malignancies (Bennett et al., 1991; Guadagnoli et al., 1990; Samet et al., 1986; Silliman, Guadagnoli, Weitberg, & Mor, 1989). In addition, a number of prospective studies explored the feasibility of medical management with Tamoxifen of primary breast cancer (Bates, Fennessy & Riley, 2001; Mustacchi et al., 1994). These studies, which demonstrated the inferior results of the medical versus the surgical treatment, diffuse feeling that cancer should be treated less aggressively in the elderly. Another indirect demonstration of this attitude comes from the Oxford meta-analysis of adjuvant trials (Early Breast Cancer Trialists Cooperative Group B, 1998), in which women aged 70 and older represented only 3% of the total population.

The implementation of new treatment strategies, such as breast preservation with partial mastectomy, lags behind in older patients compared to younger patients (Nattinger et al., 1992).

The enrollment of older patients in cooperative clinical trials of cancer treatment lags much behind the enrollment of younger individuals. Only 10% of patients included in clinical trials of the Eastern Cooperative Oncology Group (ECOG) (Beggs & Carbone, 1992) and of the South Western Oncology Group (SWOG) (Hutchins et al., 1999) were 70 and older, while approximately 40% of all neoplasms occur in this population. Furthermore, Kemeny and Peakman (1998) reviewed the experience of the Cancer and Acute Leukemia Group B (CALGB) to examine whether older patients were as willing as younger individuals to undergo clinical trials and found that they were, but the treatment was offered to them much less frequently by the attending physician.

While it is clear that older individuals are less likely than younger ones to receive standard cancer treatment, it is not clear whether lesser treatment is always inappropriate. Guadagnoli et al. (1990) reviewed the utilization of adjuvant chemotherapy in women over 70 with breast cancer in Boston and concluded that the majority had received treatment appropriate for the clinical situation. Petrisek, Laliberte, Allen, and Mor (1997) reached the opposite conclusion in reviewing the treatment received by a group of women of the same age in Rhode Island. Given the incertitude of retrospective studies, this controversy should not surprise. As already stated in different chapters of this book, the older population is characterized by a high degree of diversity in function, comorbidity, cognition, and social and emotional resources. The evaluation of this diversity through a comprehensive geriatric assessment is essential to individualize cancer treatment according to life expectancy, susceptibility to treatment complications, as well as personal values and desire (Exterman et al., 1998; Repetto & Balducci, in press; Repetto, Fratino, & Audisio, in press). In the absence of this assessment the interpretation of cancer treatment of older individuals, especially retrospective evaluation, cannot help being controversial. Several interventions may help in gathering information related to cancer treatment in the elderly. One consideration may be the adoption of a common language to classify older individuals, based on a comprehensive geriatric assessment; this language should be used both in clinical practice and in prospective clinical trials (Balducci & Yates, 2000). The enrollment of older individuals in ongoing clinical trials (Hutchins, 1998; Kemeny & Peakman, 1998) specifically designed for older cancer patients continues to be less than optimal. Particularly needed are clinical trials for the management of frail patients with metastatic cancer. Frailty is a condition in which functional reserve of most organ systems is exhausted (Balducci & Stanta 2000; Fried et al., 2001). Though frailty is associated with increased susceptibility to stress, including cancer treatment, the median survival of a frail person is far from negligible: it is in excess of two years (Rockwood et al., 1999). A number of older women with breast cancer metastatic to the bones; and of older men with prostate cancer metastatic to the bones, are frail and need effective and prolonged palliation of their symptoms. The tolerance of opioids may be reduced in this group of patients, and hormonal therapy or low-dose chemotherapy may represent the best venue to effective symptom control (Cleary, 1998). With the aging of the population, the prevalence of frailty—and of the association of frailty and cancer—is likely to increase; thus prospective clinical trials in this population, with clinical benefits as main objective, are highly desirable (Gridelli et al., 1998; Hainsworth & Vokes, 1999).

ASSESSMENT OF THE OLDER CANCER PATIENT

A comprehensive geriatric assessment, as summarized in Table 2.2, is then highly desirable for providing a common language to assess the quality of cancer care received by the older person (Repetto & Balducci, in press). Arguably, the benefits of a comprehensive geriatric assessment (CGA) are much more pervasive and far-reaching than quality control (Bernabei et al., 1998; Inouye, et al.; Ruben, Frank, Hirsch, McGuigan & Maly, 1999; Tinetti et al.). In the general geriatric population the use of a comprehensive geriatric assessment resulted in reduction in hospital and nursing home admission (Bernabei et al., 1999; Ruben et al., 1999) prolongation of survival and active life expectancy (Bernabei et al., 1999); and prevention of falls (Tinetti et al., 1994) and of in-hospital delirium (Inouye et al., 1999). In older patients with cancer, the potential benefits of a comprehensive assessment have been outlined by the NCCN panel on cancer and aging (Balducci & Yates, 2000). These recommendations consider that the CGA can accomplish the following:

- Recognition and remedy of reversible health-related conditions, including comorbidity, malnutrition, polypharmacy, early memory disorders, and depression that may interfere with cancer treatment;
- Recognition and remedy of reversible social-economic conditions that may interfere with the management of cancer; of these, access to transportation and availability of the caregiver are paramount;
- Gross estimate of life expectancy;
- Gross estimate of treatment tolerance;
- Adoption of a common language to classify older cancer patient, enabling assessment of quality of care and interpretation of clinical trials.

TABLE 2.2 The elements of a Comprehensive Geriatric Assessment

Comprehensive Geriatric Assessment (CGA)	
Functional status	
Activities of Daily (ADL) and Instrumental Activities of Daily Living (IADL)	Relation to life expectancy, tolerance of chemotherapy, dependence
Comorbidity Number of comorbid conditions and comorbidity indices	Relation to life expectancy and tolerance of treatment
Mental status Folstein Minimental status	Relation to life expectancy and dependence
Emotional conditions Geriatric Depression Scale (GDS)	Relation to survival; may indicate motivation to receive treatment
Socioeconomic resources Income Living conditions Access to transportation Caregiver	Relationship to tolerance of chemotherapy; involves a number of reversible conditions
Nutritional status Mininutritional assessment (MNA)	Reversible condition; possible relationship to survival
Polypharmacy	Risk of drug interactions
Geriatric syndromes Delirium, dementia, depression, falls, incontinence, spontaneous bone fractures, Neglect and abuse, failure to thrive	Relationship to survival Functional dependence

Based on the geriatric assessment, a staging system of aging has been proposed by Hamerman (1998). Whereas the staging system was originally designed to evaluate the rehabilitative need of individual patients, it may also be used, as outlined in Table 2.3, to plan antineoplastic treatment (Balducci & Extermann, 2001). Given the benefits of the geriatric assessment, failure to perform this assessment in the majority of the older cancer patients appears as one of the most glaring deficits in the study and the management of elderly persons with cancer.

In view of the considerable amount of time the geriatric assessment takes, it should be used only in patients with clinical signs of dysfunction and comorbidity. The experience of the Senior Adult Oncology

TABLE 2.3 Stages of Aging and Consequences for Cancer Treatment

Stage	Clinical characteristics	Treatment plan
Primary	Independent in ADL and IADL; No comorbidity or geriatric syndromes	Full standard treatment, if the risk of cancer-related is likely to reduce the life expectancy, or the active life expectancy, or the quality of life of the patient
Intermediate	This stage is to some extent reversible Dependent in one or more IADL Comorbidity that interferes with regular activities Mild memory disorder or sub-clinical depression	Full treatment if the patient's dysfunction and comorbidity may be reversed; if not, and the cancer threaten the patient life expectancy, active life expectancy, or quality of life, treatment with with special precautions. These may include initial reduction of the dose of chemotherapy, provision of a live-in caregiver.
Secondary or frailty	This stage at present is irreversible. Currently, one of the following definitions of frailty may be used: One of the following criteria (Balducci and Extermann): Dependence ≥ 1 ADL ≥ 1 geriatric syndrome ≥ 3 comorbid conditions Three or more of the following (Fried et al.): Weight loss ≥ 10% over one year; Decreased grip strength; Low energy level; Difficulty in starting movement; Slow walking	Palliative treatment that may involve chemotherapy in low doses
Tertiary or near death	This stage is irreversible. Estimated life expectancy less than 6 months	Palliative treatment

program in Tampa suggests that this approach is too restrictive. Our program is directed to serve patients with different cancers aged 70 and over. Each patient undergoes a comprehensive geriatric assessment. In this population of generally wealthy and independent persons we found the following abnormalities:

Prevalence of unsuspected dementia: 18%
Prevalence of subclinical depression: 19%
Prevalence of serious comorbidity: 67%
Prevalence of IADL dependence: 70%
Prevalence of nutritional risk: 28%
Prevalence of polypharmacy: 35%

Most of these abnormalities would have been lost without a detailed geriatric assessment. In our opinion, the solution to the time burden involved in the CGA is the adoption of some creative solution, such as the use of screening instrument to select patients who may benefit from a full assessment (Balducci & Yates, 2000) (Table 2.4), or the

TABLE 2.4 Example of Screening Tests to Decide Which Patients May Benefit from a Full Assessment

Interview Domain	Question
Cognitive	Serial three (ask the patients to repeat the name of three objects named five minutes earlier)
Depression	Leading questions: Do you have the blues? Do you feel like crying?
Function	Do you need any help with eating, bathing, and dressing? Can you go where you want without help?
Geriatric Syndromes	Do you fall? Do you from time to time lose control of your bladder?
Comorbidity	Review medical record
Socioeconomic Status	Where do you live? Do you need help at home?

B: Functional tests:

Rise up from an armchair, walk 30 feet, and come back to the chair. Monitor the time employed.

employment of pre-filled questionnaires (Cohen et al., JCO, 2001). More information on the CGA is provided in Chapter 5.

OPPORTUNITIES FOR NURSING INTERVENTION

The scarcity of information related to the management of the older cancer patient should be largely imputed to the progressively shrinking space reserved to the patient in modern medical practice. The trend of modern health care appears to be the creation of specialists able to manage fewer and fewer diseases in a reduced amount of time with the help of special tests and expensive intervention. Paradoxically, the medical environment seems to follow a direction that is in direct opposition to the current demographic changes (Yancik & Ries, 2000). With the expansion of the older population, the skill to assess and manage multiple and diverse issues in different domains is essential to tailor nursing interventions to individual needs.

Fortunately, nursing has the expertise and the interest to bridge this enlarging gap. The unique expertise of nursing education consists in weaving together the expertise of different nursing and humanistic fields, to create an environment able to accommodate and foster personal growth (Jennings-Dozier & Mahon, 2000). The current problems related to the diagnosis and management of cancer in older persons present unique opportunities to both nursing practice and nursing research. Clearly, the proper management of cancer in the older aged person involves both primary and oncology nursing. We suggest two models according to the different practice settings (Figure 2.1). In primary care, nursing assessment should address both the issue of screening and that of new symptoms. If proper screening has not been performed, the patient should be directed to screening interventions; if new suspicious symptoms have been recognized, the patient should be directed to diagnostic testing. In oncology (Figure 2.2), the nurse should screen the patient for need of a comprehensive geriatric assessment and perform or obtain the assessment if the person screens positive; in addition, the nurse should obtain both a quality of life and a value history. The results of these assessments should be recorded and become part of the patient's permanent record. In both cases it behooves the nurse to provide education about the value of cancer prevention and cancer treatment even at an advanced age, and to combat ageism in the most determined terms. We recognize of course that alternative and more complex models may be formulated; we propose these models mainly as a statement of the nursing role in the management of older patients with cancer. At the same time, we do

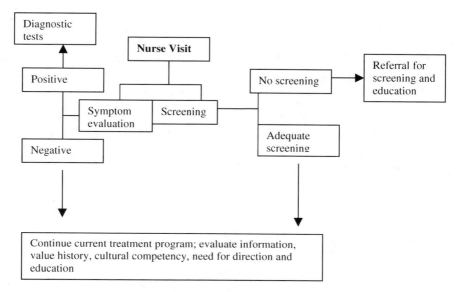

FIGURE 2.1 Nursing Model in Primary Care.

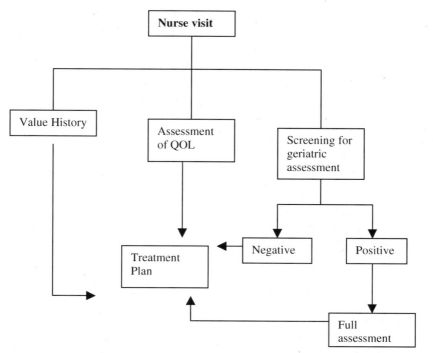

FIGURE 2.2 Nursing Model in Oncology.

recognize that the time commitment involved in this approach should be adequately compensated.

Clearly the management of cancer in the older aged person presents a host of nursing research opportunities. Because of his/her specific training in the holistic approach to the patient, the nurse is in the best position to carry on these research projects, whose complexity may elude the specialist focus of modern nursing. A list of all possible projects is beyond the scope of this chapter. We list the projects that are key to understanding the management of cancer in the older aged person:

- Adoption of a common language, including a common staging system to describe the older person, both with and without cancer;
- Interaction of geriatric and oncology nursing in the planning of the treatment of the older person with cancer. This interaction would be most useful to avoid duplications and redundancy, as well as for case-management purposes;
- Fine-tuning of the geriatric screening instrument to improve the sensitivity and specificity of the instrument;
- Case management in the older cancer patient;
- Educational techniques to overcome ageism and to promote life-saving interventions;
- Criteria for the assessment of quality of care of the older cancer patient;
- Standardization of nursing interview to elicit the description of early symptoms of cancer and to recognize conditions that may hinder timely care.

CONCLUSIONS

Aging is associated with changes in the pattern of cancer care in two areas; delayed diagnosis of cancer, due to reduced utilization of screening interventions and failure to recognize early symptoms and signs of cancer; and decreased utilization of diagnostic tests and of treatment intervention.

Whereas it is not clear whether late diagnosis and under-treatment of cancer may be appropriate in individual circumstances, firm criteria to assess effectiveness and quality of care are missing. To explore these issues, enrollment of additional older persons in clinical trials of cancer prevention and cancer treatment, clinical trials geared uniquely to older patients, and the adoption of a common language to describe older patients are essential. In addition, an intense effort of professional and public education to combat the prejudices related to ageism are essential. Thanks to an orientation toward managing the whole person, the nurse is in an ideal position to lead and conduct these investigations.

REFERENCES

Ahacic, K., Parker, M. G., & Thorslund, M. (2000). Mobility limitations in the Swedish population from 1968–1992: age, gender and social class differences. *Aging, 12*(3), 190–198.

Bain, R. P., Greenberg, R. S., & Whitekar, J. P. (1986). Racial differences in survival in women with breast cancer. *Journal of Chronic Disease, 39*, 631–642.

Balducci, L. (1994). Perspective on quality of life of older patients with cancer. *Drugs & Aging, 4*, 313–324

Balducci, L., & Extermann, M. (2000). *Management of the frail person with advanced cancer. Critical Reviews of Hematology and Oncology, 33*(2), 143–148.

Balducci, L., & Extermann, M. (2001). A practical approach to the older patient with cancer. *Current Problems in Cancer, 25*, 1–76

Balduci, L., Extermann, M., & Carreca, I. (2001). Management of breast cancer in the older woman. *Cancer Control, 8*(5), 431–441.

Balducci, L., Hardy, C. L., & Lyman, G. H. (2001). *Current Opinion in Hematology.*

Balducci, L., Silliman, R. A., & Diaz, N. (in press). Breast cancer: an oncological perspective. In L. Balducci, G. Lyman, & W. B. Ershler (Eds.), *Comprehensive geriatric oncology* (2nd ed.). London, England: Harwood Academic Publishers.

Balducci, L., & Stanta, G. Cancer in the frail patient: a coming epidemic. *Hematology/Oncology Clinics of North America, 2000, 14*, 235–250.

Balducci, L., & Yates, G. (2000). General guidelines for the management of older patients with cancer. *Oncology NCCN Proceedings*, 221–227.

Bates, T., Fennessy, M., & Riley, D. L. (2001). Breast cancer in the elderly: surgery improves survival. The results of a breast cancer campaign trial. *Proceedings of the American Society of Clinical Oncology, 20*, 1533.

Bates-Jensen, B. M. (2001). Quality indicators for prevention and management of pressure ulcers in vulnerable elders. *Annals of Internal Medicine, 135*, 744–751.

Bausell, R. B. (1986). Health-seeking behavior among the elderly. *Gerontologist, 26*, 556–559.

Begg, C. B., & Carbone, P. (1983). Clinical trials and drug toxicity in the elderly. The experience of the Eastern Cooperative Oncology Group. *Cancer, 52*, 1986–1992.

Bennett, C. L., Greenfield, S., Aronow, H., Ganz, P., Vogelzang, N. J., & Elashoff, R. M. (1991). Pattern of care related to men with prostate cancer. *Cancer, 67*, 2633–2641.

Berger, D. H., & Roslyn, J. J. (1997). Cancer surgery in the elderly. *Clinical Geriatric Medicine, 13,* 119–141.

Bergman, L., Kluck, H. M., van Leeuwen, F. E., Crommelin, M. A., Dekker, G., Hart, A. A., & Coebergh, J. W. (1992). The influence of age on treatment choice and survival of elderly cancer patients in South Eastern Netherlands: a population-based study. *European Journal of Cancer, 28A,* 1475–1480.

Bernabei, R., Gambassi, G., Lapane, K., Landi, F., Gatsonis, C., Dunlop, R., Lipsitz, L., Steel, K., & Mor, V. (1998). Randomised trial of impact of model of integrated care and case management for older people living in the community. *British Medical Journal, 316,* 1348–1351.

Chafetz, P. K. (2001). Response to ageism in gerontological language. *Gerontologist, 41*(3), 410.

Cleary, J. F. (1998). Management of pain in the older patient. In L. Balducci, G. H. Lyman, & W. B. Ershler. (Eds.), *Comprehensive geriatric oncology* (pp. 744–753). Amsterdam: Harwood Academic Publishers.

Cohen, H., *Journal of Clinical Oncology,* 2001.

Drucker, D. J. (2001). Development of glucagon-like peptide-1–based pharmaceuticals as therapeutic agents for the treatment of diabetes. *Current Pharmacology, 7*(14), 1399–1441.

Early Breast Cancer Trialists' Collaborative Group A: Tamoxifen for early breast cancer: an overview of the randomized trials. *Lancet, 351,* 1451–1467.

Early Breast Cancer Trialists' Collaborative Group B: Polychemotherapy for early breast cancer, an overview of the randomized trials. *Lancet, 352,* 930–942

Extermann, M., Overcash, J., Lyman, G. H. et al. (1998). Comorbidity and functional status are independent in older cancer patients. *Journal of Clinical Oncology, 16*(4), 1582–1587.

Extermann, M., Balducci, L., & Lyman, G. H. (2000). What threshold for adjuvant therapy in older breast cancer patients? *Journal of Clinical Oncology, 18,* 1709–1717.

Fox, S. A., Siu, A. L., & Stein, J. A. (1994). The importance of physician communication on breast cancer screening of older women. *Archives of Internal Medicine, 154,* 2058–2068.

Fox, S. A., Roetzheim, R. G., & Kington, R. S. (1999). Barriers to cancer prevention in the older person. *Clinical Geriatric Medicine, 13,* 79–95.

Fox, S. A., Stein, J. A., Sockloskie, R. J., & Ory, M. G. (2001). Targeted mail materials and the Medicare beneficiary: increased mammogram screening among the elderly. *American Journal of Public Health, 91,* 55–61.

Fried, L. P., Storer, D. J., King, D. E., & Lodder, F. (1991). Diagnosis of illness presentation in the elderly. *Journal of the American Geriatric Society, 39,* 117–123.

Fried, L. P., Tangen, C. M., Walston, J., Newman, A. B., Hirsch, C., Gottdiener, J., Seeman, T., Tracy, R., Kop, W. J., Burke, G. & McBurnie, M. A. (2001). Frailty in older adults: evidence for a phenotype. *Journal of Gerontology, 56A,* M146–M156.

Goss, P. E., & Strasser, K. (2001). Aromatase inhibitors in the treatment and prevention of breast cancer. *Journal of Clinical Oncology, 19,* 881–894.

Greenfield, S., Blanco, D. M., & Elashoff, R. M. (1987). Pattern of care related to age in breast cancer patients. *Journal of the American Medical Association, 257,* 2766–2770.

Gridelli, C., Perrone, F., Gallo, C., Rossi, A., Barletta, E., Barzelloni, M. L., Creazzola, S., Gatani, T., Fiore, F., Guida, C., & Scognamiglio, F. (1999). Single-agent gemcitabine as second-line treatment in patients with advanced non small cell lung cancer (NSCLC): a phase II trial. *Anticancer Research, 19*(5C), 4535–4538.

Guadagnoli, E., Weitberg, A., Mor, V., Silliman, R. A., Glickman, A. S., & Cummings, F. J. (1990). The influence of patient age on the diagnosis and treatment of colorectal cancer. *Archives of Internal Medicine, 150*(7), 1485–1490.

Hainsworth, J. D., & Vokes, E. E. (1999). Docetaxel (Taxotere) in combination with radiation therapy and the potential of weekly administration in elderly and/or poor performance status patients with advanced non–small cell lung cancer. *Seminars in Oncology, 28*(1 Suppl 2):22–27.

Hamerman, D. (1999). Toward an understanding of frailty. *Annals of Internal Medicine, 130,* 945–950.

Hamerman, D. (1998). Aging: a global theme issue. *Journal of the American Geriatrics Society, 46*(5), 656.

Hillner, B. E., Penberthy, L., Desch, C. E., McDonald, M. K., Smith, T. J., & Retchin, S. M. (1996). Variation in staging and treatment in local and regional breast cancer in the elderly. *Breast Cancer Research and Treatment, 40,* 75–86.

Holly, K., Valavaara, R., & Blanco, G. (2000). Safety and efficacy results of a randomized trial comparing toremifene and tamoxifen in patients with node-positive breast cancer. *Journal of Clinical Oncology, 18,* 3487–3494.

Holmes, F. F. (1994). Clinical course of cancer in the elderly. *Cancer Control, 1,* 108–114.

Hutchins, L. F., Unger, J. M., Crowley, J. J., Coltman, C. A., & Albain, K. S. (1999). Underrepresentation of patients 65 years of age and older in cancer treatment. *New England Journal of Medicine, 341,* 2061–2067.

Inouye, S. K., Bogardus, S. T., Charpentier, P. A., Leo-Summers, L., Acampora, D., Holford, T. R., & Cooney, L. M. (1999). A multicomponent intervention to prevent delirium in hospitalized older patients. *New England Journal of Medicine, 340,* 669–676.

Kemeny, M., & Peakman, M. (1998). Recent advances. Immunology. *Bone Marrow Journal, 316*(7131), 600–603.

Kerlikowske, K., Salzmann, P., Phillips, K. A., Cauley, J. A., & Cummings, S. R. (1999). Continuing screening mammography in women aged 70 to 79 years. *Journal of the American Medical Association, 282,* 2156–2163.

Kurtz, J. M., Jacquemier, J., Amalric, R., Brandone, H., Ayme, Y., Hans, D., Bressac, C., Spitalier, J. M. (1990). Why are local recurrences after breast-conserving therapy more frequent in younger patients. *Journal of Clinical Oncology, 10,* 141–152.

Jennings-Dozier, K., & Mahon, S. M. (2000). Introduction: cancer prevention and early detection—from thought to revolution. *Oncology Nurse Forum, 27*(9), 3–6.

Jezewski, M. A., & Finnell, D. S. (1998). The meaning of DNR status: oncology nurses' experiences with patients and family. *Cancer Nursing, 21*(3), 212–221.

Lagergren, M. (2001). ASIM: a system for monitoring and evaluating the long-term care of the elderly and disabled. *Health Service Research, 28*(1), 27–44.

Lipton, A., Theriault, R. L., Hortobagyi, G. N., Simeone, J., Knight, R. D., Mellars, K., Reitsma, D. J., Heffernan, M., & Seaman, J. J. (2000). Pamidronate prevents skeletal Complications and is effective palliative treatment in women with breast carcinoma and osteolytic bone metastases: long-term follow-up of two randomized placebo-controlled trials. *Cancer, 88,* 1082–1090.

Mackey, H. T. (2001). Nurses in all practice settings will benefit from cancer prevention and early-detection supplement. *Oncology Nurse Forum, 28*(5), 993–994.

MacLean, C. H. (2001). Quality indicators for the management of osteoarthritis in vulnerable elders. *Annals of Internal Medicine, 16,* 711–721.

Mahon, S. M. (2000). Principles of cancer prevention and early detection. *Clinical Journal of Oncology Nursing, 4*(4), 169–176.

Mandelblatt, J. S., Wheat, M. E., Monane, M., Moshief, R. D., Hollenberg, J. P., & Tang, J. (1992). Breast cancer screening for elderly women with and without comorbid conditions. *Annals of Internal Medicine, 116,* 722–730.

Mathews, H. F., Lannin, D. R., & Mitchell, J. (1994). Coming to terms with advanced breast cancer: black women's narratives from eastern North Carolina. *Social Science and Medicine 38*(6), 789–800.

Monfardini S., & Carbone, A. (1998). Non-Hodgkin's lymphomas. In L. Balducci, G. H. Lyman & W. B. Ershler (Eds.), *Comprehensive geriatric oncology* (pp. 577–595). Amsterdam: Harwood Academic Publishers.

Mor, V., Guadagnoli, E., Masterson-Allen, S., Silliman, R., Glicksman, A. S., Cummings, F. J., Goldberg, R. J., & Fretwell, M. D.(1988). Lung, breast and colorectal cancer: the relationship between stage of disease and age at diagnosis. *Journal of the American Geriatrics Society, 36,* 873–876.

Mor, V., Masterson-Allen, S., Goldberg, R., Guadagnoli, E., Wool, M. S. (1990). Pre-diagnostic symptom recognition and help seeking among elderly patients. *Journal of Community Health, 15,* 253–266.

Muss, H. (2001). Older age—not a barrier to cancer treatment. *New England Journal of Medicine, 345*(15), 1127–1128.

Mustacchi, G., Milani, S., Pluchinotta, A., De Matteis, A., Rubagotti, A., & Perrota, A. (1994). Tamoxifen or surgery plus tamoxifen as primary treatment for elderly patients with operable breast cancer: The G.R.E.T.A. Trial Group for Research on Endocrine Therapy in the Elderly. *Anticancer Research, Sep-Oct,* 14.

Nattinger, A. B., Gottlieb, M. S., Veum, J., Yahnke, D., & Goodwin, J. S. (1992). Geographic variation in the use of breast-conserving treatment for breast cancer. *New England Journal of Medicine, 326,* 1102–1107.

Nixon, A. J., Neuberg, D., Hayes, D. F., Gelman, R., Connolly, J. L., Schnitt, S., Abner, A., Recht, A., Vicini, F., & Harris, J. R. (1994). Relationship of patient's age to pathologic features of the tumor and prognosis for patients with stage I or II breast cancer. *Journal of Clinical Oncology, 12,* 888–894.

Olivotto, I., & Levine, M. (2001). Clinical practice guidelines for the care and treatment of breast cancer: the management of ductal carcinoma in situ. *Canadian Medical Association Journal, 165*(7), 912–913.

Overcash, J., Extermann, M., Parr, J., Perry, J., & Balducci, L. (in press). Validity and reliability of the FACT-G scale for use in the older person with cancer. *American Journal of Clinical Oncology, 24*(6), 591–596.

Pearson, M. L., Lee, J. L., Chang, B. L., Elliott, M., Kahan, K. L., & Rubenstein, L. V. (2000). Structured implicit review: a new method for monitoring nursing quality. *Medical Care, 38*(11), 1071–1091.

Petrisek, A. C., Laliberte, L. L., Allen, S. M., & Mor, V. (1997). The treatment decision-making process: age differences in a sample of women diagnosed with non-recurrent early-stage breast cancer. *Gerontologist, 37,* 598–608.

Repetto, L., Fratino, L., & Audisio, R. A. (in press). The comprehensive geriatric assessment adds to the ECOG performance status in elderly cancer patients. *Journal of Clinical Oncology, 20*(2), 494–502.

Repetto, L., & Balducci, L. (in press). A case for geriatric oncology. *Lancet.*

Reuben, D. B., Frank, J. C., Hirsch, S. H., McGuigan, K. A., & Maly, R. C. (1999). A randomized clinical trial of outpatient geriatric assessment (CGA), coupled with an intervention, to increase adherence to recommendations. *Journal of the American Geriatrics Society, 47*(3):371–372.

Rhew, D. C. (2001). Quality indicators for the management of pneumonia in vulnerable elders. *Annals of Internal Medicine, 135,* 735–743.

Rockwood, K., Stadnyk, K., MacKnight, C., McDowell, I., Hebert, R., & Hogan, D. B. (1999). A brief clinical instrument to classify frailty in elderly people. *Lancet, 353,* 205–206.

Roetzheim, R. G., Fox, S. A., & Leake, B. (1995). Physician-reported determinant of screening mammography in older women: the impact of physician and practice characteristics. *Journal of the American Geriatrics Society, 43,* 1398–1402.

Samet, J. M., Hunt, W. C., & Goodwin, J. S. (1990). Determinant of cancer stage: a population-based study of elderly New Mexicans. *Cancer, 66,* 1302–1307.

Samet, J., Hunt, W. C., Key, C., Humble, C. G., & Goodwin, J. S. (1986). Choice of cancer therapy varies with age of patient. *Journal of the American Medical Association, 255,* 3385–3390.

Samet, J. M., Hunt, W. C., Lerchen, M. L., & Goodwin, J. S. (1988). Delay in seeking care for cancer symptoms: a population-based study of elderly New Mexicans. *Journal of the National Cancer Institute, 80,* 432–438.

Schostak, Z. (1991). Ethical guidelines for the treatment of the dying elderly. *Journal Halacha Contemporary Society, 22,* 62–86.

Seidman, A. D., Fornier, M. N., Esteva, F. J., Tan, L., Kaptain, S., Bach, A., Panageas, K. S., Arroyo, C., Valero, V., Currie, V., Gilewski, T., Theodoulou, M., Moynahan, M. E., Moasser, M., Sklarin, N., Dickler, M., D'Andrea, G., Cristofanilli, M., Rivera, E., Hortobagyi, G. N., Norton, L., & Hudis, C. A. (2001). Weekly Trastuzumab and paclitaxel therapy for metastatic breast cancer with analysis of efficacy by HER2 immunophenotype and gene amplification. *Journal of Clinical Oncology, 19,* 2587–2595.

Silliman, R. A., Guadagnoli, E., Weitberg, A. B., & Mor V. (1989). Age as a predictor of diagnostic and treatment intensity in recently diagnosed breast cancer patients. *Journal of Gerontology, 44,* M46–M50.

Spielberger, R. T., Stiff, P., & Emmanouilides, C. (2001). Efficacy of recombinant human keratinocyte growth factor (rHuKGF) in reducing mucositis in patients with hematologic malignancies undergoing autologous peripheral blood progenito cell transplantation after radiation-based conditioning. Results of a Phase 2 trial. *Proceedings of the American Society of Clinical Oncology, 20,* 7a, Abstr 25.

Tinetti, M. E., Baker, D. I., McAvay, G., Claus, E. B., Garrett, P., Gottschalk, M., Koch, M. L., Trainor, K., & Horwitz, R. I. (1994). A multifactorial intervention to reduce the risk of falling among elderly people living in the community. *New England Journal of Medicine, 331,* 821–827.

Treacy, J. T., & Mayer, D. K. (2000). Perspectives on cancer patient education. *Seminars in Oncology Nursing, 16*(1), 47–56.

Valentinis, B., Silvestrini, R., and Daidone, M. G. (1991). 3H-Thymidine labeling index, hormone receptors and ploidy in breast cancer from elderly patients. *Breast Cancer Research and Treatment, 20,* 19–24.

Zambrana, R. E., Breen, N., Fox, S. A., & Gutierrez-Mohamed. M. L. (1999). Use of cancer screening practices by Hispanic Women: analysis of a subgroup. *Prevention Medicine, 29,* 466–477.

Yancik, R., & Ries, L. A. G. (2000). Aging and cancer in America: demographic and epidemiological perspectives. *Hematology/Oncology Clinics of North America, 14,* 17–24.

CHAPTER THREE

Cancer Screening and Prevention in the Older Cancer Patient

Michael A. Silverman, Scott D. Barnett, Patricia Ryan, Adam Golden, and Neil Nusbaum

EPIDEMIOLOGY OF PREVENTION

Preventive medicine can be thought of as three chronologically distinct topics. The goal of primary prevention is to promote a healthy lifestyle to reduce the number of new cases of disease (incidence) in healthy individuals. The goal of secondary prevention is to detect asymptomatic (occult) disease. (Greenberg, Daniels, & Flanders, 1993) Tertiary prevention seeks to decrease the future additional effects of disease once it has already been diagnosed.

Secondary cancer prevention strategies rely on screening, the application of an accepted test or method to identify unrecognized cancer. Cancer screening tests sort out those individuals who are more likely to have the disease, and they can then be studied more closely for the presence of occult cancer. Four characteristics of a disease have been cited as requirements for making it suitable for screening and are seen in Table 3.1 (Wilson & Jungner, 1964).

Results of screening fall into two categories—positive and negative. Sensitivity of a screening test is the probability that an individual with a disease will test positive. Sensitivity thus reflects the proportion of positive tests in all those individuals with the disease. The specificity of a given test is the probability that an individual who is disease-free will test negative. Specificity thus reflects the proportion of negative

TABLE 3.1 Characteristics of a Suitable Test for Screening

The disease should have serious consequences.

The disease must have a treatment once a diagnosis is made.

The detectable preclinical phase of the disease should have a high prevalence; otherwise, too few cases would be detected to justify the expense of a screening program.

The test must also be available at a reasonable cost.

tests in all those individuals free of disease. A false-positive test is said to occur when a disease-free person tests positive. A false-negative test is seen when a person with disease tests negative.

The positive predictive value (PPV) of a screening test is the probability that an individual has the disease given that the test is positive. The negative predictive value (NPV) of a screening test is the probability that an individual is disease-free given that the test is negative. The mathematical relationship of sensitivity and specificity is such that an increase in one necessitates a decrease in the other. When screening for cancer in the elderly, a low specificity leads to a large number of false positives, which is concomitant with an increase in diagnostic tests at increased cost and with the potential for the risks of unnecessary examinations.

It is important to recognize that screening tests have potential limitations. For example, the apparent increase in survival due to early detection (lead-time bias) may lead to no real increase in the patients' life expectancy. Additionally, screening does not fare well with aggressive cancer. Those individuals appearing to live longer after early detection tend to have less-aggressive cancers compared to individuals dying immediately after the detection of an aggressive cancer (length-time bias). Furthermore, there will always be some proportion of individuals that will be "over diagnosed" (Black, 2000). These individuals have preclinical detectable cancer that would remain stable or progress too slowly ever to become clinically apparent in their lifetime.

GERIATRIC ISSUES IN SCREENING

The use of screening for the early detection of cancer in the elderly poses a challenge for health care providers (Silverman et al., 2000). Many health care providers feel that there is a lack of time and monetary reimbursement for providing preventative health services. In addition, the recommendations for screening that are advocated by different organizations are often contradictory or do not address screening in the elderly. Many investigations utilizing new technology are performed by skilled experts in academic centers, making extrapolation difficult for primary care providers. These studies often report only survival data. They do not address issues such as quality of life and functional outcomes. (Bennahum, Forman, Vellas, & Albarede, 1997). The presumed benefits of screening in identifying occult disease must be counterbalanced by possible negative consequences of any further diagnostic or therapeutic interventions resulting from positive screen findings. The life expectancy of the person to be screened must be considered in any decision regarding screening, but age alone cannot be used as the single determining factor when making decisions regarding screening (Walter & Covinsky, 2001). Understanding the needs and desires of a well-informed patient is at the heart of the decision making process.

BREAST CANCER

INCIDENCE

Breast cancer is the second leading cause of cancer death in women, with 40,800 deaths in 2000 (Greenlee et al., 2001). The incidence of breast cancer increases with age. Forty-three percent of all new breast cancer cases are in women 65 years and older.

PATHOLOGY

Breast cancer in older women is thought to be less aggressive, with a larger percentage of estrogen-receptor (ER) positive cells and more favorable biologic characteristics (Diab, Ellege, & Clark, 2000).

RISK FACTORS

The major risk factor for breast cancer is age older than 60 years (McCarthy et al., 1998). Additionally, breast cancer is an important diagnostic consideration even if the older woman has no family history of the disease. Many other risk factors have been identified including first degree relative with breast cancer diagnosed when younger than 40, postmenopausal body mass index greater than 35, menopause at 55 or older, menarche before the age of 12 (Collaborative Group on Hormonal Factors in Breast Cancer, 1997).

Hormone replacement therapy with estrogen has been implicated in postmenopausal women as a risk factor for breast cancer (Clemons & Goss, 2001). The combination of estrogen-progesterone therapy may cause a rise in cancer risk, which is more than for estrogen alone. It has been shown, however, that the breast cancers found in women taking HRT may have a low biologic aggressiveness (Holli, Isola, & Cuzick, 1998).

DIET

The association between fat intake and breast cancer remains controversial. Recent studies have also been unable to confirm any association between fruit and vegetable consumption and breast cancer risk (Smith-Warner, Spiegelman, & Yaun, 2001).

CHEMOPREVENTION

The FDA has approved tamoxifen for primary or contralateral breast cancer risk reduction (Lippman & Brown, 1998). Tamoxifen also has positive results when used in patients with ductal carcinoma in situ (DCIS).

Tamoxifen increases the risk of endometrial cancer, especially in women 50 years and older (Bergman, Beelen, & Gallee, 2000). Risk benefit assessment of tamoxifen is not defined in African-American women and other minority women. The decision regarding the use of tamoxifen in older women must be individualized and take into account the potential for an increase in stroke, pulmonary embolism, and deep vein thrombosis (The American College of Obstetricians and Gynecologists, 1996). The selective estrogen response modifier raloxifene might also significantly reduce the risk of breast cancer in postmenopausal women and is currently under study (Cummings et al. 1999).

SCREENING

The preclinical period in which breast cancers are detectable is long and has been shown to increase with age (Robinson & Beghe, 1997). This tumor behavior and effective treatments make breast cancer a good candidate for screening. The methods used for breast cancer detection are breast self-examination (BSE), clinical breast examination (CBE) and mammography (Nusbaum, 2001).

In older women, the diagnosis of breast cancer is made in 90% by the findings of a breast mass, and there are those who advocate CBE alone as screening for elderly women even though mammography is more sensitive for finding smaller lesions (Kerlikowske, Grady, & Rubin, 1995).

Empirical data regarding the optimal approach to screening women aged 70 and older is limited. Older women, especially African Americans, are less likely to be screened than younger women because of cultural, economic, provider, spiritual, and religious reasons (American Geriatrics Society, 2001).

RECOMMENDATION

The American Cancer Society recommends a yearly mammogram for women starting at age 40 (Smith, Meitlin, Davis, & Eyre, 2000). Clinical breast examination supplements the mammogram. Whether screening women over 70 is beneficial is undetermined; it has been advocated in those elders with an anticipated survival (apart from breast cancer) of at least five years, so that they are likely to derive clinical benefit from a diagnosis of occult breast cancer. A recent consensus statement from a panel of gerontologists and cancer specialists called for self breast exam monthly, clinical breast exam yearly, and mammography every two years (American Geriatrics Society Clinical Practice Committee, 2000). Decisions on screening must be based on an informal agreement between provider and patient and should taken into account a consideration of life expectancy, comorbidities, and quality of life (Satariano & Ragland, 1994).

A recent review of the randomized controlled trials of screening by (Gotsche, P. C.; Olsen, O.: Is screening for breast cancer with mammography justifiable? *The Lancet, 2002, 355,* 12934), has cast coubts on the effectiveness of mammography as a strategy. This view, howevere, has been rejected by the majority of scholars and clinical investigators. The most authoritative rebuttal came from the Cochrane foundation (Cochrane Breast Cancer Group: setting the record straight, *The Lancet, 2002, 359,* 9304). The major guidelines organizatiaons, including the United States Preventive Service Task Force (USPSTF), the National Cancer Institute, The American Geriatric Society, and the American Cancer Society, still support periodical screening mammography as a way to reduce the mortality related to breast cancer in the general population.

CERVICAL CANCER

INCIDENCE

In 2000 the number of new cases of invasive cervical cancer was 12,600 with 4,600 deaths (Greenlee, 2001). The 5–year survival for early-stage disease is 88%; for advanced cancer only 13%.

TABLE 3.2 Risk Factors for Cervical Dysplasia and Cervical Cancer

Intercourse at any age
Multiple sexual partners
History of human papilloma virus (HPV)
Tobacco use
Lower socioeconomic status
History of sexually transmitted disease
History of cervical dysplasia or cervical cancer and infection for human
immunodeficiency virus

Risk Factors

There are a number of risk factors described for cervical dysplasia and cervical cancer that are listed in Table 3.2 (Schiffman & Brinton, 1995).

Screening

The sole practical means of early detection is through cervical cytology (Sawaya, Brown, & Washington, 2001). Since screening for cervical cancer with the cervical cytology screening was begun, there has been a decline in incidence rates of about 80%. This manual technique allows the early detection of cells that have been obtained from the squamocolumnar junction. Despite the effectiveness of this screening methodology, between 28% and 64% of American women 65 years and older have never sought a Pap smear or have not had one performed within the previous three years. This phenomenon may help explain the relatively high rate of disease noted in older women with abnormal screens.

Method of Obtaining Specimen

The older woman not uncommonly has an atrophic or small cervical os, which makes access to the cells of the squamocolumnar junction difficult. Women with musculoskeletal abnormalities may need to be placed in the left lateral position when obtaining a specimen.

The American Geriatrics Society's position in older women is to address barriers and to stop screening beyond age 70, if the woman has been regularly screened and shows no abnormality. In addition, two negative Pap smears one year apart should be obtained in women never screened. (ACOG Committee Opinion No. 247, 2000.)

ENDOMETRIAL CANCER

There were approximately 36,100 cases of cancer of the uterine corpus in 2000 with 6,500 deaths. (Greenlee et al., 2001). The incidence of endometrial cancer climbs with age and peaks in women 70 to 75 years.

RISK FACTORS

Risk factors include age, nulliparity, early menarche, late menopause, diabetes mellitus, obesity, history of breast or colon cancer, and tamoxifen use (Parazzini, LaVechia, Bocciolone, & Franceschi 1991). In addition, the use of estrogen without progesterone for hormone replacement therapy is also a risk factor for endometrial cancer.

RECOMMENDATIONS

There are no current recommendations for endometrial screening.

OVARIAN CANCER

In the United States cancer of the ovary is the fifth leading cause of death among women and has the highest mortality rate of all gynecological cancers. The annual incidence rate is estimated to be 26,000 new cases in 2000 with 14,000 deaths (Greenlee et al., 2001). Women whose cancer is found at Stage 1 are three times more likely to survive than women with widespread disease (80% versus 10% 5-year survival for Stage I and Stage IV, respectively) (Whiltemore, Harris & Itnyre, 1992). The incidence increases with age, with the majority of disease seen in postmenopausal women with a median age of 63. Risk declines with increased parity, oral contraceptive use, and breast-feeding. Risk is increased in women with a family history of ovarian cancer, use of fertility drugs, and estrogen replacement therapy.

SCREENING

A bimanual pelvic examination has a low sensitivity of 5% and is not a useful screening method. The two tests employed for ovarian cancer screening are the serum CA-125 level and transvaginal ultrasound (Runowicz & Fields, 1999). The CA-125 is a tumor-associated antigen that has its greatest use for monitoring patients already diagnosed with an ovarian malignancy (Rosenthal & Jacobs, 1998). The sensitivity is low, as is the specificity for CA-125. The CA-125 level can be elevated by fibroids, menstruation, endometriosis, gastrointestinal disease, other malignancies, and a host of systemic conditions. The transvaginal ultrasound, however, uses Doppler imaging and has a reported sensitivity of up to 90% (Sato, Yokoyama, Sekamoto et al., 2000). There presently are no guidelines for routine screening for ovarian cancer.

LUNG CANCER

INCIDENCE

Lung cancer is the number one cause of cancer death among men and women in the United States with 156,900 deaths in 2000 (Greenlee et al., 2001). The 5–year survival is a dismal 13%, with most persons presenting with advanced disease.

PRIMARY PREVENTION

It is never too late to benefit from quitting. Older smokers are able to quit, as are younger smokers (Baillie, Mattick, Hall, & Webster, 1994). The elderly can achieve major benefit from quitting. To overcome many years of smoking, proven cessation programs must focus on two fronts: one, behavioral patterns and two, physical addiction. Recent pharmacotherapy trials have been encouraging (Hughes, Goldstein, Hurt, & Schiffman, 1999). The use of nicotine gum, transdermal patches, or bupropion has demonstrated effectiveness in smoking cessation programs.

DIET

Although antioxidant effects appear to protect tissue from oxidative damage in humans, one trial found that the use of supplemental betacarotene and vitamin A actually increased the risk of cancer mortality in smokers and employees exposed to asbestos (Omenn, Goodman, & Thornguist, 1996).

SCREENING

Since the 1950s investigators have pursued a screening test that can lead to a decrease in disease–specific mortality (Patz, Goodman, & Bepler, 2000). Counseling about stopping smoking and patient education may be more important than routine lab tests and x-rays. Some investigators, however, are strong advocates of lung cancer screening, especially for high-risk former smokers (= 30 pack years) or those who have lung disease air flow obstruction (Petty, 2000). Newer techniques of detecting cancer at an earlier stage, such as spiral computed tomography, fluorescence bronchoscopy, sampling sputum and bronchiolar lavage (for genetic mutations such as p53 and K-ras, telomerase activity, and abnormal DNA methylation) are being studied (Ahrendt et al., 1997). Currently, there are no recommendations for routine screening for the detection of lung cancer.

PROSTATE CANCER

INCIDENCE

In North American men, prostate cancer is the most common cancer with 180,000 new cases in the United States during 2000 with 31,900 deaths (Greenlee et al., 2001). Prostate cancer is responsible for 32% of all cancer in men and for 14% of cancer-related deaths, second only to lung cancer. Cancer of the prostate rates increase until the age of 80 when the cancer plateaus and then decreases.

RISK FACTORS

The most important risk factors for prostate cancer are age, family history, and being African American (Parker et al., 1998). The incidence in African American men is 40% higher than in white men. Risk is not increased by benign prostatic hypertrophy.

DIET

There is currently a debate concerning evidence associating dietary fat and red meat in the development and progression of prostate cancer (Fair, Fleshner, & Heston, 1997).

CHEMOPREVENTION

Finasteride is a 5 alpha reductase inhibitor that is currently under study as a chemo-preventative agent (Bologna et al., 1995). No data are yet available concerning its preventive role.

SCREENING

Prostate cancer has a relatively slow doubling time, usually three years or more, making it amenable to early detection. Potential curative approaches for disease exist and include both radical prostatectomy or radiotherapy (D'Amico et al., 1998). Controversy however exists regarding both screening and treatment. A number of low-grade prostate cancers are nonprogressive over many years (Lu Yao & Yau, 1997). Asymptomatic cancers have been found at autopsy or after surgery for bladder cancer in 30%–40% of men 50 to 60 years old. The two methods for cancer screening are digital rectal examination (DRE) and measurement of serum prostate-specific antigen (PSA). Positive screening by either method leads to biopsy of the prostate in many cases. The simplest and most inexpensive test for cancer screening is digital rectal examination (DRE) but many of the cancers found on DRE are at advanced stage (Barry, 2001). DRE alone has not been shown in routine annual screening to reduce prostate cancer mortality.

PROSTATE-SPECIFIC ANTIGEN

The prostate produces prostatespecific antigen (PSA), a serine protease which is secreted in the serum (Carter, 2000). Measurement of the PSA has been used as a screening test for prostate cancer and has been found to have the highest positive predicted value (PPV). The PSA is affected by a number of conditions and interventions; including acute urinary retention, benign prostatic hypertrophy, prostate needle biopsy, prostatitis, cystoscopy, and transurethral resection of the prostate. Ejaculation may cause a slight transient rise in the PSA, but a rectal examination has no clinically significant effect (Catalona, Ramos, Carvahal, & Yan, 2000).

The effect of PSA screening on prostate cancer mortality has not yet been definitely answered. Its potential as a screening tool has been suggested by case control studies using serum bank specimens. Elevated PSA levels greater than the cutoff values of 4.0 ng/ml can predict cancer with a sensitivity of 71% at 5 years (Carter, 2000). Some have recommended lowering the PSA cutoff level of 4.0 ng/ml to 3.0 ng/ml (Babaian et al., 2001; Catalona et al., 2000). Investigations are looking at other ways to improve the sensitivity and specificity of PSA in prostate cancer screening. These approaches include measuring the rate of increase of PSA over time, the PSA density, and the fraction of PSA that is circulating as free PSA versus complexed PSA, and using higher cutoff values for PSA testing in older men.

Several studies have shown a declining trend in the incidence and mortality of metastatic prostatic cancer, which has been attributed to the current widespread PSA testing of the population (Roberts et al., 2001). There is no direct evidence from population based prospective trials as to the effects of PSA screening on mortality. The use of screening to identify prostate cancer in older men is controversial. The over-whelming majority of men diagnosed with and dying of this disease are elderly. This is of relevance in terms of screening because of the multiple chronic diseases and associated functional decline seen in older men (Litman, 1999). More than 50% of U.S. men by the age of 80 suffer from at least two chronic diseases. Thus even though prostate cancer is a frequent condition of older men, the high prevalence of comorbidities together with prostate cancer's relative slow growth in older men often points to competing causes of death in prostate cancer patients.

One of the major criticisms regarding PSA-based screening is that it leads to over-diagnosis and subsequent increased testing, unnecessary treatment, and morbidity from these procedures. The cancers detected on screening will include indolent lesions that would not have affected the patient for years into the future, and so not within the life expectancy of many of the men in whom they are detected. In one cohort of men followed for 15 years, almost 90% of the deaths were thought to be from etiologies other than prostate cancer (Johansson et al., 1997).

The American Cancer Society recommends annual screening with PSA testing and DRE for males older than 50 years (Smith et al., 2001). The American College of Physicians does not recommend routine screening for prostate cancer (American College of Physicians, 1997). Health care providers must take into account QOL (quality of life) and life expectancy and patient and family priorities (Etzion et al., 1998). Investigators should not screen unless an individual has a life expectancy of at least 10 years. No randomized trials of prostate cancer have yet demonstrated evidence to support routine screening for asymptomatic older men.

COLON CANCER

INCIDENCE

There were an estimated 130,200 new cases of colorectal cancer diagnosed in 2000, with 56,300 deaths (Greenlee et al., 2001). Despite declining mortality rates in both men and women over the past 20 years, it is still the second most common cause of cancer death in the United States. The rates of colorectal cancer, however, rise significantly after 50 years old and are a major cause of cancer death in the older population (Ries et al., 1999). Early detection and improved surgical techniques, adjuvant therapy, and radiation therapy have led to an improvement in survival rates. Patients with local disease have a 5–year survival rate of 86.7% versus 5.35% for those with advanced disease (Potter, Slattery, Bostick, & Gapstar, 1993). Colorectal cancer is thought to be a preventable disease and is amenable to screening. The mean age of presentation for colorectal cancer is in the middle of the seventh decade for both men and women.

RISK FACTORS

Most colorectal cancers are sporadic and are caused by a combination of genetic and environmental factors. The DNA damage initiates the development of abnormal epithelial cells, which progress to adenomas and eventually to colorectal cancer (Bedenne et al., 1992).

PRIMARY PREVENTION

There is substantial interest in the incidence of colorectal cancer and lifestyle (Giovannucci et al., 1994). Red meat and alcohol consumption have been associated with an increased risk of colorectal cancer. For many years, it has been reported and accepted that a diet high in fiber, fruits, and vegetables is associated with a decreased risk of colorectal cancer. Fiber has been shown to decrease transit time, lower pH, and produce short chain fatty acids, which are anticarcinogenic. Using seasoning fats such as olive oil has been reported to be of benefit (Braga et al., 1998). Recent investigations, however, have questioned these findings. Alberts et al. was unable to demonstrate that a high fiber cereal supplement decreased the risk of recurrent adenomas (Alberts et al., 2000). Calcium has shown a measurable, but not statistically significant reduction, in the risk of adenoma recurrence in patients using it as a diet supplementation (Bonithon et al., 2000). Nonsteroidal anti-inflammatory drugs and aspirin have been demonstrated to decrease the incidence and mortality from adenoma and colon cancer (Steinbach et al., 2000). The risk of colon cancer may be decreased by Hormone Replacement Therapy (HRT). Smoking may be a modifiable factor in the development of colorectal cancer.

SECONDARY PREVENTION

Because of its high prevalence, long asymptomatic phase, and the presence of treatable precancerous lesions (adenomas), colorectal cancer is an ideal candidate for screening. Secondary prevention thus is the major emphasis in the prevention of colorectal cancer and involves breaking the adenoma-carcinoma sequence. There are screening tests and diagnostic tests that are safe and effective and include fecal occult blood tests (FOBT), flexible sigmoidoscopy, barium enema, and colonoscopy.

FECAL OCCULT BLOOD TEST (FOBT)

FOBT screening detects cancer at an early stage and reduces mortality by up to 30% to 40% (Towler et al., 1998). FOBT screening may have an effect on incidence rates although its ability to detect adenomas is less sensitive than its detection of asymptomatic early cancer. In the elderly the question of benefits versus risks is paramount. It is difficult to answer, however, because specific data is scarce; published rates of complications may not necessarily reflect those encountered in the community. Since the time it takes for a polyp to transform into a malignancy is calculated at about 10–15 years, many polyps found by screening would not be expected to become malignant during an older patient's lifetime. Many persons would be put through expensive and potentially harmful interventions with no specific benefit. For instance, a FOBT, which has a low predictive value (2%-11% for cancer and 20%-30% for adenomas) when positive, exposes many frail elderly patients to procedures such as colonoscopy. Benefits to the individual might not be seen unless the person has at least a 3–5 year life expectancy. Cost analyses indicate that all methods of screening for colorectal cancer are cost-effective. FOBT may reduce the incidence of colorectal cancer (Mandel et al., 2000). It is not very sensitive to detect polyps, but will detect those that are large, and are more likely to bleed and become cancerous. Three randomized controlled trials and observational studies have concluded that both annual and biennial screening for occult blood significantly decrease the rate of death from colorectal cancer (Kronborg, Fenger, Olsen, Jorgensen, & Sondergaard, 1996; Mandel, Church, Ederer, & Bond, 1999). The FOBT can yield either false-positive or false negative results.

Case control studies provide the evidence that proctosigmoidoscopy lowers mortality from cancer with protection that lasts up to 6 to 10 years (Sutton et al., 2000). The sensitivity of flexible sigmoidoscopy is between 44% and 64%. The sensitivity improves with the 60 cm sigmoidoscope rather than the 25 cm–35 cm scope.

Biopsies are required for small polyps. If hyperplastic, no further action is needed. Colonoscopy is indicated for adenomatous polyps. The National Polyp Study concluded that a three-year interval between examinations versus a one-year interval was effective for prevention of advanced adenomas and was cost-effective (Winawer et al.,

1993). Colonoscopy may be undertaken every 5 years for patients with only a single small tubular adenoma after one negative follow-up at three years. If the complete removal of all polyps is uncertain, additional colonoscopy may be required in 3 to 6 months. Colonoscopy for preoperative evaluation of colorectal cancer is performed to ensure removal of all synchronous polyps and cancers. The major objective of follow-up colonoscopy is to detect additional cancer because people with a history of colon cancer are at risk for further colon cancer lesions.

The procedure of choice for assessing patients for symptoms or for a positive screening test and for surveillance is colonoscopy. No convincing data is yet available for the use of colonoscopy as a screening tool and its effects on lowering mortality. One would deduce, however, that since it can detect more proximal disease than does sigmoidoscopy, it would be superior in reducing mortality. A barium enema can be used as an alternative screening test to flexible sigmoidoscopy in low-risk individuals. Patients with polyps seen on barium enema should undergo a colonoscopy. Indications for colonoscopy are listed in Table 3.3.

Colonoscopy allows for immediate removal or biopsy of suspicious lesions. It is considered safe and well tolerated (Zubarik et al., 1991). Bleeding or perforation is reported in 10–30/10,000 examinations with death in 1 patient per 10,000 colonoscopies (Lieberman et al., 2000).

The USPSTF recommends fecal occult blood testing yearly starting at 50 years. Sigmoidoscopy screening is an alternative to FOBT. The evidence is insufficient to recommend screening with DRE, barium enema, or colonoscopy (United States Preventive Services Task Force, 1996). The ACS recommends for average risk persons over the age of 50, yearly FOBT plus flexible sigmoidoscopy every 5 years, colonoscopy every 10 years (USPSTF Recommendation, 2000). DRE should be performed simultaneously. No upper age limit is given.

TABLE 3.3 Indications for Colonoscopy in Cancer Screening

Prior colorectal cancer
Prior colonic adenomas
Ulcerative pancolitis of 8 years' duration
Left sided colitis greater than 15 years' duration
Familial adenomatous polyposis
Hereditary nonpolyposis colorectal cancer (HNPCC)
First-degree relatives with colorectal cancer

REFERENCES

ACOG Committee Opinion No. 247. (2000). *Routine Cancer Screening.* Washington, DC: American College of Obstetricians and Gynecologists.

Ahrendt, S. A., Yang, S. C., Wu, L., Westra, W. H., Jen, J., Califano, J. A., & Sidransky. (1997). Comparison of oncogene detection and telomerase activity for the molecular staging of non-small cell lung cancer. *Clinical Cancer Research, 3,* 1–14.

Alberts, D. S., Martinez, M. E., Roe, D. J., Guillen-Rodriquez, J. M., Marshell, J. R., van Leeuwen, J. B., Reid, M. E., Ritenbaugh, C., Vargus, P. A., Bhattacharyya, A. B., Earnst, D. L., & Sampliner, R. E. (2000). Lack of effect of a high-fiber cereal supplement on the recurrence of colorectal adenomas. *New England Journal of Medicine, 342,* 1156–1162.

American College of Physicians. (1997). Guidelines for screening for prostate cancer. *Annals of Internal Medicine, 126,* 480–484.

American Geriatrics Society Clinical Practice Committee. (2000). Breast cancer screening in older women. *Journal of the American Geriatrics Society, 48,* 842–844.

American Geriatrics Society. (2001). Screening for Cervical Carcinoma in Older Women. *Journal of the American Geriatrics Society, 49,* 655–657.

The American College of Obstetricians and Gynecologists Guidelines for Women's Health Care. (1996). Washington, DC: American College of Obstetricians and Gynecologists. 104.

Babaian, R. J., Johnston, D. A., Naccarato, W., Ayala, A., Bhadkamkar, V. A., Fritsche, H. A. (2001). The incidence of prostate cancer in a screening population with a serum prostate antigen between 2.5 and 4.0 ng/ml. relation to biopsy strategy. *Journal of Urology 2001, 165,* 757–760.

Baillie, A., Mattick, R. P , Hall, W., & Webster, P. (1994). Meta-analytic review of the efficacy of smoking cessation interventions. *Drug Alcohol Review, 13,* 157–170.

Barry, M. S. (2001). Prostate-specific-antigen testing for early diagnosis of prostate cancer. *New England Journal of Medicine, 344,* 1373–1377.

Bedenne, L., Faivre, J., Boutron, M. C., Piard, F., Cauvin, J. M., & Hillon, P. (1992). Adenoma-carcinoma sequence on 'denovo' carcinogenesis? *Cancer, 69,* 883–888.

Bennahum, D. A., Forman, W. B., Vellas, B., & Albarede, J. L. (1997). Life expectancy, comorbidity, and quality of life: A framework of reference for medicine decisions. *Clinical Geriatric Medicine, 13,* 33–53.

Bergman, L., Beelen, M. L., Gallee, M. P., Hollema, H., Benraadt, J., & van Leeuwen, F. E. (2000). Risk and prognosis of endometrial cancer after tamoxifen for breast cancer. *Lancet, 356,* 811–817.

Black, W. C. (2000). Overdiagnosis: An under-recognized cause of confusion and harm in cancer screening. *Journal of the National Cancer Institute, 92,* 1280–1282.

Bologna, M., Muzi, P., Biordi, L., Festuccia, C., & Vicentini, C. (1995). Finasteride dose dependently reduces the proliferation rate of the Ln Cap human prostatic cancer cell line in vitro. *Urology, 45,* 282–290.

Bonithon-Kopp, C., Kronoborg, O., & Giacosa, A. (2000). Calcium and fibre supplementation in prevention of colorectal adenoma recurrence: a randomized intervention. *The Lancet, 356,* 1300–1306.

Braga, C., LaVecchia, C. L., & Franceschis, S. (1998). Olive oil, other seasoning fats, and the risk of colorectal cancer. *Cancer, 82,* 448–453.

Carter, H. (2000). A PSA threshold of 4.0 ng/ml for early detection of prostate cancer: the only rational approach for men 50 years old and older. *Urology, 55,* 796–799.

Carvahal, G. T., Smith, D. S., & Mager, D. E. (1999). Digital rectal examination for detecting prostate cancer at PSA levels 4 ng/ml or less. *Journal of Urology, 161,* 835–839.

Catalona, W. J., Ramos, C. G., Carvahal, G. F., & Yan, Y. (2000). Lowering PSA cutoffs to enhance detection of curable prostate cancer. *Urology. 55,* 791–795.

Clemons, M., & Goss, P. (2001). Estrogen and the risk of breast cancer. *New England Journal of Medicine, 344,* 276–285.

Collaborative Group on Hormonal Factors in Breast Cancer and Hormone Replacement Therapy. (1997). Collaborative re-analysis of data from 51 epidemiologic studies of 52,705 women with breast cancer and 108,411 without breast cancer. *Lancet, 350,* 1047–1059.

Colon Cancer Screening (USPSTF Recommendation). (2000). *Journal of the American Geriatrics Society, 48,* 333–335.

Cummings, S. R., Eckert, S., Krueger, K. A., Grady, D., Powles, T. J., Cauley, J. A., Norton, L., Nickelson, T., Bjarnason, N. H., Morrow, M., Lippman, M. E., Black, D., Glusman, J. E., Costa, A., & Jordan, V. C. (1999). The effect of raloxifene on risk of breast cancer in post-menopausal women: Results from the MORE Randomized Trial. *Journal of the American Medical Association, 281,* 2189–2197.

D'Amico, A. V., Whittington, R., Malkowicz, S. B., Weinstein, M., Tomaszewski, J. E., Schultz, D., Rhude, M., Rocha, S., Wein, A., & Richie, J. P. (1998). A biochemical outcome after radical prostatectomy, external beam radiation therapy, or interstitial radiation therapy for clinically localized prostatic cancer. *Journal of the American Medical Association, 95*(2), 969–974.

Diab, S. G., Ellege, R. M., & Clark, G. M. (2000). Tumor characteristics and clinical outcome of elderly women with breast cancer. *Journal of the National Cancer Institute, 92,* 550–556.

Essink-Bot, M. L., de Koring, H. J., Nijs, H. G., Kirkels, W. J., van der Mass, P. J., & Schroder, F. H. (1998). Short-term effect of population based screening for prostate cancer on health related quality of life. *Journal of the National Cancer Institute, 20,* 925–931.

Etzion, R., Cha, R., Feuer, E. J., & Davidov, O. (1998). Asymptomatic incidence and duration of prostate cancer. *American Journal of Epidemiology, 148,* 775–785.

Giovannucci, E., Rimm, E. B., Stompfer, M., J., Colditz, G. A., & Willett, W. C. (1994). Aspirin use and the risk for colorectal cancer and adenoma in male health professionals. *Annals of Internal Medicine, 121,* 241–246.

Greenberg, R. S., Daniels, S. R., & Flanders, W. D. (1993). *Diagnostic testing in medical epidemiology.* Norwalk, CT: Appleton and Lange. 63–65.

Greenlee, R. T., Hill Harman, M. B., Murray, T., & Thun, M. (2001). Cancer Statistics 2001. *California Cancer Journal for Clinicians, 51,* 15–36.

Holli, K., Isola, J., & Cuzick. J. (1998). Low biologic aggressiveness in women using hormone replacement therapy. *Journal of Clinical Oncology, 16,* 3115–3120.

Hughes, J. R., Goldstein, M. G., Hurt, R. D., & Schiffman, S. (1999). Recent advances in the pharmacotherapy of smoking. *Journal of the American Medical Association, 281,* 72–76.

Johansson, J. E., Holmberg, L., Johansson, S., Bergstom, R., & Adami, H. O. (1997). Fifteen-year survival in prostate cancer. *Journal of the American Medical Association, 277,* 467–471.

Kerlikowske, K., Grady, D., Rubin, S. M., Sandrock, C., & Ernster, V. L. (1995). Efficacy of screening mammography: A meta-analysis. *Journal of the American Medical Association, 273,* 149–154.

Kronborg, O., Fenger, C., Olsen, J., Jorgensen, O. D., & Sondergaard, O. (1996). Randomized study of screening for colorectal cancer with faecal occult blood test. *The Lancet, 348,* 1467–1471.

Lieberman, D. A., Weiss, D. G., Bond, J. H., Ahnen, D. J., Garawal, H., & Cheifec, G. (2000). Use of colonoscopy to screen asymptomatic adults for colorectal cancer. Veterans Affairs Cooperative Study Group 380. *New England Journal of Medicine, 343,* 162–168.

Lippman, S. M., & Brown, P. H. (1999). Tamoxifen prevention of breast cancer: An instance of the fingerpost. *Journal National Cancer Institute, 91,* 1809–1819.

Litman, M. S. (1999). Health related quality of life in older men without prostate cancer. *Journal of Urology, 161,* 1180–1184.

Lu Yao, G. L., & Yau, S. L. (1997). Population-based study of long-term survival in patients with clinically localized prostate cancer. *Lancet, 349,* 906–910.

Mandel, J. S., Church, T. R., Bond, J. H., Ederer, F., Geisser, M. S., Mongin, S. J., Snover, D. C., & Schuman, L. M.. (2000). The effect of fecal occult blood screening on the incidence of colorectal cancer. *New England Journal of Medicine, 343,* 1603–1607.

Mandel, J. S., Church, T. R., Ederer, F., & Bond, J. H. (1999). Colorectal cancer mortality: effectiveness of biennial screening for faecal occult blood. *Journal of the National Cancer Institute, 91,* 434–437.

McCarthy, E. P., Burs, R. B., & Coughlin, S. S. (1998). Mammography use helps to explain differences in breast cancer stage at diagnosis between older black and white women. *Annals of Internal Medicine, 128,* 729–736.

Nadler, R. B., Humphrey, P. A., Smith, D. S., Catalona, W. J., & Ratliff, T. L. (1995). Effect of inflammation and benign prostatic hyperplasia on elevated serum prostate specific antigen levels. *Journal of Urology, 154,* 407–411.

Nusbaum, N. (2001) Role of the clinical breast examination in breast cancer screening. *Journal of the American Geriatrics Society, 49,* 991–992.

Omenn, G. S., Goodman, G. E., & Thornquist, M. D. (1996). Risk factors for lung cancer and for intervention effects in CARET, the Beta-Carotene and Retinol Efficacy Trial. *Journal of the National Cancer Institute, 88*:1550–1559.

Parazzini, F., LaVecchia, C., Bocciolone, L., & Franceschi, S. (1991). The epidemiology of endometrial cancer. *Gynecological Oncology, 41*, 1–16.

Patz, E. F., Goodman, P. C, & Bepler, G. B. (2000). Screening for lung cancer. *New England Journal of Medicine, 343*, 1627–1633.

Petty, L. P. (2000). Screening strategies for early detection of lung cancer. *Journal of the American Medical Association, 284*, 1977–1980.

Potter, J. D., Slattery, M. L., Bostick, R. M., & Gapstar, S. M. (1993). Colon cancer, a review of the epidemiology. *Epidemiological Review, 15*, 499–545.

Ries, L., Kosary, C., Hankey, B., Feuer, E. J., Merrill, R. M., Clegg, L. X., & Edwards, B. K. (1999). *SEER cancer statistics review, 1973–1996.* Bethesda, MD: National Cancer Institute.

Roberts, R. O., Bergstralh, E. J., Katusic, S. K., Lieber, M. M., & Jacobsen, S. L. (1999). Decline in prostate cancer mortality from 1980 to 1997 and an update on incidence trends in Olmsted County, Minnesota. *Journal of Urology, 16*, 529–533.

Robinson, B., & Beghe, C. (1997). Cancer screening in the older patient. *Clinics in Geriatric Medicine, 13*, 97–188.

Rosenthal, A. N., & Jacobs, I. J. (1998). The role of CA-125 in screening for ovarian cancer. *International Journal of Biological Markers, 13*, 216–220.

Runowicz, C. D., & Fields, A. L. (1999). Screening for gynecologic malignancies: a continuing responsibility. *Surgical Oncology Clinics of North America, 8*, 703–723.

Satariano, W. A., & Ragland, D. R. (1994). The effect of comorbidity on 3–year survival of women with primary breast cancer. *Annals of Internal Medicine, 120*, 104–110.

Sato, J., Yokoyama, Y., Sekamoto, T., Futagami, M., & Saito, Y. (2000). Usefulness of mass screening for ovarian carcinoma using transvaginal ultrasonography. *Cancer, 89*, 582–588.

Sawaya, G. F., Brown, A. D., Washington, A. E., & Garber, A. M. (2001). Current approaches to cervical cancer screening. *New England Journal of Medicine, 344*, 1603–1607.

Schiffman, M. H., & Brinton, L. A. (1995). The epidemiology of cervical carcinogenesis. *Cancer, 76*, 1888–1901.

Silverman, M. A., Zaidi, U., Barnett, S., Robels, C., Khurnan, V., Marten, H., Barnes, D., Chu, L., & Roos, B. A. (2000). Cancer screening in the elderly population. *Hematology/Oncology Clinics of North America, 14*, 89–112.

Smith, R. A., Meitlin, C. J., Davis, K. J., & Eyre, H. (2000). American Cancer Society guidelines for the early detection of cancer. *CA Cancer Journal for Clinicians, 50*, 49.

Smith, R. A., von Eschenbach, A. C., Wender, R., Levin, B., Byers, T., Rothenberger, D., Brooks, D., Creasman, W., Cohen, C., Runowics, C., Saslow, D., Cokkinides, V., & Eyre, H. (2001). American Cancer Society guidelines for the early detection of cancer, update of early detection guidelines for prostate, colorectal, and endometrial cancers. *CA Cancer Journal for Clinicians, 51,* 38–75.

Smith-Warner, S. A., Spiegelman, I., & Yaun, S. (2001). Intake of fruits and vegetables and risk of breast cancer. *Journal of the American Medical Association, 285,* 769–776.

Steinbach, G., Lynch, P. M., Phillips, R. K., Wallace, M. H., Hawk, E., Gordon, G. B., Wakabayashi, N., Saunders, B., Shen, Y., Fujimura, T., Su, L. K., & Levin, B. (2000). The effect of celecoxib, a cyclooxygenase-2 inhibitor, in familial adenomatous polyposis. *New England Journal of Medicine, 342,* 1946–1952.

Sutton, S., Wardle, J., Taylor, T., McCaffery, K., Williamson, S., Edwards, R., Cuzick, J., Hart, A., Northover, J., & Atkin, W. (2000). Predictors of attendance in the United Kingdom flexible sigmoidoscopy screening trial. *Journal of Medical Screening, 7,* 99–104.

Towler, B., Irwig, L., Glasziou, P., Weller, D., & Kewenter, J. (1998). A systematic review of the effects of the screening for colorectal cancer using the faecal occult blood testing hemoccult. *British Medical Journal, 317,* 559–565.

United States Preventive Services Task Force. Routine Cancer Screening. (1996). *Screening for colorectal cancer: guide to clinical preventive services, 2ⁿᵈ Ed.* Baltimore: Williams & Wilkins.

Walter, L. C., & Covinsky, K. E. (2001). Cancer screening in elderly patients. *Journal of the American Medical Association, 285,* 2750–2757.

Whiltemore, A. S., Harris, R., & Itnyre, J. (1992). Characteristics relating to ovarian cancer risk: Collaborative analysis of 12 US controlled studies. II. Invasive epithelial cancer in white women. Collaborative Ovarian Cancer Group. *American Journal of Epidemiology, 136,* 1184–1203.

Wilson, J. M. G., & Jungner, G. (1964). *Principles and practices of screening for disease.* Public Health Paper No. 34. Geneva, World Health Organization.

Winawer, S. J., Zauber, A. G., Ho, M. N., O'Brien, M. J., Gottlieb, L. S., Stemberg, S. S., Waye, J. D., Schapiro, M., Bond, J. H., & Panish, J. F. (1993). Prevention of colorectal cancer by colonoscopic polypectomy: The National Polyp Study Workgroup. *New England Journal of Medicine, 329,* 1977–1981.

Zubarik, R., Fleischer, D. E., Mastropietro, C. , Lopez, J., Carroll, J., Benjamin, S., & Eisen, G. (1999). Prospective analysis of complications 30 days after outpatient colonoscopy. *Gastrointestinal Endoscopy, 50,* 322–328.

SECTION TWO

Management of Care

Kathy's Treatment

Kathy Clark found it difficult to get out of bed. She slept fitfully most of the night, but just as morning approached she finally dropped off to sleep. The cats were curled up at her feet in peaceful slumber. Kathy wanted this day to be over. She wanted to know the extent of her cancer and possible treatments. "I can deal with anything, as long as I know what it is," Kathy thought as she turned on the shower.

Kathy reached the doctor's office and surprisingly found herself ushered into the exam room. A very pleasant nurse greeted her, and introduced herself as Emily Goodman. She asked Kathy some questions about her health history. Ms. Goodman had hardly left the room when a young man entered the room and introduced himself as Dr. DeRon. Dr. DeRon had what seemed to be her chart with several loose papers that looked like the glossy texture of a fax.

"Well, let's get right to the reports. Your pathology report suggests breast cancer. It was a fairly big tumor and it looks like we need to operate. I may be able to preserve your breast with a lumpectomy; however, I would prepare yourself for a mastectomy. We will also need to take some lymph nodes from under your left arm to make sure the tumor has not spread," directed Dr. DeRon, not looking up from the mangled papers on the exam room counter.

Kathy felt numb. She sat quietly overwhelmed, with a barrage of thoughts flooding her mind.

"OK, when should we schedule the surgery?" snapped Dr. DeRon as he raised his face to look at her.

Kathy heard herself reply, "As soon as possible."

"OK, how about Friday?"

"Sounds good."

"The nurse will be in with all the directions and things you need to do to prepare. See you Friday," said the doctor as the tail of his lab coat fluttered through the closing door.

Emily Goodman returned and began going over how to prepare for surgery. She told Kathy about not eating before surgery, not taking aspirin prior to the procedure, and what seemed like a million other things that Kathy could not comprehend. The nurse had given her a packet of papers that she didn't realize she had until she found herself in her car. Kathy dropped her things down on the counter, feeling overwhelmed and angry with all the information which had just been thrown at her.

"I don't remember a thing anyone told me," thought Kathy as she fumbled for the card Ms. Goodman had given her while exiting the exam room. Kathy dumped out her purse, found the card, and began dialing the number in hopes of having the information re-explained to her.

It seemed like an eternity, but Friday finally came. Mary came to the door at 5:00 A.M. on the dot. A forced smile accompanied a worried expression as Mary walked though the door to kiss her mother.

"Ready?" asked Mary nervously.

"Yes, let me just put the curtains up for the cats," said Kathy as she walked over to her front window.

"OK, I got everything. Let's go and get this over with," said Kathy as she locked the door.

Kathy awakened from surgery in the recovery room. "You did just fine in surgery," said the OR nurse. Kathy wanted to ask about her breast, but felt herself drift back to sleep. Later that afternoon, Kathy awakened to find Mary asleep by the bedside.

"Hey, who's the patient here? I'm the one who is supposed to be sleeping," said Kathy in hopes of making Mary more at ease.

"So how'd ya do?" asked Mary under the haze of sleep.

"Great, piece of cake," joked Kathy.

"So what's the damage?" asked Kathy quite seriously.

"Mom, they had to take the whole breast, and they found . . .

At that time Dr. DeRon appeared through the doorway. "Ahh . . . I see you're awake."

"Yes. Give me the news," said Kathy impatiently.

"OK, well, we had to do the mastectomy. The tumor was fairly big and I made the decision to take the entire breast. The preliminary test on your lymph nodes shows that 2 of the 12 nodes we resected were involved with cancer. I am going to refer you to Dr. Davis and she can help you decide what further steps you need to take to make sure this cancer never comes back. See you in two weeks," said Dr. DeRon as he hurried out of the room.

Kathy recovered quickly from her surgery. A thick white dressing took the place of her left breast. Kathy had not been too eager to look at the surgery site. For a time after surgery, Kathy found herself significantly dependent on Mary. This was a new experience for Kathy, as she was typically the caregiver for her family. Mary prepared meals, kept the house, and practically moved in to be a source of continuous support. Kathy accepted the help and was sincerely glad for Mary's support, but was ready to resume her independent lifestyle. After a week, Kathy was done being sick.

After a two week recovery from surgery, she was scheduled to meet with her oncologist. Mary accompanied Kathy to the visit at Kathy's request. After the last experience at the doctor's office, Kathy wanted to make sure she had more ears to collect information. Mary rarely misses anything and will surely understand everything the doctor says, Kathy thought.

Dr. Davis entered the examination room. She was a large woman with big teeth and tightly pulled back hair.

"I reviewed your reports and we have several options," said Dr. Davis in a soft, kind voice.

"Because your tumor is hormone receptive positive, you may benefit from a medicine called tamoxifen." Dr. Davis spent the next several minutes explaining the side effects of the medication. Mary was diligently recording the information on her notepad. Kathy felt like an observer while much of the explanation was occurring. She really didn't have the energy to engage actively in this conversation. "Mary will explain it to me when I get home anyway," thought Kathy.

"The next thing we need to talk about is chemotherapy," said Dr. Davis, leaning forward in her chair, patting Kathy's knee.

"Chemotherapy!" exclaimed Kathy. "I thought surgery would be enough. How much can I possibly go through?."

"I'm sorry," said Dr. Davis, shaking her head. "Because two lymph nodes were positive, it is very important to try to prevent the cancer from returning and that's what chemotherapy does. Once cancer returns, it does not return to the breast. It can go to the bone, lung, liver, or other places." Dr. Davis spent the next 45 minutes explaining the two different types of chemo that might be helpful. One type of chemo would cause hair loss and the other would not. One type of chemo caused . . . The words became incomprehensible to Kathy so she began tuning out the entire oration.

Mary was furiously taking notes.

"We can start next week," suggested Dr. Davis.

"Go ahead and schedule us for next week to have chemo and Mom and I will decide what chemotherapy to take," asserted Mary.

Kathy and Mary left the doctor's office silent. The drive home too was silent. After some discussion, Kathy and Mary decided on which chemotherapy to take. Kathy went for the shorter duration of chemo, but this would mean her hair would fall out.

"I just want this to be over with," Kathy said to Mary as they watched their favorite shows on TV that night.

Kathy took her chemotherapy and had good health for the next year. During that time she experienced the birth of her grandchild. Life was wonderful. Matthew was growing and becoming a little boy. Kathy loved being a grandmother and frequently kept the baby while Mary worked. Over the year, Kathy made the decision to sell her home and move to Florida with Mary. This would enable her to start fresh. She could get away from her ex-husband and the memories that still lingered in the house, help Mary with Matthew (actually she couldn't stand to be apart from the child), and possibly escape the breast cancer. Cindy, Kathy's oldest daughter, lived in Sarasota, and Mary and Kathy would be moving about 15 minutes from her house. Kathy thought optimistically that it would be nice to have her family together again—minus her ex-husband of course!

Before the move Kathy stopped by Dr. Davis's office for her routine checkup. Kathy hadn't worried about the cancer returning. She had actually put it out of her mind, especially since Matthew was born. Dr. Davis came through the door looking tired. She had in her hand Kathy's chest x-rays performed two days ago.

"Kathy, some spots have shown up on your x-rays. I will need to get some other tests to make sure the cancer has not spread. Do you have any time this week?"

"Yes," replied Kathy as she sat shocked that this ordeal was not over. "Spots, where?"

"In your lungs," said Dr. Davis emphatically.

"I thought this cancer thing was behind me. Now as I'm finally moving with my life, here it comes again. I survive a divorce, a diagnosis of cancer, I have a beautiful grandson and am looking forward to a move to Florida to be with both my daughters and you tell me the cancer is back?"

Kathy drove herself home, dreading telling her daughter the news. Her daughter was actually one of the few people she had told of the diagnosis. Certainly Cindy, her other daughter knew, and her ex-husband, but none of her friends. Kathy did not want to have to deal with the "I'm sorrys" or the pitiful expressions so many of her friends had directed to those wearing the badge of cancer. Since Kathy had received her diagnosis, she had accepted her illness and moved on with her life. She did not want the cancer to be her identity. She wanted to remain the fun-loving, 74-year-young, on-the-move grandmother that she felt she was. For the first time since her diagnosis of breast cancer she was frightened. "What's going to happen now? Will I be here in six months?"

Kathy pulled in the drive; she noticed the daylilies were blooming with their characteristic yellow color. The irises she had planted several months ago were also beginning to bloom. Spring in California was wonderful. The air was crisp in the morning and fairly warm in the afternoon. "I will certainly miss this when I get to Florida," thought Kathy as she collected her purse from the backseat. Florida is where people go to . . . " Kathy stopped herself in mid-thought before saying the word "die". "Enough," Kathy barked out loud to herself as she opened the door. "I am not going to bury myself yet. I've come too far in my life and I'm finally enjoying myself."

Kathy's evening went about as she had anticipated. Mary wept as Kathy told her the news. Kathy remained strong for her daughter and tried to protect her from the bad news (a role she played for her family her entire life). Kathy assured Mary everything would be all right and that they were to proceed with their plans to move to Florida. Reassuring Mary made Kathy feel stronger to the point that she too believed everything would be fine.

A week passed as Kathy continued her normal routine. She conscientiously did not allow herself to think about the advancing breast cancer. She continued to garden, meet with friends, and play with Matthew. The day finally came when she was to meet with the doctor. All the tests had been performed and Dr. Davis would have the results. Kathy hated getting the tests, especially the ones for which she was required to drink the contrast material.

When she reached Dr. Davis's office, she was instructed that she would be seeing Dr. Coleman. Dr. Davis was out unexpectedly and she would be back next week. Dr. Coleman was a young physician who, several years ago, had completed his fellowship at Memorial Sloan-Kettering. The giggly young receptionist told Kathy he was "brilliant" and had a great "bedside manner," so Kathy awaited the entrance of this young dynamo. Dr. Coleman entered the exam room wearing a crisp lab coat and warmly smiling. He greeted Kathy, then sat down to look at her chart. All at once, he leaned forward in his chair and touched Kathy's hand.

"I am so sorry for you," said Dr. Coleman as he mustered up a very concerned, quasi grieving expression.

"Sorry for me? Why?" Kathy sternly asked.

"Because of your cancer," responded Dr. Coleman, looking shocked that Kathy would even question his concern.

"You don't even know me—it's the first time you ever met me. I would like to know the results of the tests and what options I have. I do not need a down attitude. I have to live with this breast cancer." Kathy must have responded rather sharply, because Dr. Coleman stumbled over the results of the diagnostic exams and his rough sketch of a plan. The only plan Kathy wanted was to see Dr. Davis when she returned.

Kathy left the office feeling more emotional then she did when she originally received the news the cancer had spread. Later that day, Kathy called the office of her doctor to have all her records sent to the cancer center in Florida where she was planning to receive treatment. Kathy called and made herself an appointment for the following Friday with any available doctor. She was no longer going to think about her cancer until she saw another physician. Today was box packing day.

The move went well. All survived, including the cats, who required vast amounts of sedatives to complete the cross-country excursion. The caravan reached the apartment Kathy had rented over the phone. It was clean and close to the beach. Kathy loved the beach and the sun and the ocean. She knew at this very moment that she would love her new life in Florida.

CHAPTER FOUR

Atypical Presentation of Cancer in the Elderly

Katherine K. Stanley and Janice T. Hoff

T he purpose of this chapter is to provide practical information and the useable tools necessary for the professional nurse to be instrumental in the diagnosis of cancer. The information presented is meant to assist the nursing professional in identifying clinical and psychosocial issues faced by the patient and family when a cancer diagnosis is made. Skill in this area is essential in promoting a confidence level for professionals as they work with this population.

When given the magnitude of cancer and how it affects the patient and family unit, one must consider and address many issues. A discussion of the physical presentation of cancer as well as other issues including social, financial, educational, and emotional will be presented. The authors' hopes are that the reader will develop a greater understanding of the professional nurse's responsibility and influence in the lives of the patient and family members who must deal with the diagnosis of cancer.

NORMAL CHANGES OF AGING

As people age, they become more unique and each situation must be individually evaluated. Acute illness in older individuals often presents with vague, nonspecific symptoms. Usual signs and symptoms of acute disease may be absent or delayed. Often, nonspecific symptoms that represent severe illness in older adults include confusion, falling, incontinence, anorexia, and self-neglect (Ham & Sloane, 1997,

p. 30). Likewise, symptoms of cancer may be missed or dismissed due to the vagueness of the complaints. Assuming that vague symptoms and/or complaints are related to old age can lead to a delay in the diagnosis of cancer and other serious illnesses. As the nurse completes a head-to-toe assessment, differentiating normal changes of aging from serious symptoms is critical to the overall patient management and care. The following information is intended to be an overview of the common age related changes and their implications for cancer presentations. Additional information may be obtained from various geriatric assessment tools and guidelines (Leukenotte, 1998).

Several explanations are available of why the presentation of illness is modified in old age. Altered central processing can occur due to reduced cognitive functioning or because of unrecognized dementia. The brain is very sensitive, and a change in mental status is frequently a presenting symptom of acute illness in older adults. Because there is a general feeling of negativity about aging in our society, older adults may deny or ignore symptoms, limit activities, or accept symptoms as signs of old age. Fear of illness and treatment, and especially nursing home placement, are contributing factors to patient and family behaviors that deny or ignore symptoms of illness. Many older adults suffer from depression, which can reduce the individual's motivation to seek treatment for a treatable illness (Ham & Sloan, 1997, p. 31).

There are some common denominators that emerge in age-related physiologic changes. A decrease in blood supply to various tissues occurs due to deposition of calcium and fat in the intima of blood vessels. A reduction in circulation of blood volume is a factor, as well as a decrease in endocrine function. Alterations in tissue elasticity, fat distribution, gastrointestinal and renal function, muscle and bone changes, immunity, and mental functioning contribute to the overall changes of aging. In addition, wear and tear of the body over time through injuries and accidents contributes to decreased functioning (Ebersole & Hess, 1998, p. 86).

Facial changes occur due to a decrease in skin thickness, decreased elasticity, and the loss of bone mass, particularly in the mandible. A decrease in visual acuity occurs due to progressive changes in the eye structures of the cornea, lens, retina, and vitreous and aqueous humor. Senile ptosis occurs due to the loss of tissue elasticity. The inability to hear is a significant deterrent to communication and can lead to isolation and frustration. Auditory changes occur due to changes in the external, middle, and inner ear structures. The gradual hearing loss of aging is termed presbycusis. A buildup of earwax can also be a contributing factor in hearing loss. Atrophy of the taste buds and a decrease in olfactory sensitivity result in changes in taste perception. Crude taste consists of differentiating sweet and sour and is controlled by the taste buds. Fine taste is mediated by the sense of smell. In the healthy older adult, taste changes are usually moderate although the quality of taste may vary. Smoking and medications can alter taste perception as well (Ebersole & Hess, 1998, p. 97–100). Older adults are more prone to dry mouth due to decreased saliva production. Dry mouth is also a side effect of many medications and predisposes the elder to periodontal disease. Twenty-three percent of the elderly have severe periodontal disease and thirty percent of those over age 65 are edentulous. Regular dental care is often neglected in this population. Oral and pharyngeal cancers are primarily diagnosed in the elderly and can often be identified by an oral exam (Baldwin, 2001).

Age-related changes of the respiratory system include a decrease in chest wall compliance and loss of elasticity. These changes result in the decreased efficiency of gas exchange and ventilatory capacity. Residual capacity increases due to decreased inspiratory and expiratory muscle strength. Decline in muscle strength can result in a decreased cough response, which when combined with other structural changes and impairments such as dysphagia can contribute to problems with obstruction and chronic or frequent infection. Environmental factors, such as exposure to toxins and smoking, contribute to a decrease in the respiratory reserve. Repeated inflammatory injuries, decreased immune response, diminished capability for tissue repair, structural changes, and environmental factors contribute to airway problems in the elderly. Underlying chronic obstructive pulmonary disease, including bronchitis and asthma, are medical conditions that can lead to life-threatening situations in the elderly. In addition, pneumonia is prevalent and is a leading cause of death for this population (Ebersole & Hess, 1998, p. 92–94).

Cardiovascular changes of aging include a decrease in the work response of the left ventricle at rest that results in a decrease in cardiac output. Delayed contractile recovery and heart muscle irritability are also present in the older heart. Under normal, non-stressful conditions, the older heart can maintain adequate function; however, stresses such as infection, pain, or bleeding can result in a poor cardiac response due to limited cardiac reserve. Underlying atherosclerotic heart disease and valvular disease further limit the cardiac reserves in older adults. A decrease in the elasticity of the arteries contributes to decreased blood flow to vital organs. Veins and arteries exhibit changes in the intima, which result in loss of flexibility and increased peripheral resistance. Resulting problems with hypertension influence the degree of cardiac and renal dysfunction. Because of a loss of elasticity in the venous system, pooling of blood often occurs in the lower extremities, resulting in venous insufficiency. Sinus rhythm is the normal rhythm for older adults. Arrhythmias and damage to the conduction system can occur from myocardial damage either directly from impaired blood flow or indirectly from valvular insufficiency (Ebersole & Hess, 1998, p. 90–91).

Renal changes also occur with age. The size and function of the kidney decrease with age with as much as 50% loss of nephrons. The large renal vessels begin to develop sclerosis and preglomerular arterioles can become destroyed, resulting in decreased blood flow. By the age of 80, the blood flow through the kidneys decreases to half that of a young adult. This in turn affects the glomerular filtration rate and affects creatinine clearance. The decrease in urine creatinine clearance is an important factor in determining drug therapy in the older adult (Ebersole & Hess, 1998, p. 94).

Endocrine changes occur due to organ atrophy with a resulting decrease in hormone secretion. Glands can become more active, less active, or non-active because of gradual changes in functioning. The pancreas continues to secrete insulin via the beta cells throughout life. Decreased tissue sensitivity to insulin, also termed insulin resistance, is the age-related change. Higher levels of circulating proinsulin and alteration in insulin receptor sites are factors that make insulin less effective in the older adult. The thyroid gland tends to decrease with age and becomes fibrotic. Adrenal gland function and secretion of cortisol, epinephrine, norepinephrine, and dopamine decrease in varying degrees. The pituitary gland decreases in volume by 20%. Gonadotropic, estrogenic, and andrenogenic hormones decrease and result in physiologic changes such as atrophy of ovaries, vaginal tissues, and testes, and benign prostatic hypertrophy (Ebersole & Hess, 1998, p. 95).

Changes in other organ systems affect the gastrointestinal system as well as pathological conditions such as diabetes, vascular compromise, and neurological changes. Dental health is an important adjunct to good gastrointestinal functioning. Many elderly individuals are edentulous or dependent on dentures. Muscle strength and motility of the gastrointestinal structures decrease with age, resulting in diminished peristaltic action. Relaxation of the lower esophageal sphincter also occurs, resulting in a slowed emptying of the esophagus and dilatation. Sixty percent of those over age 70 develop hiatal hernias. Changes also occur in the number of parietal and chief cells in the stomach, resulting in a decreased production of hydrochloric acid (HCL) and pepsin. The stomach pH increases, predisposing the aged to gastric irritation. Changes in small bowel motility, epithelial membranes, perfusion, and gastrointestinal membrane transport affect the absorption of nutrients and vitamins. Large intestine atrophy, decreased mucus secretions, and loss of muscle tone predispose the elderly to problems in bowel evacuation. A slowing of neural impulses lessens awareness of the need to evacuate the bowel and can result in incontinence or constipation. Weakness of the intestinal walls may also result in multiple diverticula, which may be asymptomatic (Ebersole & Hess, 1998, p. 96–97).

Physiologic changes of the brain associated with aging include brain atrophy, loss of neurons, a decrease in the number of receptors, and decrease in neurotransmitter synthesis (Lang, 2001). Neurofibrillary tangles are associated with Alzheimer's disease but may also be found in non-Alzheimer's brains. Central processing functions begin to slow down, resulting in the older individual taking longer to complete tasks (Ebersole & Hess, 1998, p. 97). In the absence of dementia, memory deficit is limited to the acquisition and retrieving of new information. Other cognitive functions remain intact (Small, 1999).

Age related changes of the skin, hair, and nails also occur. Replacement of epidermal cells is slowed and the dermis becomes thinner due to a decrease in subcutaneous fat. Melanin synthesis increases, resulting in pigment spots that can enlarge or increase depending upon light exposure. The sweat glands decrease in size, number, and activity with resulting difficulty adjusting to temperature changes. Oral temperature tends to range from 95 to 97 degrees Fahrenheit. A low-grade temperature is significant for illness in the elderly. Thinning of the hair occurs in both sexes although this varies due to ethnic background. Nail growth decreases and the nail plate thickens (Ebersole & Hess, 1998, p. 87–88).

The musculoskeletal system undergoes changes with the normal aging process, which include calcium loss from the bones and atrophy of cartilage and muscle. Vertebral disks thin and cause shortening of the trunk that results in a forward bent stance. The maintenance of bone mass is a dynamic process of constant resorption and renewal of bone. Excess loss of calcium results in osteoporosis and is more prevalent in older women although men may develop this condition (Ebersole & Hess, 1998, p. 86–87).

THE NATURE OF CANCER

Cancer is usually thought of as one disease when in fact it includes more than 200 different diseases such as skin cancer, lung cancer, leukemia, and lymphoma (Dollinger, Rosenbaum, & Cable, 1991). When one looks simply at the description of cancer it can be termed as an uncontrolled cell growth. Uncontrolled cell growth, resulting from cellular damage, may occur as a result of injury to a cell from an internal source like a genetic predisposition or an external source such as tobacco use. During cell division or mitosis, the deoxyribonucleic acid (DNA) replicates itself and forms two new cells. During the replication process a mutation could occur which would lead to an alteration in the cellular structure. As cellular division and replication continue, a pattern would develop which would lead to an abnormal type of cell being replicated. If the cellular feedback mechanism does not correct the defect, the abnormal cells proliferate. It is the proliferation of these abnormal cells that is termed a cancer. These may form a solid tumor, a skin lesion, or an abnormality in the blood or lymph system. A compromised immune system may lead to a proliferation of cancer as evidenced by the many cancers that are prevalent in individuals with the human immunodeficiency virus (HIV) or those who are on immunosuppressive therapy following an organ transplant surgery (Wyngaarden, Smith, & Bennett, 1992).

CANCER IN THE ELDERLY

The annual report to the nation on the status of cancer published in the May 15, 2000 issue of *Cancer* indicates that the overall rate of cancer cases and deaths for all cancers has declined from 1990 to 1997 (National Cancer Institute, 2000). However, some believe the number of cancer cases diagnosed will increase as the population escalates and ages. Sixty percent of new cancer cases and two thirds of cancer deaths occur in persons greater than 65 years of age (Beers & Berkow, 2000). It is thought that repetitive exposure to environmental carcinogens as well as the decrease in the body's ability to repair itself along with a relaxed immune system response all contribute to the increased number of cancer cases in the elderly. One can also be predisposed to certain types of cancers through genetics. For example, one can have a genetic predisposition to breast cancer if it is present in the family bloodline. Beers and Berkow (2000) explore theories for why cancer incidence increases with age. These include a lifetime of carcinogenic exposure, increased susceptibility of cells to carcinogens, the body's decreased ability to repair DNA, oncogene activation or amplification (accumulation), decreased tumor-suppressor gene activity, microenvironment alterations, including hormonal alterations or exposure, and decreased immune surveillance due to immune senescence.

THE SYMPTOMS REVIEW

There are many factors to consider when performing an assessment of the elderly patient, which are outlined below. A more comprehensive discussion of assessment is provided in the next chapter. One point the examiner must remember is that the patient is not an island. The family, caregiver, or significant other may be an important source of information regarding external symptoms or performance status, especially if the patient demonstrates short-term memory loss or dementia. Keep in mind a patient is generally able to tell the examiner if there are any bothersome symptoms such as shortness of breath or pain. A head-to-toe format may be followed by the examiner. Use the following questions as a guide.

Do you have headaches or dizzy spells?
Do you have difficulty swallowing or chewing your food?
Do you have indigestion, nausea, or vomiting?
Do you have shortness of breath? (Evaluate if they are winded with
    conversation.) What type of activity can you normally perform?
How much did you smoke?
Do you have chest pain or an irregular heart beat that you can feel?
Do you have constipation or diarrhea?
Do you have urinary symptoms such as burning, frequency, pain, or
    trouble starting or stopping your stream?
Do you have aches or pains in your muscles or joints?
Do you have trouble sleeping?
Do you have changes in your appetite or weight?
Do you have sores on your skin? Unusual lumps or bumps?
How is your energy level? Do you have night sweats?
What type of surgeries did you have and why?
Do you have any questions or anything else to add?

Generally this brief line of questioning will lead the examiner to the beginning point of the physical assessment. Always pursue areas that need further questioning as indicated by the responses.

THE PHYSICAL ASSESSMENT

The objective part of the physical assessment is important for the detection of cancer in an elderly patient. This chapter will provide a brief overview of the physical assessment and factors to consider when looking for cancer in the elderly. Following the physical assessment narrative there will be a case description that incorporates multiple factors to consider when an elderly patient is diagnosed and treated for cancer.

The examiner must always investigate further if anything is identified during the review process. For example, if the patient identifies a growth it is essential to evaluate it, at least objectively, if not microscopically. For purposes of simplicity a head-to-toe assessment will be explored. Generally documentation tools are written in a head-to-toe format and the use of a logical format may be beneficial for completeness of documentation.

In evaluating the patient keep in mind the American Cancer Society's list of Seven Early Warning Signals as reviewed by Dollinger et al. (1991):

Change in bowel or bladder habits.
A sore that does not heal.
Unusual bleeding or discharge.
Thickening or lump in breast or elsewhere.
Indigestion or difficulty in swallowing.
Obvious change in wart or mole.
Nagging cough or hoarseness.

When performing an initial assessment look at the patient, evaluate alertness and orientation, and look for subtle clues such as jaundice in the sclera, skin lesions, or dyspnea with conversation. Confusion, a recent mental status change, or a headache could indicate a brain tumor or metastatic disease to the brain from another cancer such as breast cancer. Hyponatremia or hypercalcemia are also causes of mental status changes and may indicate a cancer or metastatic disease. Evaluate the patient's oral cavity to see if there are lesions of the gum or oropharynx. Palpate the neck, axillae, and groin for any unusual swelling or nodes. Enlarged lymph nodes may indicate a lymphoma or metastatic disease from an existing cancer. In auscultation of the lungs consider the important fact that it is not always the breath sounds that are heard but those that are not heard that may be significant. A pleural effusion from a lung cancer may present in this fashion. When performing an initial assessment and if providing personal care such as bathing take the opportunity to perform a breast exam. Check the breasts and axillary lymph nodes for masses or tenderness. Breast cancer is usually diagnosed by finding a new lump in the breast tissue. Check for inversion of nipples and dimpling of the skin. Palpate the abdomen for masses or areas of tenderness. A female patient who gives the complaint of abdominal bloating with no history of hysterectomy may have an ovarian or uterine carcinoma. Evaluate the rectum by internal examination for any masses or friable areas that bleed easily as this may be the presentation for an adenocarcinoma of the rectum. The skin should always be examined for suspicious lesions and recommendations made for further evaluation. Remember the ABCD's of melanoma detection: Asymmetry—a lesion that is not symmetrical; Border—a lesion that has an irregular border; Color—a lesion that has a variegated color (black and brown or lighter); and Diameter—a lesion that is larger than six millimeters (the size of a pencil eraser). The elderly may also have actinic keratosis (AK) or seborrheic keratosis (SK). AK is a raised red somewhat scaly lesion that is generally precancerous. AK may be treated with cryosurgery. SK is a brown lesion with a stuck on appearance that also occurs commonly in the elderly. SK requires no further treatment.

COMMON CANCERS IN THE ELDERLY

In 1995 cancer was the second leading cause of death for persons greater than 65 years of age, with 22.5% recorded (Beers & Berkow, 2000). There are several types of cancers that are very common in the elderly. According to Beers and Berkow (2000), prostate cancer in men and breast cancer in women are the most common types of cancer in the population aged 55 years or greater. This is followed by lung cancer, then colon cancer, respectively.

OVERVIEW OF CANCER TREATMENT

Generally cancer treatment is based on the type of cancer, whether or not it has metastasized at the time of original diagnosis, the age and performance status of the patient, as well as social and cost considerations. Four types of cancer treatment options are commonly offered to patients at the time a diagnosis is made. Surgical resection, radiation therapy, chemotherapy, and biological therapy are all treatment options (Dollinger et al., 1991). The patient or health care surrogate and physician must decide which is most appropriate for the type of cancer being treated as well as the patient's overall situation including consideration of the family support system and financial as well as health insurance issues.

A tissue diagnosis is generally needed to study the type of cancer cells and aid the physician in offering the appropriate treatment options. A biopsy is obtained to determine the type of cancer. An interventional radiologist may do a computed tomography (CT) guided needle biopsy or a surgeon may do an open biopsy.

Surgical resection is primarily considered for tumors that are localized. This is a great option for the elderly who have an acceptable surgical risk and a good performance status because the recovery period is generally shorter compared to chemotherapy or radiation therapy.

Chemotherapy or drug therapy for cancer is generally more difficult for the elderly to undertake because of the physiological changes of the elderly. For example, the distribution of medication into the tissue and the excretion of drug through the kidneys are often different in the elderly due to the normal aging process. As research continues and newer and milder drugs are developed, chemotherapy will continue to be offered to the elderly. Some cancers are more indolent or slow growing in the elderly and a mild form of chemotherapy may be a viable treatment option (Balducci, 2001).

Radiation therapy is generally a favorable option for the elderly because the stress of recovering from surgery or side effects of chemotherapy may not have to be endured (Sanders, 2001). Radiation damages the genetic structure of the tumor cells so they can not proliferate. This also affects any healthy cells in the radiation beam; however, these cells generally are able to regenerate themselves thereby shortening the side effects associated with the radiation therapy (Dollinger et al., 1991).

Biological therapy is an accepted form of treatment for some cancers. Biological therapy consists of highly purified proteins (e.g., interferon and interleukin-2) that are given to boost the body's immune system by stimulating the lymphocytes (T-cell and B-cell) to fight foreign cells or proteins (Dollinger et al., 1991).

LUNG CANCER CASE DESCRIPTION

The following case description will demonstrate the many factors to consider in the diagnosis and treatment of cancer in the elderly. A. S. is a 77–year-old Caucasian female who has a diagnosis of Alzheimer's dementia. She is a resident in the dementia unit at a nursing home. Her son lives in the area and her daughter lives out of town. She lived with her daughter in the past and recently moved to the nursing home to be near her son so he could help share some responsibility for oversight of her care. The dementia has progressed to the point where she has no short-term memory but still recognizes her family and familiar caregivers. She is very cheerful and outgoing in her interactions with the other residents and caregivers.

Past medical history includes excisions of melanomas of the left upper extremity, left lower extremity, umbilicus, and flank. Melanoma then metastasized to the left lower lobe of the lung. She was treated with extensive chemotherapy in the 1970s and 1980s as well as a left lower lung lobectomy approximately 20 years ago. She also has chronic obstructive pulmonary disease, treated with metered dose inhalers, chronic anemia with baseline hemoglobin around 9 g/dl, chronic renal insufficiency, and gastric esophageal reflux disease with a large hiatal hernia. She has a remote history of diarrhea and polyps. She had a vaginal hysterectomy in 1960, a bilateral salpingo-oophorectomy in 1974, and a cholecystectomy in 1985. She has allergies to sulfa and tetanus. Her father died at a young age from a farming accident and her mother died at age 76 from a stroke and hypertension. She has twelve siblings; five are deceased from breast cancer and one from an unknown cancer.

A. S. ambulates independently on the dementia unit, is continent of bowel and bladder, able to feed herself, and requires supervision for activities of daily living. In September the examiner observed that A. S. was more short of breath than usual. A chest x-ray showed a pulmonary nodule in the right lower lobe. A CT scan of the thorax further evaluated the nodule. It revealed a 2.5–cm nodule, an adjacent 5–mm nodule, and some pretracheal lymph nodes, which were enlarged to 2 cm. A fine needle aspiration (FNA) was performed by an interventional radiologist using CT guidance and the pathology was interpreted as squamous cell carcinoma. A. S. was taken to her medical oncologist who sees her every six months in follow-up. Records and treatment options were reviewed and discussed with her children. The options offered included no treatment, surgical wedge resection followed by radiation therapy, radiation therapy alone, or chemotherapy. Her children elected surgical resection and a surgeon was consulted. A. S. had a cervical mediastinoscopy in November to rule out metastatic lung cancer. The pathology reported the pretracheal lymph nodes were positive for squamous cell carcinoma and A. S. was not a candidate for a right lower lung lobectomy. She was referred to radiation oncology for consideration of radiation therapy. Her son accompanied her to the appointment and took her to several radiation therapy treatments. Due to her weakened condition, continued restless type movements of her extremities, and the general overall situation, her children elected to discontinue radiation therapy treatments in December. After evaluation of A. S. in the emergency department for a syncopal episode, her children were told that she had progression of the lung cancer. Her daughter, who has durable power of attorney, continues to request full code status in spite of her overall prognosis. Her daughter plans to visit in January.

DISCUSSION

The above case description brings many issues to light regarding cancer and the elderly. Additional comorbid conditions may limit the treatment options available to the elderly. A. S. was not eligible for chemotherapy and surgery was thought to be a less favorable option because of her previous lobectomy. As it turned out she was not a candidate for surgery because of metastatic disease at the initial presentation. Transportation was a consideration because her children were responsible for providing transportation for any type of physician visits and to radiation therapy. She has metastatic lung cancer and was not able to complete the radiation therapy. Her daughter, who lives out of state and visits intermittently, continues to request full code status in spite of the advancing disease.

As the general population ages, those in the medical profession should always keep in mind that an elderly patient is not an island. As elaborated in the case description of A. S., many factors must be considered when the diagnosis and treatment of cancer is undertaken.

ACKNOWLEDGMENT

The authors would like to acknowledge the untiring assistance of Tiffany Hanley, Nancy Davis, and Denise Mabry in the preparation of this chapter.

REFERENCES

Anderson, K. (Ed.). (1994). *Mosby's medical, nursing, & allied health dictionary* (4th ed.). St. Louis, MO: Mosby-Year Book, Inc.

Annual report shows continuing decline in U. S. cancer incidence and death rates. (2000). Cancer Facts: National Cancer Institute. *http://cis.nci.nih.gov*

Balducci, L., & Beghe, C. (2001). Cancer and age in the USA. *Critical Review of Oncology Hematology, 1*(37), 137–145.

Baldwin, J. (2001). Cavities to cancer: the silent epidemic of oral disease. *Geriatric Times, 2*(2), 16.

Beers, M., & Berkow, R. (2000). *The merck manual of geriatrics* (3rd ed.). Whitehouse Station, NJ: Merck Research Laboratories.

Dollinger, M., Rosenbaum, E., & Cable, G. (1991). *Everyone's guide to cancer therapy: How cancer is diagnosed, treated, and managed day to day.* Kansas City, MO: Somerville House Books Limited.

Duthie, E., & Katz, P. (Eds.). (1998). *Practice of geriatrics* (3rd ed.). Philadelphia: W. B. Saunders Company.

Ebersole, P., & Hess, P. (1998). *Toward healthy aging human needs and response* (5th ed.). St. Louis, MO: Mosby.

Ham, R., & Sloane, P. (1997). *Primary care geriatrics* (3rd ed.). St. Louis, MO: Mosby.

Lang, M. (2001). Screening for cognitive impairment in the older adult. *Nurse Practitioner, 26* (11), 26–41.

Leukenotte, A. (1998). *Gerontologic assessment* (3rd ed.). St. Louis, MO: Mosby.

Resnick, B. (2001). Motivating older adults to engage in self-care. *Patient Care for Nurse Practitioners, 4* (9), 9–13.

Resnick, B. (2001). Promoting health in older adults: a four-year analysis. *Journal of the American Academy of Nurse Practitioners, 13* (1), 23–33.

Saunders, C. (2001). Cancer screening in older patients. *Patient Care for the Nurse Practitioner, 11,* 41–46.

Small, S., Stern, Y., Tang, M., & Mayeux, R. (1999). Selective decline in memory function among healthy elderly. *Neurology, 52,* 1392–1396.

Wyngaarden, J., Smith, L., & Bennett, J. (1992). *Cecil textbook of medicine* (19th ed.). Philadelphia: W. B. Saunders Company.

CHAPTER FIVE

Obtaining a Comprehensive Geriatric Assessment

Kathy Effingham, Julie Meyer, and Lodovico Balducci

T he management of cancer in the older aged person entails questions such as: is the patient going to die of cancer, or with, cancer (Balducci & Beghe, 2000; Balducci & Extermann, 2001)? Is the patient able to tolerate the complications of antineoplastic treatment, especially cytotoxic chemotherapy? Is the patient going to suffer cancer-related morbidity during his/her lifetime? Are there reversible conditions that may interfere with the effectiveness and safety of antineoplastic treatment? The answers to these questions require the estimate of life expectancy and risk of treatment complications. The evaluation of the patient's ability to understand the treatment, to follow instructions, and to reach the treatment center on time, are common sensical, yet vital components of a geriatric assessment. The evaluation of the willingness to receive treatment and the concomitant medical conditions (comorbidity) are necessary data to determine before cancer therapy is initiated. In addition, the assessment of patient nutrition may be pivotal in preparing the patient for cancer therapy, as malnutrition is itself associated with increased risk of therapeutic complications. Nutritional status may deteriorate during treatment, and ongoing assessment can help prevent nutritional issues such as general weight loss, nausea, and constipation.

This multidimensional evaluation is obtainable with a Comprehensive Geriatric Assessment (CGA), which is described in this chapter. The CGA examines the medical, functional, cognitive, socioeconomical, and emotional domains of the individual (Balducci, 2001; Extermann & Aapro, 2000). The value of CGA has been documented in different areas of geriatrics. Benefits have included decreased rate of hospitalization and nursing home admission (Bula et al., 1999; Reuben et al., 1999; Stuck et al., 1993; the maintenance of independence (Bula et al., 1999; Reuben et al., 1999), prevention of falls (Tinetti et al., 1994), and the prevention of delirium in hospitalized patients (Inoyoue et al., 1999). In this chapter we illustrate the benefits of a CGA in geriatric cancer patients.

EVALUATION OF THE OLDER CANCER PATIENT

Aging is multidimensional and highly individualized (Balducci & Extermann, 2001). Hence, the approach to the older person should be tailored to the patient's characteristics that may influence effectiveness and safety of care, even if they don't pertain directly to health care. The assessment of functional limitations that may impair the mobility, the independence, and the ability of self-care of the older person is often a basic component of a geriatric assessment. Compromised function is an independent risk factor for mortality (Reuben et al., 1992). Understanding whether the patient is able to perform tasks that maintain some sort of independence may provide a sense of whether the patient can withstand some of the toxicities often associated with chemotherapy. A functional assessment looks beyond the boundaries of the clinic or hospital and considers how a person lives day to day.

The assessment of a patient's social support system is also important to consider when treating the older person. Many older individuals live alone or in company of an elderly spouse, in need of supportive care himself/herself. Access to care may represent a serious problem for these individuals, especially in the case of an emergency; in addition, inadequate social support may be associated with malnutrition, depression, and cognitive deterioration.

Often besides the diagnosis of cancer, other chronic medical conditions, unrelated to cancer, may have gone neglected or unrecognized. Comorbidity may decrease the patient survival and may prevent optimal cancer treatment (for example, coronary artery disease may contraindicate cancer surgery and the administration of cardiotoxic chemotherapy) (Piccirillo et al., 1996; Satariano & Ragland, 1994).

The prevalence of dementia increases with age, which is another basic component of the geriatric assessment. Dementia may prevent understanding of treatment plans and recognition of early symptoms of toxicity. While persons with mild dementia are able to conduct an independent life in condition of homeostasis, they may not be able to cope with the increased cognitive demand imposed by the diagnosis of cancer and the institution of cancer treatment. In addition to factors not associated with malignancy, cancer treatment itself, including cytotoxic chemotherapy and radiation therapy to the brain, may enhance a pre-existing memory disorder. Dementia is an independent risk factor for survival (Bruce et al., 1995). Of interest, a number of new medications may delay the progression of dementia.

The evaluation of depression may be subtle and atypical and may lessen the motivation to receive cancer treatment, as well as the motivation to engage in health maintenance including exercise and regular food intake. Depression is also an independent risk factor for mortality (Blazer et al., 2001; Covinski et al., 1999; Lyness et al., 1997; Lyness et al., 1999).

Often reduced access to food or fresh, unprocessed food may prompt malnutrition, which in turn is a risk factor for mortality and therapeutic complications (Astani et al., 2000). Decreased access to food may have multiple and interrelated causes, including poor mobility, lack of transportation, poverty, lack of interest and forgetfulness (Hardy et al., 1986).

Polypharmacy includes over the counter and alternative medications (Corcoran, 1998) and is a term common to geriatrics that refers to numerous medications that together produce harmful interactions. Iatrogenic illnesses are highly prevalent in the older population and often present as confusion, falls, dementia, and depression (Zhan et al., 2001).

The potential benefits of the CGA in the management of cancer include (Balducci & Yates, 2000):

- Recognition and reversal of conditions that may interfere with cancer treatment, including comorbidity, malnutrition, polypharmacy, inadequate caregiver, socioeconomic restrictions, dementia, and depression, and, more in general, vulnerability to stress.
- Assessment of functional reserve, which predicts tolerance of stress, and in particular of the complications of cancer and cancer treatment.
- Assessment of life expectancy, based on functional reserve, comorbidity, emotional status, and cognitive function.
- Recognition of frailty and vulnerability. Frailty is a condition in which the functional reserve is near exhausted (Balducci & Stanta, 2000). Frail patients are candidates only for palliative cancer treatment. Vulnerability is a condition in which the functional reserve is critically reduced, but still sufficient to allow some

TABLE 5.1 Questions Related to the CGA in Oncology

Integration of function, comorbidity, and geriatric syndromes with the management of cancer.

The extent of the assessment, in particular whether some screening test would be adequate to distinguish the patients who do and don't benefit from a complete CGA.

The person or persons who should perform the assessment, whether a physician, a nurse, or a multidisciplinary team.

Cost of CGA in the management of the older patient.

Age limit beyond which the CGA should be instituted.

form of stress, if proper precautions are taken. Unlike frailty, vulnerability may be reversible to some extent (Wenger & Shekelle, 2001).

- Adoption of a common language in the assessment of the older person. This language is essential for different purposes, including quality assurance of cancer management, retrospective study of the treatment received by older cancer patients, and proper classification of patients enrolled in prospective clinical trials. Given the diversity of the geriatric population, patients enrolled in clinical trials should be classified according to their life expectancy and functional reserve, rather than chronologic age (Extermann & Balducci, 1998).

The National Cancer Center Network (NCCN), a coalition of major USA comprehensive cancer centers that issues guidelines related to cancer management, has recently recognized these benefits of the CGA and has recommended that all patients aged 70 and older receive some form of geriatric assessment (Balducci & Yates, 2000). Despite these broad agreements, a number of questions persist related to practical application of the geriatric assessment (Table 5.1). In the following section we explore the use of the CGA in oncology.

APPLICATION OF THE CGA TO THE MANAGEMENT OF CANCER

COMPONENTS OF THE CGA

Table 5.2 summarizes those domains explored by the CGA and the instruments used for each domain.

Functional status is assessed as ability to perform Activities of Daily Living (ADLs) and Instrumental Activities of Daily Living (IADLs). ADLs

TABLE 5.2 Components of the Geriatric Assessment and its Relevance to Cancer Treatment

Comprehensive Geriatric Assessment (CGA)	
Functional status	
Activities of Daily Living (ADL) and Instrumental Activities of Daily Living (IADL)	Relation to life expectancy, tolerance of chemotherapy, dependence
Comorbidity	
Number of comorbid conditions and comorbidity indices	Relation to life expectancy and tolerance of treatment
Mental status	
Folstein Minimental status	Relation to life expectancy and dependence
Emotional conditions	
Geriatric Depression Scale (GDS)	Relation to survival; may indicate motivation to receive treatment
Nutritional status	
Mininutritional assessment (MNA)	Reversible condition; possible relationship to survival
Polypharmacy	
Geriatric syndromes	
Delirium, dementia, depression, falls, incontinence, spontaneous bone fractures, neglect and abuse, failure to thrive	Risk of drug interactions Relationship to survival Functional dependence

are necessary to maintain one's viability; IADLs to maintain one's independence. ADLs include transferring, bathing, dressing, feeding, toileting, and grooming and IADLs use of transportation, shopping, banking, use of telephone, use of medications, ability to provide one's meals, laundering, and housekeeping. Dependence in one or more ADLs establishes the diagnosis of frailty, a condition in which a person's functional reserve is nearly exhausted, and which is associated with a threefold increase in short-term (2 to 3 years) mortality (Balducci & Stanta, 2000; Reuben et al., 1992). Dependence in IADLs is associated with a twofold short-term mortality and with increased risk of dementia and of chemotherapy-related complications (Reuben et al., 1992).

Not surprisingly, the risk of mortality increases with the number and the seriousness of comorbid conditions. In patients with cancer of the breast and of the upper airways, comorbidity was an independent risk of all cause mortality (Piccirillo et al., 1995; Satariano & Ragland, 1994). It is reasonable to extend these conclusions to patients with other forms of cancer, especially cancer with a chronic course (prostate cancer, low-grade non-Hodgkin's lymphoma). It is important to observe that these studies expressed comorbidity as number of pathologic conditions and did not attempt to grade the severity of each disease. A more precise estimate of the impact of comorbidity on overall mortality may be obtained with comorbidity scales accounting for the seriousness of each comorbid condition with a numeric score. As comorbidity is very sensitive to definition, the use of well validated tools is important in research and practice (59bis). Scales of common use include the Charlson index (Charlson et al., 1994) and the CIRS-G (Cumulative Illness Rating Scale-Geriatrics) (Parmelee et al., 1995), both of which proved reliable in predicting mortality. The Charlson scale is user-friendly but overlooks a number of important conditions; the CIRS-G is more time-consuming, but more comprehensive and more sensitive to variations in symptom severity. Ongoing studies are comparing the value of these scales in the practice of oncology.

Among the comorbid conditions, a special attention has recently been paid to anemia (Balducci et al., 2001), which has a prognostic significance of its own. In older individuals anemia has been associated with:

- Increased mortality (Chaves et al., 2001; Izaks et al., 1999; Kikuchi et al., 2000);
- Increased risk of functional dependence (Cleeland et al., 1999);
- Increased risk of iatrogenic complications, including myelosuppression of cytotoxic chemotherapy, and postoperative delirium (Marcantonio et al., 1997; Schjivers et al., 1999).

In most cases, anemia is reversible with administration of erythropoietin.

Decline in cognition is also associated with increased risk of mortality. In the absence of dementia, the average life expectancy of individuals aged 70 is more than 7 years in the presence of severe dementia (Bruce et al., 1992). In addition, cognitive impairment implies the need of a caregiver to assure treatment compliance and prevent complications for a patient not fully able to understand the treatment plans. The Folstein minimental status (MMS) is the test of common use for the assessment of cognition: this test is of easy administration and the scores are well standardized (Folstein et al., 1975). The main limitation of the MMS is scarce sensitivity for the early stages of dementia.

Depression, even subclinical depression, has been associated with increased risk of mortality in persons over 70 (Blazer et al., 2001). A number of recent studies have highlighted the advantages of screening populations at risk for clinical depression. Both elderly patients and cancer patients are considered at special risk. (Valenstein et al., 2001; Whooley et al., 2001.) The geriatric depression scale is a self-administered and sensitive screening test for depression in older individuals (Lyness et al., 1997).

For in the social assessment, the caregiver is pivotal (Haley et al., 1998; Weitzner et al., 2000). Is the caregiver available on a short notice to manage home emergencies, to arrange transportation of the patient to the clinics or to the hospital, and in general to support the patient during the ordeals of cancer and cancer treatment? Ideally, the caregiver should bridge the communication between the family and the provider. In this capacity, the caregiver may spare the practitioner the discordant communication with different family members and at the same time may avoid the stress of conflicting treatment decisions within the family. The choice of the caregiver may represent a serious challenge. The majority of older people, especially older men, are cared for by an older spouse, who may have health problems and functional dependence of her/his own. When the spouse is inadequate, the task befalls a child, most often a married daughter, with preexisting family and professional commitment. To assure the efficiency and the allegiance of the caregiver, the physician needs to take an active role in the choice and the training of this person, which should involve counseling about stress management and family conflicts. The management of the caregiver is one of the distinctive aspects of geriatric medicine.

In addition to recognizing malnourished persons, the importance of a nutritional assessment consists of identifying individuals at risk of malnutrition in the course of stress (such as surgery and antineoplastic chemotherapy). Preventative interventions may be effective to avoid development of malnutrition in these patients. Some of these interventions are very simple and include early dietary advice or prophylactic insertion of a gastrostomy tube in patients receiving radiation therapy to the upper airways and the esophagus. The mini-nutritional assessment (MNA) is a self-administered screening tool, of common use for this purpose (Guigoz et al., 1997).

Polypharmacy implies the assumption of more than three daily drugs (Corcoran et al., 1998). While in some cases polypharmacy may be justified by the clinical situation, polypharmacy is often an aberration

(Zhan et al., 2001). It is prudent to perform a periodic review of medications of older individuals, especially those who are cared for by different practitioners.

A number of conditions called geriatric syndromes have been recognized in recent years. The presence of one or more geriatric syndromes is generally considered a sign of frailty associated with reduced survival and negligible stress tolerance (Balducci & Stanta, 2000). The current definition of geriatric syndrome requires qualifications, however. For example, dementia is a geriatric syndrome only when it is moderate or severe and prevents a person's independent living; depression when severe and poorly controlled by medication; delirium when it complicates mild urinary or upper respiratory infection or treatment with non-psychotropic drugs (such as anticholinergics); falls when they are spontaneous and frequent (three or more in a month). Failure to thrive is absence of weight gain and functional recovery in spite of adequate nutritional support. At present, the diagnosis of failure to thrive and of neglect and abuse is trusted to a clinical impression; more precise diagnostic criteria are wanted. Both failure to thrive (Verdery, 1997) and neglect and abuse are associated with increased risk of mortality (Dyer et al., 2000).

FUNCTIONAL RESERVE AND COMORBIDITY

Function, comorbidity, and geriatric syndromes help define the life expectancy and the tolerance of cytotoxic chemotherapy by older individuals. Hamermann (1999) proposed four stages of aging reflecting a progressive decline in life expectancy and functional reserve (Table 5.3). For the purposes of cancer management the Hamermann stages may be condensed into three stages.

Standard treatment in older individuals involves special considerations:

Prophylactic use of hemopoietic growth factors is recommended for patients aged 70 and over receiving moderately toxic chemotherapy, such as CHOP for large-cell non-Hodgkin's lymphoma (Balducci & Yates, 2000), because the risk and severity of myelodepression increase after age 70 (Balducci, Lyman, & Ozer, 2001).

Hemoglobin levels should be maintained at $\geq$ 12 gm/dl with erythropoietin, to prevent chemotherapy-related toxicity as well as anemia complications (Balducci and Yates, 2000; Balducci, Hardy, & Lyman, 2001; Schjivers et al., 1999).

TABLE 5.3 Stages of Aging

Hamermann	Cancer-management related staging	Appropriate cancer management
Independent	Independent without comorbidity	Standard treatment
Independent with difficulty	Dependent in one or more Instrumental Activities of Daily Living and/or < 3 comorbid conditions	Special precautions: Initiate treatment with lower doses of chemotherapy Adjust doses of chemotherapy to kidney function Explore possibility of alternative treatment regimens Initiate treatment only when optimal social support and control of other conditions is achieved
Frail	Frail: Dependent in one or more Activities of Daily Living (ADLs) Three or more comorbid conditions or at least one serious comorbid condition One or more geriatric syndromes (delirium, dementia, severe depression, falls, incontinence, failure to thrive, neglect and abuse).	Palliative treatment only, that may include mild cytotoxic chemotherapy
Near death		

The value and safety of high-dose chemotherapy with autologous stem cell rescue has not been established in older individuals, but a number of patients aged 70 and 80 with multiple myeloma seem to have benefited from high-dose chemotherapy and autologous stem cell rescue (Badros et al., 2001).

The indications for adjuvant chemotherapy or any form of treatment whose complications are immediate whereas the benefits are hypothetical may be difficult to establish in older individuals. In the case of adjuvant therapy of breast cancer, Extermann et al., (2001) devised an interesting model based on risk of cancer recurrence and cancerrelated deaths. These authors calculated the threshold for risk of cancer-related death, above which adjuvant chemotherapy would be indicated. Not surprisingly, the threshold increased with the age of the patients; for a woman aged 70 of good health the threshold was 13%; for an 80-year-old it was 30%. The same model could be adapted to decisions related to the adjuvant treatment of colorectal, prostate and stomach cancer, and to the use of chemotherapy in low-grade lymphoma.

The staging system proposed by Hamerman (1999) should be considered a frame of reference to accommodate new information that is accruing. Probably the best defined stage is frailty. Two definitions of frailty are of common use. The classic definition holds frailty present for one or more of the following conditions (Balducci & Stanta, 2000):

- Dependence in ≥ 1 ADL;
- Presence of ≥ geriatric syndrome;
- Presence of ≥ 3 comorbid conditions.

The new definition (Fried et al., 2001) establishes the diagnosis of frailty for three or more of the following:

- Weight loss ≥ 10% of the original body weight;
- Lack of energy;
- Decreased grip strength;
- Slow movements;
- Difficulty in initiating movements.

The two definitions are not mutually exclusive and should be maintained. The classical definition is less sensitive but more specific, and allows for a more immediate diagnosis of frailty based on the general evaluation of the patient. The new definition is more sensitive, but more laborious, and should be used to investigate patients who don't qualify as frail with the classic definition. An important consideration related to diagnosis and management of frailty is that frailty is a chronic condition. A person who presents with acute changes in function and cognition but was totally independent a few days before clinical presentation should not be considered frail. That person is probably suffering an acute condition deserving emergency treatment.

Frailty does not necessarily imply near death. The average life expectancy of the frail person is longer than two years since the diagnosis of frailty (Rockwood et al., 1999). Many older women with breast cancer metastatic to the bone or older men with prostate cancer metastatic to the bone are frail and may require prolonged and effective symptom palliation. These are also the patients more susceptible to the complications of opioids. The use of chemotherapy in frail patients is feasible for palliative purposes. New agents, including taxanes in low doses, weekly Navelbine or gemcitabine, and capecitabine at reduced doses may be safely given to older individuals.

The least defined patient population in the Hamerman staging system is the population of patients intermediary between fully independent and frail. The prevalence of this stage, which includes the majority of cancer patients aged 75 to 90, increases with age. The recent defi-

TABLE 5.4 The VES 13 Scale

Domain	Score
Age:	
75–85	1
> 85	3
Self-rated health:	
Good, very good, and excellent	0
Fair and poor	1
ADL/IADL	
Assistance with:	
Bathing or showering	1
Shopping	1
Money management	1
Transfer	1
Light housework	1
Difficulty in special activities:	
Kneeling, bending, and stooping	1
Performance of heavy housework (example scrubbing the floor)	1
Reaching out and lifting upper extremities above the shoulder	1
Lifting and carrying 10 pounds	1
Walking ¼ of a mile	1
Writing or handling and grasping small objects	1

VES is a self-report measure. The higher the score the more vulnerable. These analyses are reported in Saliba, S., Elliot, M., Rubenstein, L. A., & Solomon, D. H., et al. (2001). The Vulnerable Elders Survey (VES-13): A tool for Identifying Vulnerable Elders in the Community. *Journal of the American Geriatric Society, 49,* 1691–9.

nition of "vulnerable patients" (Saliba et al., 2001; Wanger et al., 2001) allows the practitioner to recognize a group of patients at special risk of death and disability, and presumably at increased risk of treatment complications. The diagnosis of vulnerability is based on a score of 3 or higher in the VES 13 a 13-item scale that may be completely prepared by the patient prior to the clinic visit (Saliba et al., 2001) (Table 5.4). Although some of the items of the VES 13 may be sex-sensitive (inclusion of housework in the questions), overall this scale may prove extremely useful to recognize older cancer patients in need of special attention. Undoubtedly, one may expect some overlapping between extreme vulnerability and frailty. It is worthwhile remembering that the diagnosis of frailty involves full dependence in at least one of the ADLs, whereas the diagnosis of vulnerability involves partial dependence in selected ADLs.

In addition to allowing the staging of aging, the assessment of function, comorbidity, and geriatric syndromes may also reveal conditions that may be reversible or somehow ameliorated with proper intervention. Even in the frail patients, functional deterioration may be delayed with proper treatment and rehabilitation.

HOW MUCH ASSESSMENT IS NECESSARY

As a rule, the CGA evaluates function as IADLs and ADLs, comorbidity, number of diseases, or as comorbidity scores living conditions, income, caregiver status, cognition (as Folstein Minimental status), depression, with a geriatric depression scale, presence of geriatric syndromes, nutrition, and polypharmacy. All elements of the CGA are important, but clearly the time burden of the CGA may be unrealistic for a busy clinical practice of oncology. Extermann et al. (1998) explored the possibility that the evaluation of function and comorbidity be interchangeable, and found these parameters to be independent variables that cannot substitute for each other. The same study also showed that some degree of cognitive dysfunction and depression were present, albeit unsuspected in approximately 20% of patients with cancer aged 70 and older.

A number of options are available to reduce the time commitment of the CGA:

- Patient selection. Patients who are clearly frail on initial assessment do not need CGA. Likewise, patients with high degree of physical and professional function may not need CGA.

- Patient screening. A number of few item questionnaires may be used to recognize patients who need more "in depth" assessment (Lachs et al., 1990; Maly et al., 1997). It is important to add that these screening instruments have been validated in only a small number of patients and may not substitute for the CGA, at least in the research setting. Another screening test may involve functional tests, the most used of which is the time taken by a patient to get up from an armchair, walk 8 yards, come back, and sit again. Perhaps assessment of vulnerability will prove the best screening test, and the one of most clinical significance, but this hypothesis should be explored in clinical trials (Saliba et al., 2001),
- Cooperation of a primary care provider in the management of the older cancer patient.

Ideally, periodical assessments should be performed by the primary care provider based on the CGA indicating preventive measures in older individuals. Based on the geriatric assessment, the primary care provider could select the patients who might benefit most from antineoplastic treatment upon the diagnosis of cancer. This solution encounters some practical, albeit not insurmountable difficulties. Whereas in many European countries older individuals receive primary care by a geriatrician, in the USA many older people don't even have a primary care provider, and may be followed by different specialists, which results in fragmentation of care (Clarefield et al., 2001) and polypharmacy (Zhan et al., 2001). A practical mechanism of assigning each older individual to a primary care provider is needed, in the absence of Universal Health Care. The primary care providers, especially the geriatricians, tend to overestimate the risks and underestimate the benefits of cancer treatment and may not keep abreast with the new form of cancer treatment with very limited toxicity.

Perhaps a better solution would be that older patients with newly diagnosed cancer be referred to a cancer specialist, provided a CGA, and the oncologist and the oncology nurses should be able to interpret the CGA as a base of treatment-related decisions. These different models of practice are summarized in Figure 5.1. Realistically, a combination of the three models according to different situations appears the most practical solution in the USA. It is also important to remember that recent studies have shown that patient-reported information is highly reliable (Ingram et al., 2002). The mailing of a questionnaire to the patient may save a substantial portion of clinic time.

Irrespective of the model of care, the critical role of nursing cannot be overemphasized. Nursing is on the front line of patient manage-

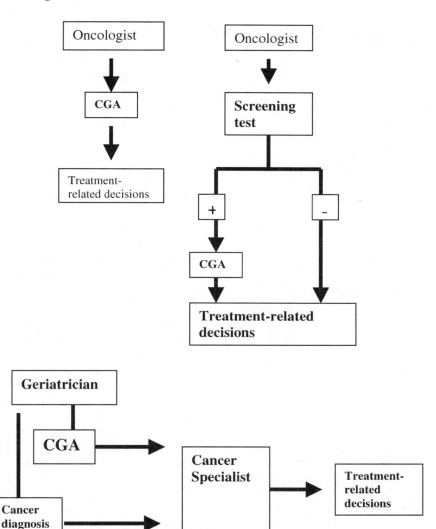

FIGURE 5.1 Different Practice Models for the Management of the Older Person with Cancer.

ment, both in the geriatrician and in the oncologist office. The nurse has a unique opportunity to implement the geriatric assessment. One can construct the nursing role by stating that the quality of care of older cancer patients hinges on nursing care. The nursing profession has been responsible almost single-handedly for the installment of new and more effective principles of symptom management within medical practice, for introducing the central role of quality of life as treatment outcome, and for the development of terminal care. It is not unreasonable then to expect the nurses to take the lead in advocating a holistic approach to the management of older individuals.

An advocacy role is also implicit in nursing. This role can only be satisfied when the growing population of older cancer patients has received the full attention it deserves. Fragmentation of care is a major problem in the management of the elderly in North America. The most desirable solution to that problem is competent case management, another activity developed and embraced by nursing.

WHO SHOULD PERFORM THE CGA

According to the model illustrated in Figure 5.1 the management of cancer in the older aged person presents a real opportunity for the collaboration of oncologists and primary care physicians. Whereas some form of CGA is recommended for older persons with cancer, this assessment is most reliable when performed by a professional with specific training and skills. A number of approaches to this issue include:

- Training of oncologists in the management of older persons. This approach was recently embraced by the Hartford Foundation in the USA, which offers a number of experimental fellowships training in geriatrics and oncology (Muss et al., 2000).
- Assignment of primary care provider with training in geriatrics to all persons aged 70 and older who seek medical attention. This provider would refer older patients to the specialists with a clear outline of their condition based on geriatric assessment. This obviously would be the most comprehensive approach, but would incur a number of difficulties including: Medicalization of aging, which would make of every older person a virtual patient; and imposition of a primary care physician, which would restrict the patient's free choice.

COST OF CGA

Undoubtedly, the addition of the CGA to the evaluation of the older cancer patient would increase the cost of the evaluation. The CGA would not necessarily increase the cost of the care of the older person, however, and might even decrease substantially the total cost, should the CGA result in prevention of functional dependence, which is economically devastating. In assessing the cost of the CGA, as well as of any other medical intervention, it is necessary to adopt a global perspective, embracing the different costs involved in patient care . This perspective needs to distinguish between two cost-related questions: what is the total cost of caring, and how should this cost be divided among the society, the patient, and the health care system? This cost analysis is needed. In the meantime it is recognized that even if it would add to the cost of care, the cost effectiveness of CGA would be of the same order as that of other interventions that are commonly accepted, such as the screening of women over 50 for breast cancer with serial mammography (Stuck et al., 1993).

THE FUTURE OF THE GERIATRIC ASSESSMENT

Two factors will determine the evolution of geriatric assessment:

- New insights into the biological, medical, social, and emotional issues of aging.
- New medical discoveries, especially in the field of preventive intervention, which may delay age-related decline in functional reserve.

Simpler and more objective measurements of aging are likely to become available in the near future. Of special interest are laboratory assessments of aging, in which two major advances deserve mentioning. First, the definition of "somatopause" (Martin, 1999) is as a condition involving the decreased secretion of growth hormone and of insulin-like growth factor 1, associated with increased concentration of catabolic cytokines (interleukin-6 and tumor necrosis factor) (Hamerman et al., 1999). Somatopause appears as a prevalently catabolic status in which the balance between the accrual of new lean tissue and its destruction is negative. It is not clear whether somatopause may be reversible to some extent. From an oncological viewpoint somatoapuse may have two important consequences: decreased tumor growth rate and decreased tolerance of cytotoxic chemotherapy (Astani et al., 2000). The clinical implications of somatopause at present are not clear. Several key questions still require an answer:

- Is the occurrence of somatopause predictable, as is menopause during the reproductive life of a woman, or instead does somatopause occur over a wide range of years making any prediction impractical?

- What is the average life expectancy after somatopause?
- What is the relationship of somatopause and frailty? Are they equivalent? Are all frail patients in somatopause or can you be frail without somatopause, or can you be in somatopause without being frail?
- What is the relationship of somatopause and malnutrition? Is protein-calorie malnutrition associated with transient somatopause, not unlike the administration of cytotoxic chemotherapy may cause temporary menopause?

With these important limitations, somatopause promises to become a milestone of aging that can be assessed with laboratory values.

Secondly, with respect to laboratory determinants of aging, recently, Cohen et al. established that frailty is associated with increased circulating concentration of interleukin-6 and D-Dimer (Cohen et al., 2001). This combination seems to have a high positive predictive value and may be used in the clinical and research setting to establish the diagnosis of frailty according to laboratory criteria. Equally important, these tests may be used to study the reversibility of frailty with medical intervention and may represent themselves a target of interventions aimed to reverse frailty.

On the clinical assessment standpoint, the definition of vulnerability appears particularly useful to identify non-frail patients who are nonetheless at risk for treatment complications and overall mortality. Also, the CGA has highlighted the need for case management in the majority of older individuals. In a pilot study conducted by the Senior Adult Oncology Program (SAOP) we found that seemingly healthy women with breast cancer had an average of five problems each that could have endangered their welfare and put them at risk for treatment complications. Even more astonishing was the fact that one third of them did not have a primary care provider able to coordinate their care.

The current knowledge of aging affords us the opportunity both to test research hypotheses and to establish golden standards for the validation of new clinical and biological information. Testable hypotheses that may be explored at present include:

- Value of repeated geriatric assessment in supporting functional independence of older cancer patients.
- Cost-saving value of the geriatric assessment.
- Development of more sensitive and effective screening instruments.
- Interrelation of frailty, vulnerability, and somatopause.
- Implications of clinical and laboratory frailty.

- Prognostic value of cancer assessment in management of cancer.
- Testing of nursing-based coordination of care models.
- The CGA remains the gold standard of geriatric assessment and the benchmark for new interventions.

CONCLUSIONS

The management of the older person with cancer should be individualized according to the results of a CGA. The nursing profession is positioned ahead of any other profession to promote the implementation of the CGA and to study the CGA in the research arena. In addition, the nursing profession is best positioned for an advocacy and educational role, involving both public and professional education.

REFERENCES

Astani, A., Smith, R. C., & Allen, B. J. (2000). The predictive value of body proteins for chemotherapy induced toxicity. *Cancer, 88,* 796–903.

Badros, A., Barlogie, B., Siegel, E., Roberts, J., Langmaid, C., Zangari, M., Desikan, R., Shaver, M. J., Fassas, A., McConnell, S., Muwalla, F., Barri, Y., Anaissie, E., Munshi, N., & Tricot G. (2001). Autologous stem cell transplantation in elderly multiple myeloma patients over the age of 70 years. *British Journal of Haematology, 114,* 600–607.

Balducci, L. (2000). Geriatric oncology: challenges for the new century. *European Journal of Cancer, 36*(14), 1741–1754.

Balducci, L., & Beghe, C. (2000). The application of the principles of geriatric medicine to the older person with cancer. *Critical Reviews in Oncology/Hematology, 35,* 147–154.

Balducci, L., & Stanta, G. (2000). Cancer in the frail patient: a coming epidemic. *Hematology/Oncology Clinics of North America, 14,* 235–250.

Balducci, L., & Yates, G. (2000). Guidelines for the management of the older person with cancer. *Oncology, 14,* 11A, 221–227.

Balducci, L., & Extermann, M. (2001). A practical approach to the older patient with cancer. *Current Problems in Cancer, 25,* 1–76.

Balducci, L., Hardy, C. H., & Lyman, G. H. (2001). Hematopoietic growth factors in the older cancer patient. *Current Opinion in Hematology, 8,* 170–187.

Balducci, L., Lyman, G. H., & Ozer, H. (2001). Patients aged ≥ 70 are at high risk for neutropenic infection and should receive hemopoietic growth factors when treated with moderately toxic chemotherapy. *Journal of Clinical Oncology, 19,* 1583–1585.

Blazer, D. G., Hybels, C. F., & Pieper, C. F. (2001). The association of depression and mortality in elderly persons: a case for multiple independent pathways. *Journal of Gerontology, 56a,* M505–M509.

Bruce, M. L., Hoff, R. A., Jacobs, S. C., & Leaf, P. J. (1995). The effect of cognitive impairment on 9–year mortality in a community sample. *Journal of Gerontology,* 50B, P289–296.

Bula, C. J., Berod, A. C., Stuck, A. E., Alessi, C. A., Aronow, H. U., Santos-Eggimann, B., Rubenstein, L. Z., & Beck, J. C. (1999). Effectiveness of preventive in-home geriatric assessment in well functioning, community dwelling older people: secondary analysis of a randomized trial. *Journal of the American Geriatrics Society,* 47, 389–395.

Charlson, M., Szatrowski, T. P., Peterson, J. et al. (1994). Validation of a combined comorbidity index. *Journal of Clinical Epidemiology,* 47, 1245–1251.

Chaves, P. H., Volpato, S., Fried, L. (2001). Challenging the world health organization criteria for anemia in the older woman. *Journal of the American Geriatrics Society,* 49, S3, A10.

Clarfield, M. A., Bergmann, H., & Kane, R. (2001). Fragmentation of care for frail older people—an international problem. Experience from three countries: Israel, Canada and the United States. *Journal of the American Geriatrics Society,* 49, 1714–1721.

Cleeland, C. S., Demetri, G. D., Glaspy, J. et al. (1999). Identifying hemoglobin levels for optimal Quality of Life. Results of an incremental analysis. *Proceedings of the American Society for Clinical Oncology,* 16, Astr 2215.

Cohen, H. J., Pieper, C. F., & Harris, T. (2001). Markers of inflammation and coagulation predict decline in function and mortality in community-dwelling elderly. *Journal of the American Geriatrics Society,* 49, S1, A3.

Corcoran, M. B. Polypharmacy in the older patient. (1998). In: L. Balducci, G. H. Lyman, & W. B. Ershler. *Comprehensive geriatric oncology* (pp. 525–532). London: Harwood Academic Publishers.

Covinsky, K. E., Kahana, E., Chin, M. H., Palmer, R. M., Fortinsky, R. H., & Landefeld, C. S. (1999). Depressive symptoms and three year mortality in older hospitalized medical patients. *Annals of Internal Medicine,* 130, 563–569.

Dyer, C. B., Pavlick, V. N., Murphy, K. P. et al. The high prevalence of depression and dementia in elder abuse or neglect. *Journal of the American Geriatrics Society,* 48, 205–208.

Extermann, M., Balducci, L. (1998). Practical proposals for clinical protocols in elderly patients with cancer. In L. Balducci, G. H. Lyman, & W. B. Ershler. *Comprehensive geriatric oncology* (pp. 263–270). London: Harwood Academic Publishers.

Extermann, M., Overcash, J., Lyman, G. H., Parr, J., & Balducci, L. (1998). Comorbidity and functional status are independent in older cancer patients. *Journal of Clinical Oncology,* 16, 1582–1587.

Extermann, M., & Aapro, M. (2000). Assessment of the older cancer patient. *Hematology/Oncology Clinics of North America,* 14, 63–78.

Extermann, M., Balducci, L., & Lyman, G. H. (2000). What threshold for adjuvant therapy in older breast cancer patients? *Journal of Clinical Oncology,* 18, 1709–1717.

Folstein, M. E., Folstein, S. E., & McHugh, P. R. (1975). A Mini Mental State: a practical method for grading the cognitive status of patients for the clinician. *Journal of Psychiatric Research,* 12, 189–198.

Fried, L. P., Tangen, C. M., Walston, J. et al. (2001). Frailty in older adults. Evidence for a phenotype. *Journal of Gerontology MS, 56A,* M146–M156

Guigoz, Y., Vellas, B., & Garry, P. J. (1997). Mininutritional assessment: a practical assessment tool for grading the nutritional state of elderly patients. In *Facts, research, interventions in geriatrics* (pp. 15–20). New York: Serdi Publishing Company.

Haley, W. E., Ehrbar, L., & Schonwetter, R. S. (1998). Family caregiving issues. In L. Balducci, G. H. Lyman, & W. B. Ershler (Eds.). *Comprehensive geriatric oncology* (pp. 805–812). London: Harwood Academic Publishers.

Hamerman, D. (1999). Toward an understanding of frailty. *Annals of Internal Medicine, 130,* 945–950.

Hamermann, D., Berman, J. W., Albers, G. W. et al. (1999). Emerging evidence for inflammation in conditions frequently affecting older adults: report of a symposium. *Journal of the American Geriatrics Society, 47,* 995–999.

Hardy, C. H., Wallace, C., Khansur, T., Vance, R. B., Thigpen, J. T., & Balducci, L. (1986). Cancer, nutrition and aging. *Journal of the American Geriatrics Society, 34*(3), 121–126.

Ingram, S. S., Seo, P. H., Martell, R. E. et al (in press). Comprehensive assessment of elderly cancer patients: The feasibility of self-report methodology. *Journal of Clinical Oncology.*

Inouye, S. K., Bogardus, S. T., Charpentier, P. A. et al. (1999) A multicomponent intervention to prevent delirium in hospitalized older patients. *New England Journal of Medicine, 340,* 669–674.

Izaks, G. J., Westendorp, R. G. J., & Knook, D. (1999). The definition of anemia in the older person. *Journal of the American Medical Association, 281,* 1711–1714.

Kikuchi, M., Inagaki, T., & Shinagawa, N. (2000). Five-year survival of older people with anemia: variation with hemoglobin concentration. *Journal of the American Geriatrics Society, 49,* 1226–1228.

Lachs, M. S., Feinstein, A. R., Cooney, L. M. Jr. et al. (1990) A simple procedure for general screening for functional disability in elderly. *Annals of Internal Medicine, 112,* 699–706.

Lyness, J. M., Ling, D. A., Cox, C., Yoediono, Z., & Caine, E. D. (1999). The importance of subsyndromal depression in older primary care patients. Prevalence and associated functional disability. *Journal of the American Geriatrics Society, 47,* 647–652.

Lyness, J. M., Noel, T. K., Cox, C. et al. (1997). Screening for depression in elderly primary care patients: a comparison of the Center for Epidemiologic Studies Depression Scale and the Geriatric Depression Scale. *Archives of Internal Medicine, 157,* 449–454.

Maly, R. C., Hirsch, S. H., & Reuben, D. B. (1997). The performance of simple instruments in detecting geriatric conditions and home-dwelling older people for geriatric assessment. *Age and Ageing, 26,* 223–231.

Marcantonio, E. R., Flacker, J. M., Michaels, M. et al. (2000). Delirium is independently associated with poor functional recovery after hip fracture. *Journal of the American Geriatrics Society, 48,* 618–624.

Martin, F. (1999). Frailty and the somatopause. *Growth Hormone IGF Research, 9,* 3–10.

Muss, H., Cohen, H., & Lichtman, S. (2000). Clinical research in the older cancer patient. *Hematology/Oncology Clinics of North America, 14,* 283–291.

Parmelee, P. A., Thuras, P. D., Katz, I. R., & Lawton, M. P. (1995). Validation of the cumulative illness rating scale in a geriatric residential population. *Journal of the American Geriatrics Society, 43,* 130–137.

Piccirillo, J. F., & Feinstein, A. R. (1996). Clinical symptoms and comorbidity: significance for the prognostic classification of cancer. *Cancer, 77,* 834–842.

Reuben, D. B., Franck, J., Hirsch, S. et al. (1999). A randomized clinical trial of outpatient geriatric assessment (CGA), coupled with an intervention, to increase adherence to recommendations. *Journal of the American Geriatrics Society, 47,* 269–276.

Reuben, D. B., Rubenstein, L. V., Hirsch, S. et al. (1992). Value of functional status as predictor of mortality. *The American Journal of Medicine, 93,* 663–669.

Rockwood, K., Stadnyk, K., Macknigt, C. et al. (1999). A brief instrument to classify frailty in elderly people. *Lancet, 353,* 205–206.

Saliba, D., Elliott, M., Rubenstein, L. Z. et al. (2001). The vulnerable elderly survey: a tool for identifying vulnerable older people in the community. *Journal of the American Geriatrics Society, 49,* 1691–1699.

Satariano, W. A., & Ragland, D. R. (1994). The effect of comorbidity on 3–year survival of women with primary breast cancer. *Annals of Internal Medicine, 120,* 104–110.

Schijvers, D., Highley, M., DuBruyn, E. et al. (1999). Role of red blood cell in pharmakinetics of chemotherapeutic agents. *Anticancer Drugs, 10,* 147–53.

Stuck, A. E., Siu, A. L., Wieland, D., Adams, J., & Rubenstein, L. Z. (1993). Comprehensive geriatric assessment: a meta-analysis of controlled trials. *Lancet, 342,* 1032–6.

Tinetti, M. E., McAvay, G., Claus, G. et al. (1994). A multifactorial intervention to reduce the risk of falling among elderly people living in the community. *New England Journal of Medicine, 331,* 821–827.

Valenstein, M., Vijan, S., & Zeber, J. E. (2001). The Cost/Utility of screening for depression in primary care. *Annals of Internal Medicine, 134,* 345–360.

Verdery, R. B. (1997). Failure to thrive in old age: follow-up on a workshop. *Journal of Gerontology, 52,* M333–336.

Weitzner, M. A., Haley, W. E., & Chen, H. (2000). The family caregiver of the older cancer patient. *Hematology/Oncology Clinics of North America, 14,* 269–282.

Wenger, S., & Shekelle, P. G. (2001). Assessing care of vulnerable elders: ACOVE project overview. *Annals of Internal Medicine, 135,* 642–646.

Whooley, M. A., & Simon, G. E. (2000). Primary care: managing depression in medical outpatients. *New England Journal of Medicine, 343,* 1942–1950.

Yancik, R. M., & Ries, L. (2000). Aging and cancer in America: demographic and epidemiologic perspectives. *Hematology/Oncology Clinics of North America, 14,* 17–23.

Zhan, C., Sangl, J., Bierman, A. S. et al. (2001). Potentially inappropriate medication use in community-dwelling elderly. *Journal of the American Medical Association, 286,* 2823–2829.

CHAPTER SIX

Understanding Patient Preferences

Hongbin Chen

A n area that tends to be often overlooked is the input from the patient perspective in the medical decision making process. With an increasing awareness of the importance of individual autonomy and consumer rights, many changes have occurred in medical practice over the past several decades. This is largely reflected in the emphasis on the provision of information to patients and the involvement of them in the treatment decision making process. For example, most physicians in the United States in the 1950s would not reveal the diagnosis to their cancer patients (Oken, 1961). By the late 1970s, however, the reverse was true (Novack et al., 1979). As a result, more active participation, information seeking, open communication, full disclosure, informed consent, preference eliciting, and joint decision-making have been gradually incorporated into physician and patient (including older patient) interaction during the medical encounter (Putman, 1996).

Medical decisions have become more and more complex tasks, with competing and conflicting issues presented to health care providers, patients, and their families. The goal is to provide adequate and appropriate quality health care. However, evidence has shown that older patients are less likely to receive cancer treatments that are considered definitive or potentially curative than younger patients (Schrag et al., 2001; Yancik et al., 2001). A better understanding of the patient's perspective can help clinicians improve their clinical practice by appropriately incorporating them, without either overemphasizing or underestimating, into treatment decision-making considerations.

PATIENT PREFERENCES

Concerns about treatment efficacy and the tolerance level of side effects in older patients come from both physicians and patients. Patient preferences, however, were not always sought. Critical therapeutic choices should not be based solely on rigid, formal guidelines, but need to be individualized and take into account patients' preferences (Ravdin et al., 1998). Good clinical decisions require a better understanding of how *patients* view certain treatment procedures and outcomes that affect their well-being. Incorporating patients' preferences into medical decisions also helps to establish a more collaborative partnership between physician and patient.

Kassirer (1995) listed some of the circumstances under which identifying patients' preferences is particularly relevant. They include: when there are major differences in the kinds of possible outcomes (e.g., death versus disability); when there are major differences between treatments in the likelihood and impact of complications; when choices involve trade-offs between near-term and long-term outcomes; when the apparent difference between options is marginal; or when a patient is particularly averse to taking risks. Obviously, cancer treatment requires important decisions in older adults. Choice of treatment may influence disease-free and overall survival (e.g., systemic adjuvant therapy for breast cancer) or toxicity level (e.g., hormonal therapy versus chemotherapy), but may still have comparable outcomes with regard to local relapse (e.g., mastectomy versus breast conservation therapy followed by radiation). For advanced cancers, palliative chemotherapy or supportive care may be offered, but the relative value of these two options is less well documented. When treatments are roughly equivalent in outcome or equivalency is unknown, patients' treatment preferences concerning quality of life (QOL) and their perception of the efficacy of treatment ought to play a role in making decisions about treatment (Siminoff & Fetting, 1991). Therefore, the nature of the benefits and risks associated with different treatment options is likely to affect preferences of patients.

Patient preference research can provide information to help patients and oncologists make selections from various treatment alternatives that offer only small differences in survival but substantial differences in toxicity. Response, toxicity, time to treatment failure, and survival data are becoming better defined for current therapies of most cancers. Just like any other medical intervention, cancer treatment inevitably has side effects as a result of killing tumor cells as well as damaging normal cells in the body. Treatment-related toxicity can range from mild fatigue and weakness, physical limitation, body image change, nausea and vomiting, mouth sores, hair loss, decreased appetite, and suppressed immune function, to severe events such as cardiac toxicity or even death. It can occur from any form of available cancer treatment, including a radical operation, chemotherapeutic regimen, radiation therapy, hormone therapy, or even more cutting-edge immuno-biological therapy. When older cancer patients are presented with a treatment option, which can be a combination of several therapies, potential side effects of the treatment emerge as one of the major concerns and risks for them to consider. Some previous studies have found that a substantial proportion of older cancer patients would trade off anything for longer survival time regardless of potential side effects (Brundage et al., 1997; Hamel et al., 2000; Navari et al., 2000), while other studies revealed that a considerable number of older cancer patients still put more value on their current health status by choosing a less toxic treatment or rejecting any kind of cancer treatment even though they might have to sacrifice the potential chance of prolongation of life (Bremnes et al., 1995; Newcomb & Carbone, 1993; Yellen et al., 1994).

Although determinants of decision making in cancer patients are still not fully explored and understood, it has been suggested that patient treatment decisions do not appear to be the result of purely rational evaluation of all relevant information, but are influenced by individual, situational, and interpersonal factors (Lindley et al., 1998; Petrisek et al., 1997; Siminoff & Fetting, 1991; Silliman et al., 1997; Ward et al., 1989; Yellen et al., 1994). Along this line, factors that are associated with treatment preferences can be summarized under three general categories—those of patients' characteristics such as age, education, marital status, social support, attitudes and values, and current health status including comorbid conditions and functional disability; disease (cancer)-specific and treatment-related concerns such as cancer status, previous treatment experience, prognosis and side effects; and contextual factors during the medical encounter such as information provision and physician influence (Table 6.1). Current data suggest that preferences for cancer treatment in adult cancer patients are most likely the products of a group of factors all exerting various degrees of influence in shaping the final treatment choices.

Despite the contemporary advocacy toward a more active role for patients in medical decisions, it has been well documented that older cancer patients are more likely to assume traditional, less-participatory, passive roles. Earlier studies (Blanchard et al., 1988; Cassileth et al., 1980) of information and participation preferences among cancer patients showed that although the majority preferred all the detailed information, only 60–70% (30-40% did not want to participate) preferred to participate in therapeutic decisions. Significant age trends

TABLE 6.1 Factors that Influence Treatment Preferences in Older
Cancer Patient

Patient Characteristics
Age
Education
Marital Status
Social Support
Health Status (Comorbid Conditions and Functional Status)

Disease Characteristics
Prognosis
Cancer Status
Treatment Toxicity
Previous Treatment Experience

Contextual Characteristics
Information Provision
Physician Influence

were noted: those who sought less detailed information and who wanted to leave decisions up to the doctor were older. This type of preference for a more authoritative relationship with their oncologists in older cancer patients is still a rather predominant phenomenon in recent studies among women with breast cancer (Bilodeau & Degner, 1996; Petrisek et al., 1997).

Age-related differences exist not only in decision-making style of cancer patients, but also in the choices they make. In a study by Yellen and colleagues (1994), when cancer patients were asked to make hypothetical decisions about treatment given with respect to varying levels of disease stage and treatment toxicity, older adults did not differ from their younger counterparts in terms of acceptance of treatment (chemotherapy in this case). However, when treatment was presumed, they differed in willingness to trade survival for current quality of life. Older age predicted less willingness to accept severe toxicity in exchange of survival time, found in both early-stage disease and advanced-disease vignettes. Similar results were reported in another study (Bremnes et al., 1995) regarding the willingness to accept toxic chemotherapy for an insignificant level of benefits such as chance of cure, prolongation of life, and relief of symptoms was inversely related to age. For instance, cancer patients over the age of 60 demanded a minimal chance of cure of 50% in order to make a toxic hypothetical chemotherapy acceptable, compared with 10% in patients under 50 years old and 7% in those under 40 years old. A recent study further confirmed these findings (Silvestri et al., 1998) in that older patients tend to demand greater benefits before accepting chemotherapy when severe toxicity is presented.

Since none of these studies examined the comorbid conditions or functional status of the patients, it is not clear whether the observed age differences in treatment preference were actually due to these two factors among senior adult patients. It is very possible that these two clinical factors, which correlate with patients' general health status, play a role in their consideration of tolerating such treatment-related toxicity. Older patients who had more medical conditions (in addition to cancer) that limited their functional capacity and thus perceived themselves in a worse state of health than younger, healthier patients could opt to reject a toxic treatment or require more benefit from the treatment in order to accept it. Thus, it seems logical to expect that patients' preferences for aggressive cancer treatment would be affected or down-regulated by their awareness and consideration of their own comorbidity and functional status—an uneasy situation similar to that physicians also face as discussed in the previous section.

It was not until fairly recently that researchers made efforts to explore the demographic and clinical factors that may influence treatment preferences in older cancer patients. For instance, a retrospective study conducted by Petrisek et al. (1997) attempts to obtain greater insight into *how* and *why* therapy selection differs by patient age. This is one of the most comprehensive studies on this subject because age differences were explored concurrently in the context in which decisions are made, the style of patient decision-making, and factors considered by patients when choosing treatment options. Self-reported data were collected from a sample of 179 women recently diagnosed with nonrecurrent, early-stage breast cancer. Patients were asked to rate the importance of 15 factors in making their treatment decisions, including those aspects related to their personal needs and concerns about treatment and its outcome.

A large majority of participants rated physician recommendation, not having the problem return, family opinion, and same experience of others as very or somewhat important. Only fear of recurrence was significantly related to age, with women over the age of 70 (still as high as 86%) less likely than others (96%) to have this issue as an important consideration. Although no significant age difference was found, over 40% of patients aged 70 and over considered physiological aspects of treatment important, including length and side effects of treatment as well as physical limitation. While younger patients rated items like body image or sexuality and role maintenance important, older patients (30%, versus 12% in younger patients) were significantly more concerned about transportation difficulties. Over one-third of those 70 years and older also worried about paying for treatment. In interpreting the results of the study, it is not surprising that older women were less concerned about the effects of treatment on family responsibilities and employment opportunities since they are involved in fewer caregiving and employment activities. Their concerns about extraneous factors affecting treatment such as transportation and payment are rather understandable. In addition, the authors suggest that older patients may decide that the marginal benefits of certain types of therapy are not sufficient to justify the burdens associated with the treatment, so that fear of recurrence becomes a less compelling reason to undergo therapy.

A similar study investigated the relative importance of different factors on the trade-off between two outcomes of medical treatment of cancer: QOL and LOL (length of life) (Kiebert et al., 1994). Patients were asked to rate seven factors if they had to choose between two treatment options that differed in these two expected outcomes. The results showed that patients rated six factors as of considerable importance to them. They include, in descending order, disease-related chance of survival, baseline level of QOL (health status), presence of children, having a partner, age at the time of decision, and the nature of the side effects. Fifty-one percent of the 199 patients were 51 to 75 years old, but those over 75 years were excluded from the study. Further analysis of the relationship between these importance ratings and personal characteristics revealed significant age and education differences in several factor's rankings. The older the patients, the greater the importance of the nature of the side effects, the disease-related life expectancy and patients' baseline level of QOL. In addition to the latter two factors, the presence of children was also very important for persons with a lower level of education in making a decision.

It seems that when gains and losses have to be balanced, a cluster of factors regarding the disease and treatment as well as personal and social context are of important consideration to cancer patients. Older people may assign different weights to the relative importance of different factors that may affect their treatment preferences. Of particular interest are studies that examine the relationships among various clinical and nonclinical factors. In a study examining the impact of age, marital status, and physician-patient interactions on the care of older patients with early-stage breast carcinoma (Silliman et al., 1997), older women, unmarried women, and women with whom treatment options were discussed infrequently were found less likely to receive definitive therapy. These associations persisted after control for health status and tumor characteristics. The older unmarried women in this study were found to be more concerned about treatment-related problems that they might experience after surgery and the out-of-pocket costs of their care, which may have led them to choose less intense regimens.

The above study noted the importance of physician-patient discussion regarding treatment options. Physicians and nurses are still regarded as the major information source patients rely on in making a decision. The kind and amount of information seeking and provision during physician-patient interaction is influential in the treatment preference and decision making process. Examining the information priorities of cancer patients involved in treatment decision making can be very helpful in understanding this contextual variable. Studies have shown that the overwhelming majority of cancer patients want detailed information not only about diagnosis, but also about treatment and outcome (Bilodeau & Degner, 1996; Blanchard et al., 1988; Davison et al., 1995). Information items regarding the accomplishment of potential treatment including likelihood of cure, probability of survival and recurrence, and possible side effects are highly desired by patients of all ages. Older patients also care more about self-care issues, and it is suggested that information related to situational variables such as status of disease and treatment outcome was deemed more important than other aspects such as physical and emotional impact of the disease on family and friends. Cautions should be taken, however, as a desire for information and a desire for full participation in decision-making may not always be equated.

An interesting aspect of information provision as a contextual factor is the format and labeling of information presented to patients and its effect on the preference of cancer treatment. This is an important methodology issue in dealing with the elicitation of preferences in cancer patients. Several studies published in the late 1980s compared the effect of a positive frame, in which outcomes were expressed as the probability of surviving, a negative frame, in which outcomes were expressed as the probability of dying, and a mixed frame, in which both probabilities were given (O'Connor, 1989; O'Connor et al., 1985; O'Connor et al., 1987). The results showed that preferences were not significantly dependent on rater variables such as age or sex, nor on the medium used for elicitation, computer terminal or pencil-and-paper questionnaire. Instead, the importance of the way decision problems were framed was confirmed, as the presence or absence of the word "survive" in the outcome description became a main source of framing bias. The participants preferred a toxic cancer chemotherapy that afforded better survival to a less toxic treatment with poorer survival to a significantly greater extent in the positive frame than in the negative frame. The level of probability that was presented also influenced cancer patients' preferences. This probably suggests that a negative frame or low probability level might stimulate a "dying mode" type of value system in which QOL becomes more salient in decision making than LOL. It may have implications in clinical practice when outcome data are presented to a cancer patient in a realistic but hopeful manner rather than a negative format in order to convince the patient to accept the therapy, although some ethical concerns are raised by doing so in describing clinical trial entry.

Informed decision making may also be dependent on the patient's knowledge and understanding of cancer and potential treatment. In this case, a patient's prior experience with the disease and its treatment can be important. Older patients who had not previously received chemotherapy (chemotherapy naïve) expressed less aggressive intent than their experienced counterparts, independent of past treatment difficulty (Yellen et al., 1994). Mazur et al. (1996) also found that older (mean age 66 years, noncancer) patients' experience with physical problems associated with prostate disease was highly correlated with whether they would accept surgery or expectant management for hypothetical localized prostate cancer.

Finally, as alluded to before, physicians' recommendations are undoubtedly viewed as absolute professional opinion and shown to be one of the most influential factors in patients' choice of a treatment option. Although it may also be a matter of attitude and trust toward health care professionals, older patients have consistently rated their physicians' recommendations as hierarchically very important among other factors (Petrisek et al., 1997; Silliman et al., 1997; Siminoff & Fetting, 1991). When presented with treatment alternatives, patients of all ages rejected those that were mentioned but not recommended by the doctor (Newcomb & Carbone, 1993). What this means for nurses in that follow-up education pertaining to the health care recommendations should be conducted for the patients and their support persons. While health care providers have knowledge of disease and treatment outcomes and side effects, their perceptions and relative expectations of these facts may be quite different from those of patients (Bremnes et al., 1995; Slevin et al., 1990). Recent findings from the SUPPORT project (the Study to Understand Prognoses and Preferences for Outcomes and Risks of Treatments) showed that adult patients (mean age 62) with late-stage cancers tend to overestimate their survival probabilities, while physicians estimated prognosis quite accurately (Weeks et al., 1998). However, these estimates may influence patients' preferences about medical therapies. Patients overestimating their prognosis were more likely to favor life-extending therapy over comfort care and to undergo aggressive treatment, compared with patients who didn't overestimate. This is a typical example of how understanding illness may be between patients and physicians and its subsequent impact on the preferences of treatment. It reflects the true complexity of medical decision making in which physicians (as well as other health care providers and families) have substantial input to the preferences of patients. The problem is that their views are not necessarily always the same as those of older patients, who usually become rather compliant to these suggestions without challenging expert opinions. When there is a disparity of opinions between the two parties involved in the medical decision making process, clinicians then face the challenge of how to effectively deliver the message to the patient regarding the prognosis and treatment information while honoring patient preferences at the same time.

CONCLUSIONS

Treatment decision making in older cancer patients is truly an ongoing process that takes place immediately after the diagnosis of cancer, continues throughout the entire disease course, and lasts until the end-of-life care. Acknowledging the great inter-individual variability of older cancer patients ready to receive any kind of treatment is the first step leading to a sound judgment. Evidence-based medicine depends on reliable measurement of comorbid conditions and functional status to guide treatment planning, unbiased. Preference-based care involves the patient in decisions concerning the care process so that improved decision making process can be achieved (Katz, 2001). Preference elicitation is an important step that can facilitate the clinical communication and decision-making process, which will eventually produce better patient care and health outcomes while increasing patients' knowledge of treatment and reducing decision conflict.

For physicians, nurse practitioners, nurses, and other health care workers who are interested in treatment decision making in older cancer patients, one thing is clear from the above review and discussion; there is no single factor that can explain the whole picture of the decision making process. No doubt comorbid conditions, functional status, patient preferences, and other factors alike, all play an important, sometimes crucial, role in choosing a therapy. But these are just some of the relevant factors that have been well recognized and investigated so far at an individual level. There may be other underlying reasons yet to be identified that have an even more powerful impact on treatment decisions in this population. At an individual level, patients' belief and value systems, spirituality, risk perception and propensity, and cognitive function deserve further investigation in the future (Balducci & Meyer, 2001). At an institutional and societal level, accessibility to, and availability of, quality health care as well as the existence of health disparities also need to be addressed (Katz, 2001; Lynn et al., 2000; Pritchard et al., 1998).

REFERENCES

Balducci, L., Extermann, M., & Carreca, I. (2001). Management of breast cancer in the older woman. *Cancer Control, 8*(5), 431–441.

Balducci, L., & Meyer, R. (2001). Spirituality and medicine: A proposal. *Cancer Control, 8*(4), 368–376.

Bennett, C. L., Greenfield, S., Aronow, H. et al. (1991). Patterns of care related to age of men with prostate cancer. *Cancer, 67,* 2633–2641.

Bilodeau, B. A., & Degner, L. F. (1996). Information needs, sources of information, and decisional roles in women with breast cancer. *Oncology Nursing Forum, 23*(4), 691–696.

Blanchard, C. G., LaBrecque, M. S., Ruckdeschel, J. C., et al. (1988). Information and decision-making preferences of hospitalized adult cancer patients. *Social Science and Medicine, 27*(11), 1139–1145.

Bremnes, R. M., Andersen, K., & Wist, E. A. (1995). Cancer patients, doctors and nurses vary in their willingness to undertake cancer chemotherapy. *European Journal of Cancer, 31A*(12), 1955–1959.

Brundage, M. D., Davidson, J. R., & MacKillop, W. J. (1997). Trading treatment toxicity for survival in locally advanced non–small cell lung cancer. *Journal of Clinical Oncology, 15*(1), 330–340.

Cassileth, B. R., Zupkis, R. V., Sutton-Smith, K. et al. (1980). Information and participation preferences among cancer patients. *Annals of Internal Medicine, 92*(6), 832–836.

Davison, J., Degner, L. F., & Morgan, T. R. (1995). Information and decision-making preferences of men with prostate cancer. *Oncology Nursing Forum, 22*(9), 1401–1408.

Extermann, M. (2000). Measuring comorbidity in older cancer patients. *European Journal of Cancer, 36*(4), 453–471.

Extermann, M., & Aapro, M. (2000). Assessment of the older cancer patient. *Hematology/Oncology Clinics of North America, 14*(1), 63–77.

Extermann, M., Overcash, J., Lyman, G. H. et al. (1998). Comorbidity and functional status are independent in older cancer patients. *Journal of Clinical Oncology, 16*(4), 1582–1587.

Finkelstein, D. M., Ettinger, D. S., & Ruckdeschel, J. C. (1986). Long-term survivors in metastatic non–small cell lung cancer: An Eastern Cooperative Oncology Group study. *Journal of Clinical Oncology, 4*(5), 702–709.

Fried, L. P., Bandeen-Roche, K., Kasper, J. D. et al. (1999). Association of comorbidity with disability in older women: The Women's Health and Aging Study. *Journal of Clinical Epidemiology, 52*(1), 27–37.

Goodwin, J. S., Hunt, W. C., & Samet, J. M. (1993). Determinants of cancer therapy in elderly patients. *Cancer, 72*(2), 594–601.

Greenfield, S., Blanco, D. M., Elashoff, R. M. et al. (1987). Patterns of care related to age of breast cancer patients. *Journal of the American Medical Association, 257*(20), 2766–2770.

Hamel, M. B., Lynn, J., Teno, J. M. et al. (2000). Age-related differences in care preferences, treatment decisions, and clinical outcomes of seriously ill hospitalized adults: Lessons from SUPPORT. *Journal of the American Geriatrics Society, 48*(5), S176–S182.

Hutchins, L. F., Unger, J. M., Crowley, J. J. et al. (1999). Underrepresentation of patients 65 years of age or older in cancer-treament trials. *New England Journal of Medicine, 341*(27), 2061–2067.

Kassirer, J. P. (1995). Incorporating patients' preferences into medical decisions. *New England Journal of Medicine, 330*(26), 1895–1896.

Katz, J. N. (2001). Patient preferences and health disparities. *Journal of the American Medical Association, 286*(12), 1506–1509.

Kiebert, G. M., Stiggelbout, A. M., Kievit, J. et al. (1994). Choices in oncology: factors that influence patients' treatment preference. *Quality of Life Research, 3*(3), 175–182.

Lindley, C., Vasa, S., Sawyer, W. T. & Winer, E. P. (1998). Quality of life and preferences for treatment following systemic adjuvant therapy for early-stage breast cancer. *Journal of Clinical Oncology, 16*(4), 1380–1387.

Lynn, J., Arkes, J. R., Stevens, M. et al. (2000). Rethinking fundamental assumptions: SUPPORT's implications for future reform. *Journal of the American Geriatrics Society, 48*(5), S214–S221.

Mazur, D. J. & Merz, J. F. (1996). How older patients' treatment preferences are influenced by disclosures about therapeutic uncertainty: Surgery versus expectant management for localized prostate cancer. *Journal of the American Geriatrics Society, 44*(8), 934–937.

Navari, R. M., Stocking, C. B., & Siegler, M. (2000). Preferences of patients with advanced cancer for hospice care. *Journal of the American Medical Association, 284*(19), 2449.

Newcomb, P. A., & Carbone, P. P. (1993). Cancer treatment and age: Patient perspectives. *Journal of the National Cancer Institute, 85*(19), 1580–1584.

Newschaffer, C. J., Penberthy, L., Desch, C. E. et al. (1996). The effect of age and comorbidity in the treatment of elderly women with nonmetastatic breast cancer. *Archives of Internal Medicine, 156*(1), 85–90.

Novack, D. H., Plumer, R., Smith, R. L. et al. (1979). Changes in physicians' attitudes towards telling the cancer patient. *Journal of the American Medical Association, 241*, 897–900.

O'Connor, A. M. C. (1989). Effects of framing and level of probability on patients' preferences for cancer chemotherapy. *Journal of Clinical Epidemiology, 42*(2), 119–126.

O'Connor, A. M. C., Boyd, N. F., Tritchler, D. L. et al. (1985). Eliciting preferences for alternative cancer drug treatments. The influence of framing, medium, and rater variables. *Medical Decision Making, 5*(4), 453–463.

O'Connor, A. M. C., Boyd, N. F., Warde, P. et al. (1987). Eliciting preferences for alternative drug therapies in oncology: Influence of treatment outcome description, eliciting technique and treatment experience on preferences. *Journal of Chronic Diseases, 40*(8), 811–818.

Oken, D. (1961). What to tell cancer patients: a study of medical attitudes. *Journal of the American Medical Association, 175,* 1120–1128.

Petrisek, A. C., Laliberte, L. L., Allen, S. M. et al. (1997). The treatment decision-making process: Age differences in a sample of women recently diagnosed with nonrecurrent, early-stage breast cancer. *Gerontologist, 37* (5), 598–608.

Pritchard, R. S., Fisher, E. S., Teno, J. M. et al. (1998). Influence of patient preferences and local health system characteristics on the place of death. *Journal of the American Geriatrics Society, 46*(10), 1242–1250.

Putman, S. M. (1996). Nature of the medical encounter. *Research on Aging, 18*(1), 70–83.

Ravdin, P. M., Siminoff, I. A., & Harvey, J. A. (1998). Survey of breast cancer patients concerning their knowledge and expectations of adjuvant therapy. *Journal of Clinical Oncology, 16*(2), 515–521.

Satariano, W. A. (1992). Comorbidity and functional status in older women with breast cancer: Implications for screening, treatment, and prognosis. *Journal of Gerontology, 47* (Special Issue), 24–31.

Satariano, W. A. & Ragland, D. R. (1994). The effect of comorbidity on 3–year survival of women with primary breast cancer. *Annals of Internal Medicine, 120* (2), 104–110.

Schrag, D., Cramer, L. D., Bach, P. B. et al. (2001). Age and adjuvant chemotherapy use after surgery for stage III colon cancer . *Journal of the National Cancer Institute, 93*(1), 850–857.

Silliman, R. A., Troyan, S. L., Guadagnoli, E. et al. (1997). The impact of age, marital status, and physician-patient interactions on the care of older women with breast carcinoma. *Cancer, 80*(7), 1326–1334.

Silvestri, G., Pritchard, R. S., & Welch, H. G. (1998). Preferences for chemotherapy in patients with advanced non-small cell lung cancer: descriptive study based on scripted interviews. *British Medical Journal, 317*(7161), 771–775.

Siminoff, I. A., & Fetting, J. H. (1991). Factors affecting treatment decisions for a life-threatening illness: The case of medical treatment of breast cancer. *Social Science and Medicine, 32*(7), 813–818.

Slevin, M. L., Stubbs, L., Plant, H. J. et al. (1990). Attitudes to chemotherapy: comparing views of patients with cancer with those of doctors, nurses, and general public. *British Medical Journal, 300*(6737), 1458–1460.

Ward, S. E., Heidrich, S. M., & Wolberg, W. (1989). Factors women take into account when deciding upon type of surgery for breast cancer. *Cancer Nursing, 12*(6), 344–351.

Weeks, J. C., Cook, E. F., O'Day, S. J. et al. (1998). Relationship between cancer patients' predictions of prognosis and their treatment preferences. *Journal of the American Medical Association, 279*(21), 1709–1714.

Yancik, R., & Ries, L. A. (1998). Cancer in older persons. Magnitude of the problem—How do we apply what we know? In L. Balducci, G. H. Lyman, & W. B. Ershler (Eds.), *Comprehensive geriatric oncology* (pp. 95–103). London: Harwood Academic Publishers.

Yancik, R., Wesley, M. N., Ries, L. A. et al. (2001). Effect of age and comorbidity in postmenopausal breast cancer patients aged 55 years and older. *Journal of the American Medical Association, 285*(7), 885–892.

Yellen, S. B., Cella, D. F., & Leslie, W. T. (1994). Age and clinical decision making in oncology patients. *Journal of the National Cancer Institute, 86*(23), 1766–1770.

CHAPTER SEVEN

Health Care Decisions: How Cancer Treatment Decisions Are Made by the Health Care Team

Janine Overcash and Lodovico Balducci

The definition of special principles for the management of cancer in the older person begs the definition of aging, which is a multidimensional and highly diverse process (Balducci and Beghe, 2001). A practical approach to this complex problem involves the analysis of decisions, and the study of the likely influences of aging on these decisions. We will follow this approach as a frame of reference for practitioners involved in the management of older individuals, for social scientists involved in public health plans, and for clinical scientists involved in clinical trials.

THE ANATOMY OF HEALTH CARE DECISIONS

We will dissect a health care decision in two sections: goal(s) and mechanisms. First, the *goals of a health care decision,* are often led by two intertwined principles: beneficence and non-malfeasance. In other words, the benefits of any medical or nursing intervention must be worth the potential risks involved (Levinsky et al., 2001). The practical application of this axiom is more complicated, however, than its pure enunciation, and hinges on the assessment of benefits and risk. A large majority of people would agree that the negligible risks of a mastectomy in a women with one year and greater life expectancy are more desirable than the substantial risk of complications from breast cancer (Balducci et al., 2002). A much smaller group of persons would agree to the substantial risks of a prostatectomy, whose benefits may be minor in a man aged 70 or older (Balducci et al., 1997). Clearly, the patient is the final arbiter of what interventions are beneficial in his/her particular case, but the patient's scope may be limited by three factors:

The patient has no direct experience of the ultimate consequences of the disease nor of the treatment; thus, the patient's decision is necessarily based on a number of personal circumstances including the recommendation of health care providers, the testimony of other patients, the wishes of significant others, and the personal observation of cancer in family members or friends.

In many situations there is no definitive clinical answer to the problem under consideration, thus, patient and practitioner need to manage uncertainty. Whereas for the practitioner this is a way of life, for the patient this experience may be both confusing and distressing. A common example of this type of intervention is the use of adjuvant chemotherapy in women aged 70 and older. Though there is no direct evidence that this intervention decreases the cancer-related mortality in women over 70, it is reasonable to offer it to women at high risk of recurrence (Goldhirsch et al., 2001).

The patient's cognitive and decisional ability may be impaired by a number of conditions, including delirium and dementia, drugs, and emotional disorders.

Age may affect each one of these aspects. Older individuals are generally more dependent on the recommendations of their provider in health care matters (Fox et al., 1997), but at the same time they may be more dependent on family and friends and in general on their "informal" support network for receiving health care. Not surprisingly, the recommendations of siblings and friends often determine the final medical decision. The management of cancer and other diseases in the older person is still uncharted water, which complicates further the assessment of risk and benefits. For example, it is a common impression that the growth rate of some cancers including breast (Balducci et al., 2002) and lung (Sheppard et al., 2002) may be more indolent in older individuals, whereas the risk of cytotoxic chemotherapy may increase (Balducci & Extermann, 2001). The benefits of adjuvant treatment may be reversed if this impression is true. The comprehension of the older person may be impaired by a number of conditions, including reduced cognition, disturbances of sight and hearing, and medications. In addition, the perspective of an older person related to death and desirability of treatment has not been investigated as thoroughly as the perspective of younger individuals has been. A caveat is that not all older people suffer from dementia or confusion (most older people are highly cognitively intact), and an assessment is vital to determine how to proceed in the health education and treatment process.

When we speak of making health care decisions, it is important not to overlook the patient and family in this process. Nursing can both make decisions as part of the plan of care and provide an environment for the patient and family to make health decisions, which hopefully they will deem satisfactory. First, it is crucial to provide education to the patient. Using the nursing process, assess the patient's current knowledge of chemotherapy and cancer. Knowledge may include misconceptions or false information associated with malignancy. For people of all ages, the notion of cancer is thought to be a death sentence and treatment is often considered cruel and incapacitating. Conversely, many older people are very empowered with educational materials often obtained via the Internet and know a great deal about their cancer and the various treatment options, including clinical trials. Sites such as the National Cancer Institute and the thousands of cancer-specific sites are frequented by people of all ages who have been challenged by a diagnosis of cancer. Obtain an understanding of how a patient feels about his or her diagnosis and his or her personal goals associated with cancer treatment. Some people may worry about body disfigurement resulting from surgery, and a plastic surgery consult is important to their plan of care. Others may want pain control as their initial priority. Assessment of patient's understanding and envisioned outcomes is the first step in the development of the nursing and medical plan, and to construct a platform for the patient to make some serious decisions about his or her health. It is important to state that nursing is responsible not only for the nursing plan of care, but for contributing to the development of medical interventions. Providing the health care team with information, such as the patient's expectations, is important to the development of the general health care plan.

The next step after the determination of patient knowledge, perceptions, and goal is to cojointly develop a plan. If the problem is a lack of information concerning the cancer diagnosis and treatment in general, a description of the pathology of the malignancy and the benefits and risks of cancer treatment is essential in simple and clear terms. Take as much time as possible to provide this teaching, and evaluate the teaching by asking the patient to repeat the key points of the presentation to make sure that the comprehension has been complete. The astute nurse will calibrate the presentation to what he/she perceives are individual characteristics; the presentation will accentuate the benefits of the intervention to patients who are unduly chagrined, and will be more somber for those who may have unrealistic expectations from treatment.

Mechanisms of a Health Care Decision

The components of a health care decision are illustrated in Figure 7.1. The expected benefits of treatment are determined by the risk that the cancer and cancer treatment represents for the survival and the quality of life of the patient, with the whole process modulated by the patient's personal desires. Some practical examples may help highlight the influence of age on this process.

Let's take the case of a 90-year-old woman, in average condition, whose life expectancy without cancer may be estimated at around three and a half years. If this person develops stage 2B breast cancer, with three positive axillary lymph nodes, most oncologists would be hard-pressed to offer adjuvant chemotherapy to her. Even assuming that the benefits of adjuvant chemotherapy are the same as they are for a younger woman, they would consist at most in a 15% reduction in her risk of dying of breast cancer, which in her case is less than 10%. The highest expected benefit would be a 1.5% absolute reduction in the risk of cancer death that is easily denied by the complications of anthracycline-containing chemotherapy in this patient. If the same woman develops stage III or IV large-cell non-Hodgkin's lymphoma, on the other hand, the majority of oncologists would offer her some form of treatment, because the lymphoma is potentially curable, may shorten her 2 to 3 years to life-expectancy, and may cause serious discomfort prior to death. The risks of the complications of chemotherapy, in this case, though increased, appear more desirable than the consequences of the untreated neoplasm.

Age may affect both components of the health care decision. The biology of some neoplasms may change with age, as described in Table 7.1 (Balducci & Extermann, 2001). The study of the table reveals

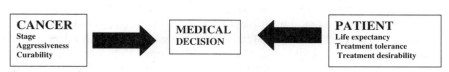

CANCER		MEDICAL		PATIENT
Stage		DECISION		Life expectancy
Aggressiveness	⟹		⟸	Treatment tolerance
Curability				Treatment desirability

FIGURE 7.1 Components of a Medical Decision.

TABLE 7.1 Aging and Clinical Behavior of Cancer

Neoplasm	Change in Prognosis	Mechanism(s)
Acute myelogenous leukemia (AML)	Worse	Higher prevalence of disease with MDR Higher prevalence of stem-cell leukemia
Non-Hodgkin's lymphoma	Worse	Increased concentration of Interleukin-6 (Il-6) in the circulation
Breast cancer	Better	Higher prevalence of hormone-receptor rich tumors Higher prevalence of well differentiated tumors Higher prevalence of slowly proliferating tumors Decreased neonangiogenesis Immune-senescence
Celomic carcinoma of the ovary	Worse	Unknown
Non–small cell lung cancer	Possibly better	Unknown

that the change in prognosis may result from two mechanisms: development of tumors that are intrinsically different from those of younger individuals, and different modulation of the tumor growth by the aging tumor host. The clinical information related to tumor stage and grade, and some specific assay of tumor cells, including the expression or lack of expression of certain genes, allow establishment with some certainty the prognosis of different tumors. For example, the expression of the Multi Drug Resistance 1 (MDR-1) gene, or of the CD 34 antigen, determine the prognosis in acute myelogenous leukemia, whereas the concentration of hormone receptors, the degree of tumor differentiation, and the over-expression of HER2/neu indicate the prognosis of breast cancer. The information related to the influence of the tumor host is much more limited. Aging is associated with a decline in the production of sexual hormones, which may delay the growth of hormone-dependent neoplasms, including prostate and breast cancer, with a reduced secretion of growth hormone and insulin-like growth factor 1, which may have a general delaying effect on the growth of most neoplasms (Martin et al., 1999). It is also associated with increased concentration of catabolic cytokines, including interleukin-6 and tumor necrosis factor (Hamerman et al., 1999), which may have different effects on different tumors. For example, interleukin 6 stimulates the growth of lymphoid neoplasms (Preti et al., 1997), but may inhibit that of solid tumors. In any case, the influence of the tumor host on the cancer prognosis cannot be assessed clinically at present. Another important observation from Table 7.1 concerns the fact that the prognosis of some neoplasms may worsen and that of others may get better with aging. Thus, the common impression that the prognosis of most tumors improves with aging is not substantiated by facts and should be corrected when expressed. This impression may prevent older individuals from receiving life-saving treatment.

Life expectancy is a function of patient age and comorbidity and can be calculated from the DEALE formula: Life expectancy = Age-related life expectancy— $(1/h1 + 1/h2 + \ldots 1/hn)$, where h1, h2, etc. represent the specific mortality for each comorbid condition (Welch et al., 1996). The age-specific life expectancy may be obtained from life tables (Table 1.1) (Overcash & Balducci, 2002). The DEALE formula represents a useful attempt to assess life expectancy, but has several limitations including:

- It may underestimate the life expectancy of healthy individuals, because the life tables represent the average life expectancy of the whole population cohort, including subjects with life-threatening diseases.
- It does not account for other conditions that may independently influence life expectancy, including function, cognitive impairment, and depression. A number of studies have shown that the 2-year mortality is doubled by dependence in IADLs, and tripled by dependence in ADLs (Ruben et al., 1992), and that it is affected by dementia (Bruce et al., 1995) and depression, even subclinical depression (Lyness et al., 1997; Lyness et al, 1999).

The tolerance of treatment may also be estimated from a geriatric assessment. Monfardini et al. (1996) reported increased risk of neutropenic infections in patients aged 70 and older who are dependent in IADLs. Furthermore, the geriatric assessment allows a staging system of aging (Table 7.2) (Hamerman, 1999). The recognition of frailty allows identification of a patient population with negligible functional reserve. For these patients, aggressive forms of cancer treatment, such as standard adjuvant therapy of breast cancer or CHOP for large cell

TABLE 7.2 Stages of Aging (modified from Hamerman, 1999)

Stage	Characteristics
Primary	No rehabilitative needs
	Functionally independent
	Minimal comorbidity
Intermediate	May be rehabilitated to full indepen-dence
	Dependent in one or more IADLs
	Comorbidity may affect functional status
Secondary or frailty	No rehabilitation
	Main goal to avoid further deterioration
	Classical criteria:
	ADL dependence
	Three or more comorbid conditions
	One or more geriatric syndrome
	Fried's criteria (at least three of the following):
	Involuntary loss of $\geq$ 10% of original body weight in one year
	Lack of energy
	Decreased grip strength
	Slow movements
	Difficulty in beginning movements
Near death	

lymphoma, are generally contraindicated. Of the two sets of criteria used to define frailty, those proposed by Fried et al. (2001) are preferable because they are more comprehensive. The more standard time-honored criteria are helpful as well (Balducci & Stanta, 2000), as they are easier to recognize in the clinical setting. If one of the standard criteria is present, the more thorough investigation of frailty with the Fried's criteria is not necessary. Frailty is discussed at length in Chapter 5, "Obtaining a Comprehensive Geriatric Assessment."

CONCLUSIONS

The main goal of health care decisions in all patients is to try to maximize the benefits and minimize the risk of interventions. In the older cancer patient the application of this principle requires special attention in the following areas:

- Assessment of benefits, which involves enhancing the comprehension of the proposed intervention with a verbal and nonverbal language that is at the same time clear to understand and respectful of the personal dignity of the patient, attention to cultural competence, and early involvement of the patient's caregiver. A value history may be extremely useful to interpret the intervention in terms of patient's desire;
- Changing biology of cancer that may involve in some cases a more indolent disease and a more aggressive one in others;
- Assessment of life expectancy, based on age, comorbidity, and functional status; of treatment tolerance, based on a staging system of aging; and of patient's desires, based on value history.

At the crossroad where medical and personal needs meet, the nurse is in a unique position to facilitate medical decisions in the older person with cancer. In addition to the assessment of the older person, the responsibility of the nurse includes the statement of the patient's aspirations and expectations emerging from the living word of the patient's daily life. The words can be expressed as much in silence, in gestures, in facial expressions, and in spontaneous reactions to pain and joy, as they are verbalized in a rational discourse.

Opportunities for nursing research include:

- Definition of cultural competence of patients from different ethnic and social background;
- Fine-tuning of the proposed staging system of aging, with special attention to the intermediate stage (see Figure 7.2), the most common in the older cancer patient;
- Application of qualitative research to the interpretation of patient's expectations from cancer and its treatment.

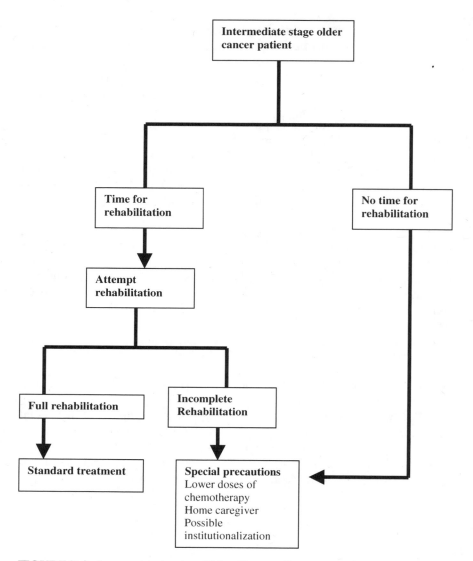

FIGURE 7.2 Approach to the Older Cancer Patient in the Intermediate Stage.

REFERENCES

Balducci, L., & Beghe', C. (2001). Cancer and age in the USA. *Critical Reviews in Hematology and Oncology, 37,* 137–145.

Balducci, L., & Extermann, M. (2001). A practical approach to the older patient with cancer. *Current Problems in Cancer, 25*(1), 6–76.

Balducci, L., Silliman, R. A., & Diaz, N. (2002). Breast Cancer: an oncological perspective. In L. Balducci, G. H. Lyman, & W. B. Ershler (Eds.), *Comprehensive geriatric oncology.* Second edition. London: Harwood Academic Publishers.

Balducci, L., & Stanta, G. (2000). Cancer in the frail patient: a coming epidemic. *Hematology Oncology Clinics of North America, 14,* 235–250.

Bruce, M. L., Hoff, R. A., Jacobs, S. C., & Leaf, P. J. (1995). The effect of cognitive impairment on 9–year mortality in a community sample. *Journal of Gerontology, 50B,* 289–296.

Fox, S. A., Roetzheim, R. G., & Kington, R. S. (1997). Barriers to cancer prevention in the older person. *Clinics of Geriatric Medicine, 13,* 79–96.

Fried, L.P., Tangen, C. M., Walston, J., Newman, A. B., Hirsch, C., Gottdiener, J., Seeman, T., Tracy, R., Kop, W. J., Burke, G., & McBurnie, M. A. (2001). Frailty in older adults: evidence for a phenotype. *Journal of Gerontology, 56*(3), M146–56.

George, M. (2001). The challenge of culturally competent health care: application of asthma. *Heart Lung, 30,* 3392–3400.

Gill, T. M., Desai, M. M., Gahbauer, E. A., Holford, T. R., & Williams, C. S. (2001). Restricted activity among community-living older persons: incidence, precipitants, and health care utilization. *Annals of Internal Medicine, 135,* 313–321.

Goldhirsch, A., Glick, J. H., Gelber, R. D. , Coats, A. S., & Senn, H. J. (2001). Meeting Highlights: International Consensus Panel on the Treatment of Primary Breast Cancer, *Journal of Clinical Oncology, 19,* 3817–3827.

Haley, W. E., Ehrbar, L., & Schonwetter, R. S. (1998). Family caregiving issues. In L. Balducci, G. H. Lyman & W. B. Ershler, (Eds.), *Comprehensive geriatric oncology* (pp. 805–812). London: Harwood Academic Publishers.

Hamerman, D. (1999). Toward an understanding of frailty. *Annals of Internal Medicine, 130,* 945–950.

Hamerman, D., Berman, J. W., Albers, G. W., Brown, D. L., & Silver, D. (1999). Emerging evidence for inflammation in conditions frequently affecting older adults: report of a symposium. *Journal of the American Geriatrics Society, 47,* 995–999.

Levinsky, N. G., Yu, W., Ash, A., Moskowitz, M., Gazelle, G., Saynina, O., & Emanuel, E. J. (2001). Influence of age on Medicare expenditures and medical care in the end of life. *Journal of the American Medical Association, 286,* 1349–1355.

Lyness, J. M., King, D. A., Cox, C., Yoediono, Z., & Caine, E. D. (1999). The importance of subsyndromal depression in older primary care patients.

Prevalence and associated functional disability. *Journal of the American Geriatrics Society, 47*, 647–652.

Lyness, J. M., Noel, T. K., Cox, C., King, D. A., Conwell, Y., & Caine, E. D. (1997). Screening for depression in elderly primary care patients: a comparison of the center for Epidemiologic Studies Depression Scale and the Geriatric Depression Scale. *Archives of Internal Medicine, 157*, 449–454.

Martin, F. (1999). Frailty and the somatopause. *Growth Hormone IGF Research, 9*, 3–10.

Monfardini, S., Ferrucci, L., Fratino, L., del Lungo, I., Serraino, D., & Zagonel, V. (1996). Validation of a multidimensional evaluation scale for use in elderly cancer patients. *Cancer, 77*, 395–401.

Overcash, J. & Balducci, L., (2003). Epidemiology of cancer and aging. In J. Overcash, L. Balducci (Eds.), *The older cancer patient.* New York: Springer Publishing.

Preti, H. J., Cabanillas, F., & Talpaz, M. (1997). Prognostic value of serum interleukin-6 in diffuse large cell lymphoma. *Annals of Internal Medicine, 127*, 186–194.

Reuben, D. B., Rubenstein, L. V., Hirsch, S. H., & Hays, R. D. (1992). Value of functional status as predictor of mortality. *American Journal of Medicine, 93*, 663–669.

Rockwood, K., Stadnyk, K., Macknight, C., McDowell, I., Hurbert, R., & Hogan, D. B. (1999). A brief instrument to classify frailty in elderly people. *Lancet, 353*, 205–206.

Sheppard, F. (2002). Lung cancer in the older patient. In L. Balducci, G. H. Lyman, W. H. Ershler (Eds.), *Comprehensive geriatric oncology.* London: Harwood Academic Publishers.

Welch, H. G., Albertssen, P., Nease, R. F., Bubolz, T. A., & Wasson, J. H. (1996). Estimating treatment benefits for the elderly: effects of competing risks. *Annals of Internal Medicine, 126*, 572–584.

CHAPTER EIGHT

Radiation Therapy of Older Persons

Linda Casey, Babu Zachariah, and Lodovico Balducci

R adiation therapy is a major treatment modality for cancer today. Approximately 60% of cancer patients will receive radiation therapy at some time during the course of their disease. Likewise, 60% of all malignant tumors occur in individuals aged 65 years or older. Radiotherapy can be an alternative to surgery or systemic chemotherapy for the older individual, particularly the more frail cancer patient. It is widely used both curatively and palliatively. However, there is limited information regarding the effectiveness, tolerance, and management of older persons treated with radiation.

Currently, older patients with cancer are evaluated and treated less aggressively than younger individuals (Farniok & Levitt, 1994). Older patients are less likely to receive combined-modality therapy (Mizushima, Noto, Cerwenks et al., 1988). Many older patients are not treated or are undertreated due to a fear of treatment related toxicities (Chin, Fisher, Smee et al., 1995; Farniok & Levitt, 1994; Greenburg & Trotti, 1992; Mizushima, Noto, Cerwenks et al., 1988; Scalliet, 1991). Approximately two thirds of younger patients are treated with multimodality therapy whereas only one third of patients aged 75 or older receive combined modality treatment (Chu, Diehr, & Feigl, 1987). As a result, radiotherapy in the older patient is worthy of further exploration and study.

RADIOBIOLOGY IN THE ELDERLY

Sensitivity of tumor cells to radiation therapy depends on a number of factors including tumor proliferation, oxygenation, and repopulation.

131

Tumor cell proliferation has been measured and found to be decreased in several tumors in older patients compared with their younger counterparts. This suggests that the sensitivity of tumors to radiation may decrease as one ages (Balzi, Becciolini, Mauri et al., 1992; Balzi, Becciolini, Zamieri et al., 1993; Balzi, Mauri, Boanini et al., 1993; Becciolini, Balzi, Boanini et al., 1993). Age-related decrease in circulation could cause tissue hypoxia also resulting in decreased tumor sensitivity. As age advances, the functional reserve of many organs declines, causing increased toxicity from treatment. A reduction in stem cell reserve in the bone marrow and in the mucosa and the associated reduced rate of cell repopulation lead to increased damage to normal tissue during radiotherapy.

RADIOTHERAPY IN THE OLDER PATIENT

Older patients with cancer should be evaluated thoroughly, with particular attention to comorbid conditions and performance status. Following proper staging, curative or palliative therapy may be offered. Special attention should be given to the quality of life and emotional needs of the older patient as treatment decisions are made. Multimodality therapy should not be withheld on the basis of age alone (Baumann, 1998; Zachariah & Balducci, 1997; Zachariah, Casey, & Balducci, 1995). However, it is important to note that mortality from radiation therapy is rare.

There are advantages and disadvantages to radiotherapy in the elderly. Advantages include organ preservation and maintenance of functional ability at as high a level as possible. Disadvantages of radiotherapy for the elderly include the long duration of treatment. Curative therapy averages 6–7 weeks and palliative treatment is 2–4 weeks. Treatment decisions include consideration of these advantages and disadvantages.

TOLERANCE OF RADIOTHERAPY BY OLDER PERSONS

Fear that advanced age may be associated with decreased tolerance of treatment is one of the obvious reasons for treating elderly and younger patients differently. The progressive reduction of functional reserve that occurs with age may enhance radiation damage of normal tissues and increase the risk of therapeutic complications. Another reason for undertreatment of older patients is the belief that tumors are more indolent in the elderly than in younger patients and have a lesser effect on life expectancy. Analyses of tumor stage distribution by age (Yancik & Ries, 1994) and of survival rates of older patients who received less aggressive therapy do not support this contention (Goodwin, Samet & Hunt, 1996). On the contrary, inadequate radiation doses may compromise the chances of cure in older patients.

One question regarding tolerance of the elderly to radiation is whether age affects the sensitivity of normal tissues to radiation and leads to increased radiation reactions. A depletion of stem cells in normal tissue as it ages may impair the ability of normal tissue to recover from radiation injury. Thus far, there is limited data addressing this issue. Animal studies (Johnson, Parkinson, Wolpert et al., 1987; Little, Nove, Strong et al., 1988; Rhudat, Dietz, Conradt et al., 1997) do not show an increase in radiosensitivity with increasing age. Several clinical studies have also shown no increase in radiation toxicity of normal tissues with advancing age. Breast cancer patients over the age of 60 years who have undergone radiotherapy showed no increased incidence of telangiectasia, subcutaneous fibrosis, arm edema, or lung fibrosis (Bentzen & Overgaard, 1993; Bentzen, Skocylas, Overgaard et al., 1996). In addition, there was no excess of other early or late skin reactions noted (Turesson, Nyman, Holmberg et al., 1996).

Several studies have examined the effect of age on acute and late reactions during and after radiotherapy. Pignon et al. (1998) reviewed 1208 patients from five different European Organization for Research and Treatment of Cancer (EORTC) studies who received chest radiation as monotherapy or in combination with surgery or chemotherapy. They compared both acute radiation reactions (esophagitis, dyspnea, weakness, weight loss, nausea and vomiting, and change in performance status) and late side effects (dysphagia, esophagitis, weakness, radiologically detected changes, spinal cord damage, and heart damage). Subjects were grouped into six age categories ranging from less than 50 years to more than 70 years old. Acute normal tissue reactions in the categories listed were not higher in the older patients than in the younger patients. However, a trend toward higher weight loss in the older patients was noted. The mean time for development of late complications, 13 months, was similar in all age groups. Forty percent of patients were free of late complications at 4 years, with no significant difference among age groups. Initially, it appeared that older patients developed more serious esophagitis; however, when adjustments were made for radiation doses, treatment fields, treatment duration, and combination chemotherapy, the difference disappeared. The same investigators reported on patients treated for head and neck and pelvic malignancies according to several EORTC protocols (Pignon, Horist, Bolla et al., 1997; Rudat et al., 1997). The results were very similar, however, older patients did not tolerate mucositis as well as younger patients. Locoregional tumor control and survival rates were also similar. Some complications of radiation to the pelvis, such as nausea, decline in performance status, and skin reactions were greater in younger patients (Pignon et al., 1997). Sexual dysfunction was more common in older patients following pelvic irradiation.

These studies had several strengths that include the collection of data prospectively with no dose adjustment for age. The patients in the studies had good performance status with little functional impairment. Other investigators have reported similar results in older patients receiving radiation therapy (Huguenin, Glanzmann, Hammer et al., 1992; Sengelov, Klintorp, Havsteen et al., 1997).

The available data on the sensitivity of normal tissues to radiation therapy in elderly patients strongly suggest that older patients with good functional status tolerate treatment as well as younger patients (August, Rea, & Sondak, 1994). Tumor response and survival rates are comparable with those of younger patients. Therefore, aggressive radiation should not be withheld from older persons based on chronological age alone.

FACTORS INFLUENCING TOLERANCE OF RADIATION BY THE ELDERLY

Functional status remains one of the most important tools in predicting the tolerance of individuals to radiotherapy. This is especially true in the elderly population.

Performance status can also be the major determining factor in recommending radiation as primary treatment (Brady & Markoe, 1986). Often comorbid factors such as cardiac or pulmonary status preclude the use of surgery and/or chemotherapy in the elderly but may not significantly affect their ability to tolerate radiation.

There are several questions to be asked when radiation therapy is being considered in the older patient (Brady & Markoe, 1986). These include:

- Can the patient's tumor be cured or palliated?
- Does the patient's age significantly influence the potential for treatment?
- Do the performance status and the degree of debility and/or fragility of the patient influence the potential for successful completion of the radiation treatment program?

- Is the tumor site as well as the stage of disease at presentation amenable to definitive or palliative therapy?
- Are there other associated medical problems such as diabetes, hypertension, kidney disease, anemia, infections etc. that would limit tolerance to radiotherapy?
- What are the potential reactions to radiation therapy in this individual?
- Does the life expectancy of the patient justify aggressive therapy?
- Are there innovative radiation therapy techniques that may improve the patient's tolerance of treatment?

Clearly, aggressive radiotherapy should not be withheld based on chronological age, but there are a number of other factors which enter into a decision to treat older persons with radiation.

PREPARING THE ELDERLY FOR RADIATION THERAPY

There are several ways to prepare the elderly to undergo radiotherapy as well as professionals to care for individuals under treatment (Sengelov et al., 1997). Professionals should possess a knowledge of the major cancers and the role of radiation in the treatment of those cancers. In addition, knowledge of the sequelae of treatment and any age-associated factors that may exacerbate treatment reactions is essential. Nurses caring for the elderly patient receiving radiation must help the patient and caregiver anticipate the side effects of treatment and manage the sequelae of therapy.

For elderly patients even a short course of external beam radiation may seem long as transportation daily to the treatment center consumes personal resources. Therefore, the elderly should be encouraged not only to express their feelings but also to report symptoms.

In addition, patient education may need to be adjusted for the elderly undergoing radiotherapy. Instructions should be written as well as verbal and may need to be repeated, particularly for patients with memory loss. Enlisting the assistance of caregivers in the educational process can provide additional reinforcement of information. Those caring for the elderly undergoing radiation, both professional and caregivers, must help the patient anticipate side effects of treatment and manage those side effects. The patient who knows what to expect is better able to tolerate therapy and to maintain optimal quality of life during treatment (Strohl, 1992).

SUPPORT OF THE ELDERLY DURING TREATMENT

According to Brady and Markoe (1986), there are multiple mechanisms available to diminish the reaction of the elderly to radiation
treatment. These include:

- Precise and careful treatment planning and dosimetry.
- Alterations in fractionation (although research supports this is
  only necessary in selected cases).
- Careful and diligent medical and nursing support of the patient and
  caregiver during the course of the radiation therapy program.
- Emphasis on nutritional support.
- Consideration of anemia and the use of products to alleviate anemia.
- Appropriate pain management.
- Management of infections.
- Management of side effects of treatment as well as adverse ef-
  fects (i.e., mucositis, weight loss, diarrhea, cystitis, esophagitis,
  dysphagia).
- Active emphasis on ongoing continuing rehabilitation, which may
  include physical exercise within the patient's capabilities.

RESULTS OF RADIATION TREATMENT OF CANCER IN OLDER PERSONS

Cancer is a significant entity in the geriatric population. It is estimated
that 60% of all malignant tumors occur in individuals 65 years of age
or older (Zacariah & Balducci, 2000). There are a number of cancers
occurring primarily in the older patient that are potential candidates
for management with radiation. These include carcinomas of the lung,
prostate, breast, colon, and rectum, and gynecologic cancers. A brief
review of results of treatment of the elderly for these malignancies
provides an overview for planning and care.

LUNG CANCER

Older persons with lung cancer are often referred for radiation therapy because the surgical mortality is significantly higher in the geriatric population (Mizushima et al., 1997). Very few older patients receive
a radical course of therapy. Patients with early stage lung cancer (T1
or T2) referred for curative therapy are often medically inoperable
because of comorbid conditions including poor cardiac or pulmonary
conditions. Noordijik et al. (1988) reported the results of radiotherapy

in a group of 50 older patients who had peripheral T1 or T2 lung lesions. All received a full course of treatment, a total of 60Gy in 6 weeks to the primary site. Complete response was achieved in 50% of patients with tumors less than 4 cm in size. Overall survival was 56% at 2 years and 16% at 5 years. These results were comparable to older patients treated surgically at the same institution. There were no serious acute or late side effects of the radiation. Radiation fibrosis was evident on chest x-ray, but was not symptomatic. The conclusion was that radiation therapy is a reasonable alternative to surgery for patients older than 70 years who had respectable lung cancer of 4 cm or less.

In some studies performance status was measured in addition to acute and late effects of radiation. Coy et al. (1980) reported that individuals with a Karnofsky performance scale (KPS) greater than 70 had similar morbidity from radiation to that of younger patients. The most common acute reaction was dysphagia. Kusumoto et al. (1986) showed that patients over 70 years with good performance status have survival rates similar to those in younger patients when radiated with or without chemotherapy.

Studies have shown that lung cancer patients with medically inoperable disease can also tolerate radiation definitive radiotherapy even in cases with significant comorbid conditions (Furuta, Hayakawa, Saito et al., 1996). However, older patients with small cell carcinoma of the lung and those with comorbid conditions are not usually considered for standard combination chemotherapy. In this subset of patients, intensive treatment is associated with substantially increased toxicity without significant survival advantages (Findlay, Griffin, Raghavan et al., 1991). A retrospective analysis of older patients who received chemotherapy with or without radiotherapy at the Ottawa Regional Cancer Center had a response and survival rate similar to those of younger patients (Gross, Logan, Maroun et al., 1992).

Those caring for older patients receiving radiation therapy for lung cancer need to be particularly attuned to their nutritional status. Dysphagia, which accompanies thoracic radiotherapy, can quickly deplete body reserves. The older patient is at greater risk of dehydration and should be assessed frequently during treatment. The resultant nutritional deficits and effect on performance status can also decrease the quality of life.

PROSTATE CANCER

Prostate cancer is primarily a disease of older men. By age 90 it is estimated that 90% of men will have prostate cancer. Several investigators have shown that most elderly patients can be treated without causing significant complications. Patterns of care studies by Hanks et al. (1994) show similar treatment outcomes in patients younger and older than 70 years who received a full course of radiotherapy for prostate cancer. No differences in serious late complications were noted between the older and younger groups. Forman, Order, Szinreich et al., 1986 and Zachariah, Balducci, Patel et al., 1998 both reported similar results when treating the elderly with radiation therapy. They demonstrated that the absence of severe complications and the incidence of moderate complications was similar to that of younger patients. A decrease in acute and late radiation reactions is obtained using three-dimensional conformal radiotherapy as compared to conventional external beam treatment, despite an 8% increase in dose of radiation.

Should the elderly experience more severe radiation enteritis, they are at risk of developing dehydration more quickly than others with more reserve. A thorough assessment at regular intervals to evaluate the severity of diarrhea is essential. In addition, patient/caregiver education regarding nutrition, dietary changes, and fluid intake can decrease the severity of enteritis.

BREAST CANCER

Breast cancer is an age related disease for women just as prostate cancer is for men. As the population ages, more cases of breast cancer will be detected in the coming years.

The standard local treatment for stage I and stage II breast cancer in older women includes modified radical mastectomy or lumpectomy plus radiotherapy. The choice of therapy depends on the health status of the individual, her preference for breast preservation, and her willingness to undergo 5–6 weeks of radiation daily. Older women are less likely than younger women to have breast-conserving surgery (Lazovitch, White, Thomas et al., 1991).

The number of patients receiving radiation after breast-conserving surgery decreases markedly with age, regardless of comorbid conditions or stage of disease (Ballard-Barbash, Potosky, Harlan et al., 1996; Bergman, Dekker, Vanderhoff et al., 1991). Women over 75 years of age are less likely to receive adjuvant radiotherapy after mastectomy. More often, this group is treated with endocrine therapy (Bergman, Dekker, Vanderhoff et al., 1991). Wide local excision and other forms of conservative surgical techniques have been used for older breast cancer patients in an attempt to improve cosmesis and decrease operative morbidity and mortality. However, treatment with breast-conserving surgery alone is associated with a significant rate of local failure (Crile, Esselstyn, Herman et al., 1973; Taggert, 1978). Multiple studies have shown that postoperative radiotherapy is well tolerated by older women and advancing age is not a contraindication for radiation following surgery.

Radiation therapy also has a major role in palliation of advanced breast cancer. However, radiation is often underutilized in older patients. Fetting et al. (1997) reported that 57% of women under 65 with metastatic breast cancer received radiation. This compares to only 46% of patients aged 65 to 74 and 29% of patients aged 75 and older. Symptoms related to metastatic breast cancer involving the brain, bone, and soft tissues can be treated palliatively with a short course of radiation in older women and those who are frail.

COLORECTAL CANCER

Radiation therapy has a major role in the treatment of patients with colorectal cancer. However, there is a lack of information regarding the tolerance of older patients to radiation and tumor response at this site. The survival rate of patients with colon cancer seems to decrease with increasing age (Chapius, Dent, Fischer et al., 1985). This could be due to less aggressive therapy in the older population (Mor, Masterson-Allen, Goldberg et al., 1985).

Older patients are at a higher risk for radiation enteritis because of preexisting conditions such as hypertension, vascular disease, diabetes, and prior abdominal surgery. However, in clinical trials, no difference in side effects from radiation was noted between younger and older patients (Farniok & Levitt, 1994). Adjustments in the volume of bowel radiated, positioning patients prone during treatment, treating with a full bladder, and using multiple fields reduced the acute effects of treatment by as much as 5%.

BRACHYTHERAPY IN THE ELDERLY

Brachytherapy (interstitial or intracavitary radioactive seed implantation) is used to treat cancer of the head and neck, breast, and genitourinary tract. There is little information regarding the tolerance and outcome of brachytherapy in the over-65 population. The data that is available indicates that older patients tolerate brachytherapy as well as younger patients; however, more age specific studies are needed in this area.

RADIATION THERAPY IN THE OLDEST OLD

Among the population over 80 years of age, radiation is the most widely used treatment modality for cancer. Patients may be denied aggressive (curative) therapy because of concerns of treatment related toxicities. Patients over 80 are usually excluded from prospective clinical trials even when they are in good general health and have a good performance status.

In recent years, investigators have reported the tolerance to and outcome of radiation in patients over 80 years of age. Zachariah, Casey and Balducci (1995) examined 203 patients over 80 years of age treated for a variety of malignancies. Ninety four percent of patients completed the planned treatment course. Side effects were comparable to those observed in younger patients. It was apparent in this study that nutritional support before and during radiation therapy and maintenance of body weight seemed to improve compliance with therapy.

SUMMARY

Radiotherapy has a major role in the multidisciplinary approach to cancer therapy. It is widely used for curative and palliative treatment of cancer. Radiotherapy is of particular benefit to older and frail cancer patients as an alternative to surgery and to systemic therapy. The available data on the sensitivity of normal tissues to radiotherapy in elderly patients strongly suggest that older patients with good performance status tolerate radiotherapy as well as younger patients and have comparable tumor response and survival rates. Aggressive radiotherapy should not be withheld from older patients because of chronological age alone.

The nurse caring for the elderly patient receiving radiation may need to monitor the patient more frequently and adjust teaching strategies for patient education. The patient who knows what to expect and is assisted through treatment is better able to tolerate therapy and to maintain optimal quality of life during treatment.

REFERENCES

August, D. A., Rea, T., & Sondak, V. K. (1994). Age related difference in breast cancer treatment. *Annals of Surgical Oncology, 1:* 45.

Ballard-Barbash, R., Potosky, A. L., Harlan, L. C., et al. (1996). Factors associated with surgical and radiation therapy for early stage breast cancer in older women. *Journal of the National Cancer Institute, 88:* 716.

Balzi, M., Becciolini, A., Mauri, P., et al. (1992). The prognostic role of thymidine labeling index in larynx carcinoma. *Cell Proliferation, 25:* 512.

Balzi, M., Becciolini, A., Zamieri, E., et al. (1993). TLI in superficial cancer of the bladder. Prognostic Evaluation. *Cell Proliferation, 26:* 464.

Balzi, M., Mauri, P., Boanini, P. et al. (1993). Multivariate analysis of prognostic value of 3H-thymidine labeling index (TLI) in laryngeal carcinoma. *International Journal of Biological Markers, 8*:42–43.

Baumann, M. (1998). Is curative radiation therapy in elderly patients limited by increased normal tissue toxicity? *Radiotherapy and Oncology, 46*:225–227.

Becciolini, A., Balzi, M., Boanini, P., et al. (1993). Cell kinetics in breast cancer. *In Vivo 7*:627–630.

Bentzen, S. M., Overgaard, M. (1993). Early and late normal tissue injury after post-mastectomy radiotherapy. In W. Hinkelbein, G. Bruggmoser, H. Frommhold et al (Eds), Acute and long term side effects of radiotherapy. *Recent Results in Cancer Research, 130*:59.

Bentzen, S. M., Skocylas, J. Z., Overgaard, M., et al. (1996). Radiotherapy-related lung fibrosis enhanced by tamoxifen. *Journal of the National Cancer Institute 88*:918–922.

Bergman, L., Dekker, G., Vankerhof, E. H. M. et al. (1991). Influence of age and co-morbidity on treatment choice and survival in elderly patients with breast cancer. *Breast Cancer Research and Treatment, 18*:189.

Brady, L., Markoe, A. (1986). Radiation therapy in the elderly. *Frontiers of Radiation Therapy and Oncology, 20*:80.

Chapius, P. H., Dent, O. F., Fischer, R. et al. (1985). A multivariate analysis of clinical and pathological variables in prognosis after resection of large bowel cancer. *The British Journal of Surgery, 72*:698.

Chin, R., Fisher, R. J., Smee, R. I. et al. (1995). Oropharyngeal cancer in the elderly. *International Journal of Radiation Oncology, Biology, Physics, 32*:1007.

Chu, J., Diehr, P., Feigl, P. (1987). The effect of age on the care of women with breast cancer in community hospitals. *Journal of Gerontology 42*:185.

Coy, P. & Kennelly, G. M. (1980). The role of curative radiotherapy in the treatment of lung cancer. *Cancer 45*:698.

Crile, G., Esselstyn, C. B., Herman, R. E. et al. (1973). Partial mastectomy for carcinoma of breast. *Obstetrical & Gynecological Surgery, 136*:929.

Farniok, K. E., Levitt, S. H. (1994). The role of radiation therapy in the treatment of colorectal cancer: Implications for the older patient. *Cancer, 74*:2154.

Fetting, J. H., Comstock, G. W., Shanon Eby, P. H. et al. (1997) The effect of aging on the utilization of chemotherapy for metastatic breast cancer. A population based study. *Cancer Investigation, 15*:199.

Findlay, M.P., Griffin, A. M., Raghavan, D. et al. (1991). Retrospective review of chemotherapy for small cell lung cancer in the elderly: Does the end justify the means? *European Journal of Cancer, 27*:1597.

Forman, J. D., Order, S. E., Szinreich, E. S. et al. (1986). Carcinoma of the prostate in the elderly: The therapeutic ratio of definitive radiotherapy. *Journal of Urology, 136*:1238.

Furuta, M., Hayakawa, K., Saito, K. S. et al. (1996). Radiation therapy for stage

I-II non small cell lung cancer in patients aged 75 years and older. *Japanese Journal of Clinical Oncology, 26*(2): 95–98.

Goodwin, J. S., Samet, J. M. & Hunt, W. C. (1996). Determinants of survival in older cancer patient. *Journal of the National Cancer Institute, 88*:1031.

Greenberg, H. M., Trotti, A. M. (1992). Radiotherapy of cancer in the older person. In L. Balducci, G. H. Lyman, & W. B. Ershler (Eds.), *Geriatric oncology* (p. 160). Philadelphia: JB Lippincott, 1992.

Gross, G. D., Logan, D., Maroun, J. et al. (1990). Chemotherapy in elderly patients with small cell lung cancer (abstract 969). *Proceedings of the American Society of Clinical Oncology 11*:25. Hanks, G. E., Hanlon, A., Owen, J. B. et al. (1994). Patterns of radiation treatment of elderly patients with prostate cancer. *Cancer, 74*:2174.

Huguenin, P. U., Glanzmann, C., Hammer, F. et al. (1992). Endometrial carcinoma in patients aged 75 years or older: Outcome and complications after post-operative radiotherapy or radiotherapy alone. *Strohleather und Onkologe, 168*:567.

Johnson, D. W., Parkinson, D., Wolpert, S. M. et al. (1987). Intracarotideal chemotherapy with 1–3 bis 2–chloroethyl, nitrosourea (BCNU) in 5% dextrose in water in the treatment of malignant blioma. *Neurosurgery, 20*:577.

Kusumoto, S., Koga, K., Tsukino, H. et al. (1986). Comparison of survival of patients with lung cancer between elderly (greater than or equal to 70) and younger (than 70) age group. *Japanese Journal of Clinical Oncology, 16*:319–323.

Lazovich, D., White, E., Thomas, D. et al. (1991). Under-utiliztion of breast conserving surgery and radiation therapy among women with stage I or II breast cancer. *Journal of the American Medical Association, 266*(4): 3433–8.

Little, J. B., Nove, J., Strong, L. C. et al. (1988). Survival of human skin fibroblasts from normal individuals after X-irradiation. *International Journal of Radiation Oncology, Biology, Physics, 54*:899.

Mizushima, Y., Noto, H., Cerwenks, H. et al. (1997). Survival and prognosis after pneumonectomy for lung cancer in the elderly. *Annals of Thoracic Surgery, 64*:193.

Mor, V., Masterson-Allen, S., Goldberg, R. J. et al. (1985). Relationship between age at diagnosis and treatment received by cancer patients. *Journal of the American Geriatrics Society, 33*:585.

Noordijk, E. M., Clement, E. P., Hermans, J. et al. (1988). Radiotherapy as an alternative to surgery in elderly patients with resectable lung cancer. *Radiotherapy and Oncology, 13*:83.

Pignon, T., Gregor, A., Schaake Koning, C. et al. (1998). Age has no impact on acute and late toxicity of curative radiotherapy. *Radiotherapy and Oncology, 46*:239.

Pignon, T., Horist, J. C., Bolla, M. et al. (1997). Age is not a limiting factor for radical radiotherapy in pelvic malignancies. *Radiotherapy and Oncology, 42*:107.

Rudat, J., Dietz, A., Conradt, C. et al. (1997). In-vitro radiosensitivity of primary human fibroblasts. Lack of correlation with acute radiation toxicity in patients with head and neck cancer. *Radiotherapy and Oncology, 43*:181.

Scalliet, P. (1991). Radiotherapy in the elderly. *European Journal of Cancer,* *27*:3.

Sengelov, L., Klintorp, S., Havsteen, H. et al. (1997). Treatment outcome following radiotherapy in elderly patients with bladder cancer. *Radiotherapy and Oncology, 44*:53.

Strohl, R. A. (1992). The elderly patient receiving radiation therapy: treatment sequelae and nursing care. *Geriatric Nursing 13*(3):153.

Taggert, R. E. B. (1978). Partial mastectomy for breast cancer: *British Medical Journal, 2*:1268.

Turesson, L., Nyman, J., Holmberg, E. et al. (1996). Prognostic factors for acute and late skin reactions in radiotherapy patients. *International Journal of Radiation Oncology, Biology, Physics, 36*:1065.

Yancik, R., Ries, L. A. (1994). Cancer in older persons. *Cancer, 74*:1995.

Zachariah, B., Balducci, L. (2000). Radiation therapy of the older patient. *Hematology/Oncology Clinics of North America, 14*:131.

Zacariah, B., Balducci, L., Patel, S. et al. (1998). Radiotherapy for prostate cancer in the older patients (abstract 148). *Annals of Oncology, 9*(suppl 3):84.

Zachariah, B., Balducci, L., Venkattarmanabalaji, G. V. et al. (1997). Radiotherapy for cancer patients aged 80 and older: A study of effectiveness and side effects. *International Journal of Radiation Oncology, Biology, Physics, 39*:1125.

Zachariah, B., Casey, L., Balducci, L. (1995). Radiotherapy of the oldest old cancer patients: A study of effectiveness and toxicity. *Journal of the American Geriatrics Society, 43*:793.

CHAPTER NINE

Chemotherapy in the Older Person

Julie Meyer and Lodovico Balducci

T he systemic treatment of cancer includes cytotoxic chemotherapy, hormonal therapy, biological therapy, and cancer-specific or targeted therapy, resulting from translational research.

CYTOTOXIC CHEMOTHERAPY

Cytotoxic chemotherapy is still the most commonly used form of systemic therapy. This form of therapy is not tumor specific, but is toxic to all replicating cells. Not surprisingly, the normal tissues with high cell renewal rate, such as the hemopoietic and the mucosal tissues, are the most vulnerable. In general the benefits of cytotoxic chemotherapy overwhelm the risks because neoplastic tissues have a higher growth fraction (percentage of replicating cells) than normal tissues. Then, each administration of chemotherapy will destroy a higher proportion of tumor than of normal cells. Cytotoxic chemotherapy is generally administered intermittently on the assumption that the time period between chemotherapy administrations is sufficiently long for the normal but not the neoplastic tissue, to recover.

Aging is associated with molecular and physiologic changes that may affect the pharmacology of cytotoxic chemotherapy. We will examine changes in pharmacokinetics, pharmacodynamics, and susceptibility of normal tissues (Figure 9.1). Absorption has special interest for older individuals, because oral drugs may reduce the number of visits to the clinics and may offer a more flexible schedule of administration (Balducci & Carreca, 2002). A number of oral agents, including oral alkylating agents, fluorinated pyrimidines, temozolamide, and

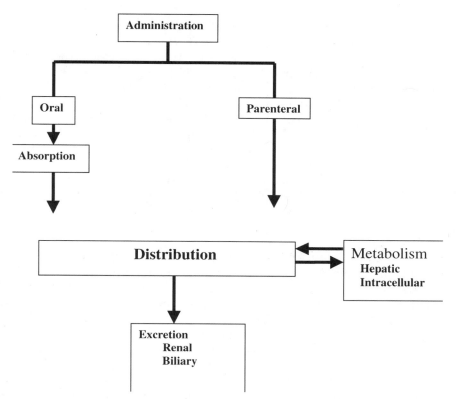

FIGURE 9.1 Overview of Pharmacokinetics.

etoposide are already available and oral derivatives of platinum, an-thracyclines, vinorelbine, taxanes, and camptothecins are undergoing clinical trials. Drug absorption may decline with age, due to reduction in the mucosal surface of the intestine and delayed gastric emptying (Gusland et al., 1997; Salzman et al., 1998). These changes do not appear to affect drug absorption up to age 80. Another problem with the administration of oral drugs is related to swallowing dysfunction which becomes more common with aging (Dejaeger, 1994).

The most consequential pharmacokinetic changes of aging are a decline in volume of distribution (Vd) for water soluble agents, and reduced glomerular filtration rate (GFR) (Vestal, 1997). The volume of distribution influences the concentration of free drug in the circula-tion and is determined by body composition, serum albumin, and red blood cell concentration (Balducci & Extermann, 2001). Aging is associated with a decline in total body water and in albumin concentration and an increased prevalence of anemia. (Balducci et al., 2001). Anemia represents an independent risk factor for the myelotoxicity of agents heavily bound to red blood cells, including anthracyclines, epipodophyllotoxins, alkaloids, and campothecins (Schjivers et al., 1999). As anemia is the only parameter of body composition that can be modified on the short range, it appears desirable to maintain hemoglobin levels ≥ 12 gm/dl in older patients during chemotherapy. Erythropoietin (Balducci et al., 2001) is preferable to red blood cell transfusions, because it ensures steadier hemoglobin levels and circumvents the risk of transfusion refractoriness, febrile reactions, and infections.

The decline in GFR (GFR) (Balducci & Extermann, 2001; Vestal, 1997) may enhance the toxicity of chemotherapy in two ways:

Reduced excretion of active drugs, such as methotrexate, bleomycin, or carboplatin. Reduced excretion of active drug metabolites, such idarubicinol from idarubicin, or daunorubicinol from daunorubicin (Table 9.1) (Doroshow et al., 1996), and of toxic metabolites such as arauridine from cytarabine in high doses (Gottlieb et al., 1987).

The consequences of GFR decline on the treatment of older persons were illustrated in a retrospective analysis of women with metastatic breast cancer of different ages (Gelman & Taylor, 1984). The toxicity of a combination of cyclophosphamide, methotrexate, and fluorouracil (CMF) was minimized, and the antineoplastic activity maintained, when the doses of methotrexate and cyclophosphamide were adjusted to the GFR in patients 65 and over.

The consequences of changes in hepatic metabolism of drugs are largely unknown. Hepatic metabolism is determined by hepatic blood flow, rate of drug extraction, hepatocyte mass, and enzymatic activity (Balducci & Extermann, 2001). Two types of drug-metabolizing reactions have been recognized. Type one reactions involve the P450 cytochrome system and may generate both active and inactive metabolites. As the activity of the P450 cytochrome system is influenced by a number of common medications, type one reactions are involved in most drug interactions. Type two reactions are conjugative reactions, which give origin to water-soluble compounds excreted through the bile or the urine. Some of the metabolites of type 2 reactions, such as the glucuronides of morphine and other opioids, may still maintain some activity; however, adverse reactions may occur when renal excretion is reduced (Shehaan & Foreman, 1997). This mechanism may account for the enhanced sensitivity of elderly individuals to opioids.

TABLE 9.1 Pharmacokinetic Parameters of Major Antineoplastic Agents

Name Parent Compound	Activity	Active Metabolite	Elimination	Dose Adjustment
A. Antimetabolites				
Methotrexate (MTX)	yes	_	Renal	yes
Fluorouracil (5FU)	—	yes	Cellular & Hepatic metabolism	no
Cytosine Arabinoside (Cytosar)	—	yes	Cellular & Hepatic metabolism	no*
Fludarabine	—	yes	Renal	yes
2–chlordeoxyadenosine (Cladribine)	—	yes	Renal	?
B. Alkylating agents Bischloroethylamines Oxazaphosphorines				
(Cyclophosphamide	—	yes	Hepatic metabolism;	yes**
Ifosfamide)			Renal	
Chlorambucil	yes	—	Hepatic metabolism; Renal	
Melphalan	yes	—	Hepatic metabolism; Renal	yes***
Aziridines Thiotepa	yes	yes	Hepatic metabolism; Renal	?
Nitrosureas	yes	yes	Hepatic metabolism	?
C. Platinum Analogues				
Cisplatin	yes	no	inactivated intracellularly and in the circulation Renal (minor)	no****
Carboplatin	yes	no	Renal	yes
D. Antibiotics Anthracyclines Daunorubicin &				
doxorubicin	yes	yes	Biliary*****	yes
Idarubicin	yes	yes	Renal	?

TABLE 9.1 *(continued)*

Name Parent Compound	Activity	Active Metabolite	Elimination	Dose Adjustment
Anthracendiones				
Mitoxantrone	yes	no	Biliary*****	yes
Mitomycins	yes******	no	Hepatic metabolism; Renal	no
E. Plant derivatives				
Epipodophyllotoxins				
Etoposide	yes	no	Mixed Hepatic and Renal Reduced CrCl	yes
Teniposide	yes	no	Mixed Hepatic and Renal	no
Vinca Alkaloids				
Vincristine				
Vinblastine	yes	no	Biliary	yes
Vinorelbine				
Taxanes				
Paclitaxel	yes	no	Hepatic metabolism	?
Docetaxel	yes	no	\Hepatic metabolism	?
F. Hydroxyurea	yes	no	Renal	?

*high doses contraindicated for Crcl<50ml/min; may also be contraindicated in patients over 60

**especially for ifosfamide

***1/2 dose for BUN>30mg/ml

****dose adjustment should be made to prevent further renal damage

*****>50% of these drugs is tissue-bound and is not accounted for in urines or stools

******spontaneously activated in hypoxic conditions and in acidic environment

The most common age-related changes in hepatic function include decline in hepatic blood flow and in hepatic mass (Balducci & Extermann, 2001) and decline in the intracellular activity of P-450 cytochrome enzymes. These changes are of consequence in the so-called frail patients, in whom the P-450 activity I is critically reduced (Vestal, 1997; Hamerman, 1999).

PHARMACODYNAMICS

Pharmacodynamics concerns the molecular effects of drugs. In normal tissues two types of age-related changes have been reported: to repair DNA damage, and to catabolize cytotoxic drugs (Balducci & Extermann, 2001; Repetto & Balducci, 2002). In neoplastic tissues, age-related changes may lead to increased resistance to chemotherapy. The best described of these changes has been increased expression of Multidrug Resistance 1 (MDR1) genel (Balducci & Corcoran, 2000) in the myeloblasts of patients aged 60 and older with acute myeloid leukemia (Leith et al., 1997). Other potential mechanisms of drug resistance include resistance to programmed cell death, (apoptosis), observed in some forms of low grade lymphomas and breast cancer (Balducci & Extermann, 2001), tumor anoxia, and decreased proliferation of tumor cells.

SUSCEPTIBILITY OF NORMAL TISSUES TO THE TOXICITY OF ANTINEOPLASTIC DRUGS

Age may influence the susceptibility of normal tissues to cytotoxic agents by at least three mechanisms:

- Decreased stem cell reserve may compromise the recovery of tissue losses . This mechanism may be responsible for the complications concerning rapidly renewing tissues, such as myelodepression or mucositis (Balducci et al., 2001; Jacobson et al., 2001).
- Decreased ability to catabolize cytotoxic drugs and to repair the cellular damage of these drugs (Rudd et al., 1995; Stein et al., 1995). This mechanism probably concerns the majority of older tissues, because the synthesis of intracellular enzymes may decline with age (Short et al., 2000).
- Critical reduction in functional tissue; so that the loss of additional tissue may lead to organ failure. This mechanism may be responsible for the increased incidence of cardiomyopathy and neurotoxicity.

The complications of cytotoxic chemotherapy that become more common in older individuals include myelodepression, mucositis, cardiotoxicity, and peripheral and central neurotoxicity (Balducci & Extermann, 2001). The issue of myelotoxicity deserves special focus, as this complication is the most common and currently the best manageable. At least six retrospective studies conducted by major cancer centers or cooperative groups failed to show higher incidence and severity of myelotoxicity in persons over 70 compared to the younger ones (Beggs & Carbone, 1983; Christmann et al., 1992; Gelman & Taylor, 1984; Giovannazzi-Bannon et al., 1994; Ibrahim et al., 2000). These studies are important as they demonstrate that age by itself is not associated with increase of risk of myelotoxicity. The generalizability of these studies is limited, because they are retrospective. Patients over 70 were underrepresented and highly selected and patients over 80 were virtually absent. A number of other studies, most of them prospective, indicate that the risk of chemotherapy-induced myelodepression increases with age. Dees et al. (2000) found that the neutrophil nadir following treatment with doxorubicin cyclophosphamide became lower with the age of the patients, and myelodepression was cumulative in those over 65 but not in younger patients. Kim et al. (2000) reported that the risk of myelotoxicity in patients with solid tumors increased with age. Perhaps the most convincing demonstration that chemotherapy—induced myelodepression is more common and severe in the aged comes from the exam of eight prospective studies of older patients with large-cell non-Hodgkin's lymphoma (LCNHL) (Table 9.2). With the exception of Armitage's, all other studies were prospective, and patients were treated with the standard combination of cyclophosphamide, hydroxydaunorubicin (doxorubicin), Oncovin, and prednisone (CHOP) or a combination of similar drug intensity. The risk of severe neutropenia was as high as 70%, the

TABLE 9.2 Incidence of Life-Threatening Neutropenia; Neutropenic Infections and Death in Older Individuals with Large Cell Non-Hodgkin's Lymphomas Treated with CHOP-like Regimens

Author (s)	Patient#	Regimen	Age	Neutropenia	Neutropenic Fever	Treatment related Deaths	Growth Factor
Zinzani	161	VNCOP-B	60+	44%	32%	1.3%	-
Sonneveld	148	CHOP	60+	NR	NR	14%	-
		CNOP	60+	NR	NR	13%	-
Gomez	26	CHOP	60+	24%	8%	0	GM-CSF
			70+	73%	42%	20%	GM-CSF
Tirelli	119	VMP	70+	50%	21%	7%	-
		CHOP	70+	48%	21%	5%	-
Bastion	444	CVP	70+	9%	7%	12%	-
		CTVP	70+	29%	13%	15%	-
Bertini	90	VEBPC	70+	44%	9%	2%	
Bjorkholm	440	CHOP/	60+	91%	47%	5%	
		CNOP	60+	91%	47%	5%	
Armitage	20	CHOP	70+	NR	NR	30%	-

risk of neutropenic infections as high as 47%, and in one study the risk of chemotherapy-related death as high as 30%. Of special interest, the study of Gomez et al. (1998) showed that two thirds of thirty chemotherapy-related deaths occurred between the first and the second course of treatment. That means that the application of current ASCO guidelines for the use of Colony Stimulating Factors, requiring a previous episode of neutropenic infection, would have not been able to prevent the death of these patients. The incidence of grade III–IV thrombocytopenia was around 20%, and the incidence of anemia was also increased.

G-CSF reduced by more than 50% the risk of severe neutropenia and of neutropenic infections in older individuals, according to four randomized and controlled studies (Bertini et al., 1996; Bjorkholm et al., 1999; Tirelli et al., 1998; Zinzani et al., 1999). Life-threatening myelodepression during induction and consolidation treatment was more frequent among patients with AML aged 60 and older than among those younger (Balducci et al., 2001; Schiffer, 1996). Depletion of normal hemopoietic stem cells might have been a consequence of AML rather than of aging hemopoiesis. Though the use of hemopoietic growth factors in older acute leukemics during induction is controversial, virtually all studies show that during consolidation colony-stimulating factors reduce the risk of neutropenic infections and the duration of hospitalization (Balducci et al., 2001).

This review clearly indicates that the risk of myelodepression and of death from neutropenic infections increases with age and is particularly pronounced after age 70, and colony stimulating factors are effective in older individuals. Anemia is also a result of myelodepression, which may have severe consequences in older individuals, including:

- Enhanced risk of complications of cytotoxic chemotherapy (Schijvers et al., 1999).
- Increased incidence of fatigue, which in turn may precipitate functional dependence (Cleeland et al., 1999). Functional dependence is very costly in terms of money and caregiver stress.
- Increased risk of drug-related complications and possibly increased risk of infections (Fried et al., 2001; Izaks et al., 1999; Marcantonio et al., 1999).

Correction and prevention of anemia are necessary to avert the risk of long-term complications, besides ameliorating the short-term risk of chemotherapy-related toxicity. The risk of mucositis increases with age. Jacobson et al. (2001) reviewed the experience of the North Central Cancer Treatment Group (NCCTG) with fluorinated pyrimidine in more than 1400 patients and showed that the risk of diarrhea and mucositis was increased for persons over 65. In some cases, mucositis led to lethal fluid depletion. The risk and severity of mucositis was increased for women aged 65 and over even in the study of Gelmann and Taylor (1984) despite dose/adjustment for methotrexate and cyclophosphamide. This finding suggests that the gastrointestinal and airway mucosas become more vulnerable by cytotoxic chemotherapy with aging. The standard management of mucositis at present includes aggressive fluid repletion. Another useful provision may involve the substitution of oral capecitabine (Balducci & Carreca, 2002) for intravenous medications. With capecitabine, the majority of the active compound is concentrated in the tumor and normal tissues may be spared. Keratinocyte growth factors for the prevention of mucositis are undergoing clinical trials and appear promising (Spielberger et al., 2001).

The risk of anthracycline cardiomyopathy increases with age but is mostly limited to patients receiving doses of doxorubicin ≥ 450 mg/m2 of body surface area. Continuous infusion of doxorubicin or administration of dexrazoxane may enhance myelosuppression and may attenuate the antineoplastic activity of doxorubicin, and the use of liposomal anthracyclines may cause palm-sole syndrome (Balducci & Extermann, 2001). These measures should be instituted only in patients for whom doses of anthracyclines above the threshold of cardiotoxicity are planned, or patients with pre-existing risk factors, such as history of ischemic cardiomyopathy or previous episodes of congestive heart failure.

The potential complications of chemotherapy on the central nervous system include cognitive decline (Schagen et al., 1999) and cerebellar toxicity (Gottlieb et al., 1987). The latter is seen with cytarabine in high doses and is related to accumulation in the circulation of ara-uridine, in presence of reduced GFR. Chemotherapy-induced peripheral neuropathy may lead to functional dependence, by compromising those fine movements that are essential for feeding or dressing. The use of drugs with low neurotoxic potential (carboplatin instead of cisplatin, docetaxel instead of paclitaxel) may be advisable in older individuals.

PREVENTION AND AMELIORATION OF CHEMOTHERAPY-RELATED TOXICITY

Table 9.3 summarizes a number of recommendations that were recently presented to the National Cancer Center Network (NCCN) (Balducci

TABLE 9.3 NCCN Recommended Guidelines for the Management of the Older Person with Cancer

Cancer patients aged 70 and older should undergo some form of geriatric assessment

Doses of chemotherapy should be adjusted to the patient's glomerular filtration rate, for persons aged 65 and older

Hemopoietic growth factors should be used prophylactically in patients aged 70 and older receiving moderately toxic chemotherapy (example CHOP; Cyclophosphamide/doxorubicin; Fluorouracil, epirubicin, cyclophosphamide)

Patients' hemoglobin should be maintained at 12 gm/dl or higher

Mucositis should be aggressively treated in older individuals, with fluid resuscitation as soon as the patient becomes unable to eat or diarrhea develops

Consider less toxic alternatives to doxorubicin for patients aged 70 and older.

& Yates, 2000). The dose-adjustment to a patient's individual GFR (Table 9.4) is recommended for patients deemed at increased risk of complication based on a comprehensive geriatric assessment. The recommendation to use prophylactic colony-stimulating factors for patients receiving treatment of dose intensity comparable to CHOP is based on the risk of myelotoxicity and neutropenic infections in patients over 70 (Table 9.2), on the substantial risk of mortality during the first course of treatment (Gomez et al., 1998), and on the demon-

TABLE 9.4 Suggested Dose Adjustment for Common Antineoplastic Agents to the GFR

Creatinine Clearance ml/min	≤ 60	≤ 45	≤ 30
Bleomycin	0.7	0.6	NR
Carboplatin	Calvert's Formula		
Carmustine	0.8	0.75	NR
Cisplatinum	0.75	0.5	NR
Cytarabine (high doses)	0.6	0.5	NR
Dacarbazine	0.8	0.75	0.7
Fludarabine	0.8	0.75	0.65
Hydroxyurea	0.8	0.75	0.7
Ifosfamide	0.8	0.75	0.7
Melphalan	0.85	0.75	0.7
Methotrexate	0.65	0.5	NR

NR = Not recommended

strated effectiveness of G-CSF in older individuals (Balducci et al., 2001). These recommendations were acknowledged by the chairman of the ASCO committee on Colony Stimulating Factors, who concurred with them (Balducci et al., 2001). Control of anemia may prevent chemotherapy-related toxicity (Schjivers et al., 1999), functional decline (Cleeland et al., 1999), and other iatrogenic complications in older individuals (Balducci et al., 2001). Of interest, anemia, even mild anemia (hemoglobin concentrations $\leq$ 13.5gm/dl), was found to be an independent risk factor for mortality in women aged 65 and over (Fried et al., 2001).

A comprehensive geriatric assessment (Balducci, Overcash & Extermann, 2002) is helpful in tailoring the treatment to the individual characteristics of the older cancer patient (Figure 9.2). The algorithm in Figure 9.2 is based on the staging of age proposed by Hamerman (1999) (Table 9.5). The frail patients have exhausted all functional reserve and are candidates only for palliative treatment unless frailty can be rapidly reversed. Some forms of low-toxicity chemotherapy, such as gemcitabine, Navelbine, weekly taxanes, oral fluorinated pyrimidines, may be used for palliation in frail individuals (Balducci & Stanta, 2000). Patients who are fully independent and without significant comorbidity should receive full treatment, with the use of growth factors if they are over 70 and the treatment dose intensity is comparable to CHOP. Patients between the extremes of frailty and full independence deserve special attention, including adjustment of the first dose of treatment to the GFR, optimal management of concomitant comorbid conditions, and home management. It is for these patients that an effective caregiver is essential. The caregiver may represent a powerful ally of the practitioner in critical management areas, including:

- Fostering treatment compliance by the patient and providing timely access to emergency care.
- Bridging the communication between the practitioner and the patient's family. Older individuals generally have several family members living in different parts of the country, all of whom may claim individual access to the practitioner. An effective caregiver may spare the practitioner the time of multiple interviews and the frustrations of miscommunication.
- Facilitating the relationship within the family. The disease of an old parent may reignite previous family conflicts. Without the intervention of the caregiver, the practitioner may inadvertently become involved in family conflicts.

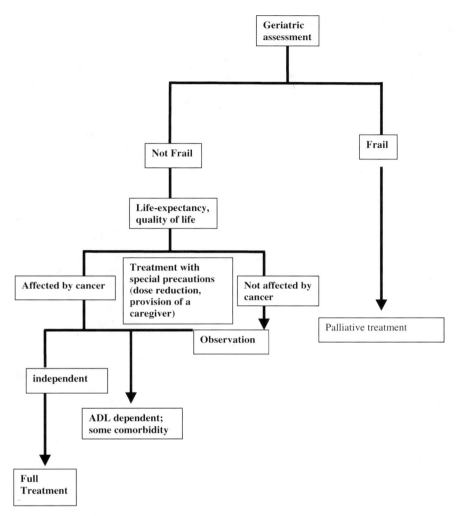

FIGURE 9.2 Algorithm for the Management of the Older Cancer Patient.

Another important aspect of treatment-related decision is the context in which chemotherapy is administered. For example, the majority of patients with advanced-stage non-Hodgkin's lymphoma or ovarian cancer will need some form of chemotherapy, as these diseases are likely to shorten their survival and cause deterioration in their quality of life. The issue of adjuvant chemotherapy is completely different in at least two respects:

TABLE 9.5 Stages of Aging and Consequences on Cancer Treatment

Stage	Clinical characteristics	Treatment plan
Primary	Independent in ADL and IADL No comorbidity or geriatric syndromes	Full standard treatment, if the risk of cancer-related is likely to reduce the life expectancy, or the active life expectancy, or the quality of life of the patient
Intermediate	This stage is to some extent reversible Dependent in one or more IADL Comorbidity that interferes with regular activities Mild memory disorder or subclinical depression	Full treatment if the patient's dysfunction and comorbidity may be reversed; if not, and the cancer threatens the patient's life expectancy, active life expectancy, or quality of life, treatment with special precautions. These may include initial reduction of the dose of chemotherapy, provision of a live-in caregiver.
Secondary or frailty	This stage at present is irreversible Currently, one of the following definitions of frailty may be used: One of the following criteria (Balducci and Stanta): Dependence ≥ 1 ADL ≥ 1 geriatric syndrome ≥ 3 comorbid conditions Three or more of the following (Fried et al.): Weight loss ≥ 10% over one year; Decreased grip strength; Low energy level; Difficulty in starting movement; Slow walking	Palliative treatment that may involve chemotherapy in low doses
Tertiary or near death	This stage is irreversible. Estimated life expectancy less than 6 months	Palliative treatment

- The patient's life is not immediately threatened;
- The treatment is beneficial to only a minority of patients.

By providing an idea of the patient's life expectancy and tolerance of treatment, the geriatric assessment provides useful indications for selecting the patients more likely to benefit from chemotherapy. Extermann et al. (2000) studied the situation in which adjuvant chemotherapy may improve the cure rate of breast cancer by at least 1%. These authors found that the risk of breast cancer death at which adjuvant chemotherapy would be beneficial increases with the age of the patient. For women aged 80, this risk should be at least 30%. This model may be useful to estimate the benefits of other forms of adjuvant chemotherapy and of treating tumors with a chronic course, such as prostate cancer, chronic lymphocytic leukemia, and low-grade lymphoma.

HORMONAL THERAPY OF CANCER

Hormonal therapy is effective in breast, prostate, and endometrial cancer. Traditionally, hormonal therapy has been preferred to chemotherapy in the older individual as safer and better tolerated. The Selective Estrogen Receptor Modulators (SERMs), tamoxifen and toremifene, have been the mainstay of the treatment of hormone-receptor rich breast cancer both in the adjuvant and the metastatic setting. An additional benefit of these compounds is prevention of osteoporosis (Balducci et al., 2002). Another SERM, raloxifene (Agnudei et al., 1999), has been recently approved for prevention of osteoporosis. Both tamoxifen and raloxifene prevent breast cancer in women at risk (Agnusdei et al., 1999; Fisher et al., 1998).

Despite their excellent record of safety, SERMs have occasionally caused life-threatening complications, which include endometrial cancer for tamoxifen and toremifene, and arterial and venous thrombosis (Fisher et al., 1998). The risk of thrombotic events increases with the age of the patient. Another problem related to the SERMs is reduced activity in tumors that over-express HER2neu in the presence of visceral metastases. The toxicity profile of the SERMs might have improved with the introduction of faslodex, a pure estrogen antagonist (Howell et al., 2000) that does not appear associated with endometrial cancer nor with thromboembolic complications, though there are concerns that this drug may promote osteoporosis. Faslodex is active in approximately 20% of patients whose breast cancer progresses during treatment with tamoxifen.

A group of drugs with an interesting profile of activity and toxicity include the new aromatase inhibitors (Santen et al., 1999). Chemically we have nonsteroidal and steroidal agents. The nonsteroidals include anastrozole and letrozole; the steroidals, sometimes referred to as aromatase inactivators, include exemestane. Though the mechanism of action of steroidals and nonsteroidals is different, it is not clear whether this difference is relevant in the clinical area. All aromatase inhibitors share the following characteristics:

- They prove more active than tamoxifen in randomized controlled study;
- HER2neu over-expression may not affect their activity;
- The risk of severe thromboembolic complications is lower that with SERMs.

A possible concern related to the long-term use of these agents is osteoporosis. The steroid structure may give two advantages to exemestane: lower incidence of hot flushes and protection from osteoporosis, but in both cases the data are very preliminary. Also, exemestane is active in about 20% of patients whose disease has progressed with the other aromatase inhibitors. The standard management of metastatic prostate cancer involves castration that may be surgical or chemical (Balducci et al., 1997). Chemical castration is obtainable with the LH-RH agonists (leuprolide and buserelin), which act by overstimulating and exhausting the pituitary, and a newly developed antagonist (Abarelix) (Stricker, H. J. 2001). The only advantage of Abarelix is to prevent the initial stimulation of tumor growth observed with the agonists.

Several issues in the management of metastatic prostate cancer need clarification. First, it is still debated whether the combination of castration and an androgen antagonist is superior to castration alone. Clearly the differences must be minimal, as the problem has not been solved by ten randomized controlled trials and at least two meta-analyses. At present the majority of practitioners would use an androgen inhibitor only during the first two weeks of treatment with an LH-RH analog, to prevent the initial tumor flare. Second, it is not clear whether intermittent treatment with LH-RH analogs is equivalent to continuous treatment. The potential advantages of intermittent treatment include substantial cost reduction, possible prevention of refractoriness to hormonal treatment, preservation of libido, at least for some periods of time, and minimization of osteoporosis, which is a serious concern when castration lasts several years. Ongoing clinical trials explore this issue. Third, it is not clear when is the best time to institute castration, whether when metastases are detected, or instead at the first rise of PSA, after surgery or radiation. Since PSA recurrences may precede by several years evidence of metastases, early castration is associated with a substantial risk of osteoporosis.

Secondary forms of hormonal treatment include aminoglutethimide and ketoconazole at high doses. Both drugs inhibit both adrenal and godanal steroidogenesis and require supplementation of corticosteroids.

In general, all forms of hormonal treatment of prostate cancer are well tolerated. The main side effects of LH-RH agonists and antagonists alike include hot flushes, controllable by low doses of progesterone, and osteoporosis, which is of special concern when castration lasts more than two years. For these men, monitoring of bone density and an osteoporosis preventative program with a bisphosphonate may be necessary.

BIOLOGICAL THERAPY OF CANCER

Despite initial promises, biological therapy of cancer is still limited to two agents: interferon and interleukin-2. At low doses, interferon seems to be well tolerated by patients of all ages, while at high doses it may be associated with a form of severe depressive psychosis, which may respond to ritalin (Jonasch et al., 2000). The experience with interleukin-2 in older individuals is limited and inconclusive.

TUMOR-TARGETED THERAPY

Perhaps the most exciting advances in cancer treatment involve the development of agents that target the neoplastic tissue and its metabolic process and largely spare normal tissues. Notwithstanding the general benefits of this approach, the elderly are likely to benefit from it more fully than is any other segment of the population. Figure 9.3 illustrates some of the most likely targets of this new form of therapy.

MONOCLONAL ANTIBODIES

This form of targeted treatment is most advanced, and several monoclonal antibodies are already available for clinical use. They may be directed against tumor antigens, against growth factor receptors, and against any of the enzymes and growth factors involved in tumor growth. Monoclonal antibodies may be free or conjugated. Free mon-

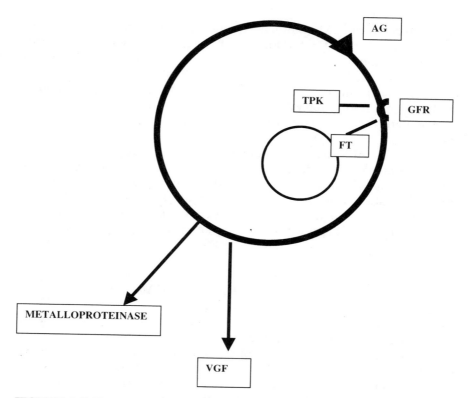

FIGURE 9.3 Targets of New Forms of Cancer Therapy.
AG = Antigen; FT = Farnesyl transferase; GFR = Growth factor receptor; TPK = Thyrosine phosphokinase; VGF = Vascular growth factor.

oclonal antibodies may act by destroying the cell after reacting with a tumor antigen (rituximab) (Borrebaeck & Carlsson, 2001), to prevent the action of growth factors by occupying the growth factor receptor (trastuzumab) (Sedman et al., 2001), and by inhibiting specific enzymes or growth factors (Cetuximab and VEGF antibody) (Raymond, et al.; Schlaeppi & Wood). Conjugated antibodies are bound to a radioisotope or to a toxin and their mechanism of action is concentrating this cytotoxic material in the neoplastic tissues (Witzig, 2001).

Currently, five monoclonal antibodies are available for clinical use in the USA. Rituximab is directed against the CD20 antigen present in most B cells. As a single agent, rituximab is active in approximately 80% of so-called low grade and in 30% of mantle cell lymphomas (Czuczman, 2001; Petryk & Grossbard, 2000). The remission duration appears longer with rituximab than with chemotherapy. In large-cell B cell lymphoma the combination of rituximab and chemotherapy was demonstrated superior to chemotherapy alone in terms of response rate, disease-free and overall survival. The main complication of rituximab is a rare allergic reaction; the initial concern about increased risk of infection has not yet proven true.

Trastuzumab (Sedman) is an antibody directed against the HER2neu (epithelial growth factor receptor). It is currently approved for the management of breast cancer and is being studied in other neoplasms including lung and prostate cancer. The main problem with this agent, which is extremely well tolerated, is the risk of cardiomyopathy, which is more common in patients previously treated with anthracyclines and in older individuals (Feldman et al., 2000). Because the cardiomyopathy is reversible, there is no reason to avoid this agent in aged persons with normal cardiac function. Campath-1 is an antibody directed against the CD52 antigen that is expressed on all monocytes and lymphocytes (Flynn & Byrd, 2000), and is effective in lymphoid malignancies. It is used primarily in chronic lymphocytic leukemia. Its administration is associated with a number of complications, including fever, hypotension, and opportunistic infections from lymphopenia and monocytopenia. Prophylactic administration of antibodies is indicated. In addition, three times per week administration makes this agent inconvenient for many older individuals.

Gentuzumab ozogamicin (Mylotarg) is directed against the CD33 antigen, found both in leukemic and normal hemopoietic precursors and is conjugated with the toxin Calicheamicin. Since the CD52 is not present in pluripotent hemopoietic stem cell, the myelotoxicity caused by mylotarg is generally reversible. This antibody is used in the management of chemotherapy refractory acute myelogenous leukemia in the elderly. The main complication is myelodepression that is substantial and prolonged (Sievers et al.).

Denileukin Diftitox (Ontak) is directed against the IL-2 receptor and is conjugated with diptherial toxin. Though very effective in the plaque stage of mycosis fungoids (Duvic, 2000), its use is associated with substantial toxicity including fluid retention and renal shutdown.

Of the monoclonal antibodies undergoing clinical trials, those conjugated with radioisotopes appear the most promising in the management of lymphoid malignancies. The risk of myelodepression however renders these agents less than ideal for older individuals (Witzig, 2001). These include Y labelled rituxam (Zavid) and I labeled tositumab (Bexxar) . Cetuximab, an inhibitor of thyrosine phospokinase, has substantial activity in cancer of the large bowel (Raymond et al., 2000).

PTK Inhibitors

PTK is essential to signal transduction. It is not surprising that that has been the focus of many inhibition attempts. Recently, Drucker et al. (2001) produced an agent, gleevec, that inhibits the specific PTK of chronic granulocytic leukemia, which is encoded by the BCR/abl oncogene. This oral agent has induced a hematologic remission in approximately 90% of patients with CGL in chronic phase, and is considered the drug of choice for the management of this disease. The toxicity is minimal even in older individuals. Inhibitors of the PTK of other tumors are undergoing clinical trials (Raymond et al., 2000).

Other Agents

Of special interest are the Farnesyl transferase inhibitors. Farnesyl transferase is also important for signal transduction, the metalloproteinase inhibitors, which may prevent metastatic spread, and the inhibitors of angiogenesis, which prevent the formation of new vessels necessary for tumor growth. The experience with these agents in older individuals is preliminary.

CONCLUSIONS

This review suggests two important conclusions:

- Cytotoxic chemotherapy may be beneficial to older individuals, when the patients who most may benefit from treatment are identified and when special precautions are taken. These include dose adjustment to renal function, initial dose reduction in patients who are not fully independent, provision of caregiver, prophylactic use of colony-stimulating factors in patients over 70 receiving moderately toxic chemotherapy, and maintenance of hemoglobin at levels ^{3} 12gm/dl.
- New advances in cancer treatment include targeted chemotherapy that may substantially reduce the risk of therapeutic complications.

REFERENCES

Agnusdei, D., Liu-lerage, S., Augendre-Ferrant, B. (1999). Results of International Clinical Trials with Raloxifene. *Annals of Endocrinology, (Paris), 60*, 342–346.

Armitage, J. O., & Potter, J. F. (1984). Aggressive chemotherapy for diffuse histiocytic lymphoma in the elderly. *Journal of the American Geriatric Society, 32,* 269–273.

Balducci, L., & Corcoran, M. B. (2000). Antineoplastic chemotherapy of the older cancer patient. *Hematology Oncology Clinics of North America,* 14, 193–212.

Balducci, L., & Extermann, M. (2001). A practical approach to the older patient with cancer. *Current Problems in Cancer, 25,* 1–76.

Balducci, L., Hardy, C. H., & Lyman, G. H. (2001). Hematopoietic growth factors in the older cancer patient. *Current Opinion in Hematology, 8,* 170–187.

Balducci, L., Lyman, G. H., & Ozer, H. (2001). Patients aged ≥ 70 are at high risk for neutropenic infection and should receive hemopoietic growth factors when treated with moderately toxic chemotherapy. *Journal of Clinical Oncology, 19,* 1583–1585.

Balducci, L., Overcash, J., Extermann, M. (2003). The care of the older cancer patient: delayed diagnosis, inadequate treatment, information gap. In J. Overcash, L. Balducci, (Eds.), *The older cancer patient.* New York: Springer Publishing Co.

Balducci, L., Pow-Sang, J., & Friedland, J. (1997). Prostate cancer. *Clinical Geriatric Medicine, 13,* 283–306.

Balducci, L., & Stanta, G. (2000). Cancer in the frail patient: a coming epidemic. *Hematology Oncology Clinics of North America, 14,* 235–250.

Balducci, L., & Yates, G. (2000). General guidelines for the management of older patients with cancer. *Oncology, NCCN Proceedings, November 2000,* 221–227.

Balducci, L., Silliman, R. A., & Diaz, N. (in press). Breast Cancer: an Oncological perspective. In L. Balducci, G. H. Lyman, W. B. Ershler (Eds.), *Comprehensive geriatric oncology. Second edition.* London: Harwood Academic Publishers.

Bastion, Y., Blay, J.Y., Divine, M., Brice, P., Bordessoule, D., Sebban, C., Blanc, M., Tilly, H., Lederlin, P., Deconinck, E., Salles, B., Dumontet, C., Briere, J., & Coiffier, B. (1997). Elderly patients with aggressive non-Hodgkin's lymphoma: Disease presentation, response to treatment and survival. A Groupe d'Etude des Lymphomes de l'Adulte Study on 453 patients older than 69 years. *Journal of Clinical Oncology, 15,* 2945–2953.

Beggs, C. B., & Carbone, P. (1983). Clinical trials and drug toxicity in the elderly. The experience of the Eastern Cooperative Oncology Group. *Cancer, 52,* 1986–1992.

Bertini, M., Freilone, R., Vitolo, U., Botto, B., Ciotti, R., Cinieri, S., DiNota. A., Di Vito, F., Levis, A., Orsucci, L., Pina, M., Rota-Scalabrini, D., Todeschini, G., & Resegotta, L. (1996). The treatment of elderly patients with aggressive non-Hodgkin's lymphomas: Feasibility and efficacy of an intensive multi drug regimen. *Leukemia & Lymphoma, 22,* 483–493.

Bjorkholm, M., Osby, E., & Hagberg, H. (1999). Randomized trial of R-methu granulocyte colony stimulating factors as adjunct to CHOP or CNOP treatment of elderly patients with aggressive non-Hodgkin's lymphoma. *Proceedings of the American Society of Hematology, 94,* 599a, Abstract 2665.

Borrebaeck, C. A., & Carlsson, R. (2001). Human therapeutic antibodies. *Current Opinion in Pharamacology, 1,* 404–408.

Christman, K., Muss, H. B., Case, D., & Stanley, V. (1992). Chemotherapy of metastatic breast cancer in the elderly. *Journal of the American Medical Association, 268,* 57–62.

Cleeland, C. S., Demetri, G. D., & Glaspy, J. (1999). Identifying hemoglobin levels for optimal Quality of Life. Results of an incremental analysis. *Proceedings of the American Society of Clinical Oncology, 16,* Astr 2215.

Czuczman, M. S. (2001). Combination chemotherapy and rituximab. *Anticancer Drugs, 12* (suppl2), s15–19.

Dees, E. C., O'Reilly, S., & Goodman, S. N. (2000). A prospective pharmacologic evaluation of age-related toxicity chemotherapy in women with breast cancer. *Cancer Investigation, 18,* 521–529.

Dejaeger, E., Pelemans, W., Bibau, G., & Ponette, E. (1994). Manofluorography analysis of swallowing in the elderly. *Dysphagia, 9,* 156–161.

Doroshow, J. H. (1996). Anthracyclines and anthracendiones. In B. A. Chabner, D. L. Longo. *Cancer chemotherapy and biotherapy.* Philadelphia: Lippincott-Raven, 409–434.

Drucker, B. J., Talpaz, M., & Resta, D. J. (2001). Efficacy and safety of a specific inhibitor of the BCR-ABL tyrosine kinase in chonic myeloid leukemia. *New England Journal of Medicine, 344,* 1031–1037.

Duvic, M. (2000). Bexarotene and DAB389IL-2(Denileukin Diftitox, ONTAK) in the treatment of cutaneous T cell lymphoma. Algorithms. *Clinical Lymphoma, 1,* Suppl 1, S51–55.

Extermann, M., Balducci, L., & Lyman, G. H. (2000). What threshold for adjuvant therapy in older breast cancer patients? *Journal of Clinical Oncology, 18,* 1709–1717.

Feldman, A. M., Lorell, B. H., & Reis, S. E. (2000). Trastuzumab in the treatment of metastatic breast cancer antitumor therapy vs cardiotoxicity. *Circulation, 18,* 102, 272–274.

Fisher, B., Costantino, J. P., Wickerham, D. L., Redmand, C. K., Kavanah, M., Cronin, W. M., Vogel, V., Robidoux, A., Dimitrov, N., Atkins, J., Daly, M., Wieland, S., Tan-Chiu, E., Ford, L., & Wolmark, N. (1998). Tamoxifen for prevention of breast cancer : report from the national adjuvant breast and bowel project. *Journal of the National Cancer Institute, 90,* 1371–1388.

Flynn, J. M., & Byrd, J. C. (2000). Campath-1H monoclonal antibody therapy. *Current Opinions in Oncology, 12,* 574–581.

Fried, L. P., Tangen, C. M., Walston, J., Newman, A. B., Hirsch, C., Gottdiener, J., Seeman, T., Tracey, R., Kop, W. J., Burke, G., & McBurnie, M. A. (2001). Frailty in older adults. Evidence for a phenotype. *Journal of Gerontology, 56A;* M146–M156.

Gelman, R. S., & Taylor, S. G. (1984). Cyclophosphamide, Methotrexate and 5Flourouracil chemotherapy in women more than 65 years old with advanced breast cancer. The elimination of age trends in toxicity by using doses based on creatinine clearance. *Journal of Clinical Oncology, 2,* 1406–1414.

Giovannozzi-Bannon, S., Rademaker, A., Lai, G., & Bensen, A. B. (1994). Treatment tolerance of elderly cancer patients entered onto phase II clinical trials. An Illinois cancer center study. *Journal of Clinical Oncology, 12,* 2447–2452.

Gomez, H., Mas, L., Casanova, L., Pen, D. L., Santillana, S., Valdivi, S., Otero, J., Rodriquez, W., Carracedo, C., & Vallejos, C. (1998). Elderly patients with aggressive non-Hodgkin's lymphoma treated with CHOP chemotherapy plus granulocyte-macrophage colony-stimulating factor: Identification of two age subgroups with differing hematologic toxicity. *Journal of Clinical Oncology, 16,* 2352–2358.

Gottlieb, D., Bradstock, K., Koutts, J., Robertson, T., Lee, C., & Castaldi, P. (1987). The neurotoxicity of high dose cytosine arabinoside is age-related. *Cancer, 60,* 1439–1441.

Guslandi, M. (1997). The aging stomach. *Gut, 41,* 425–426.

Hamerman, D. (1999). Toward an understanding of frailty. *Annals of Internal Medicine, 130,* 945–950.

Howell, A., Osborne, C. K., Morris, C., & Wakeling, A. E. (2000). ICI 187,780 (Faslodex): development of a "new" pure antiestrogen. *Cancer, 89,* 817–825.

Ibrahim, N., Frye, D. K., Buzdar, A. U., Walters, R. S., & Hortobagyi, G. N. (1996). Doxorubicin based combination chemotherapy in elderly patients with metastatic breast cancer. Tolerance and outcome. *Archives of Internal Medicine, 156,* 882–888.

Ibrahim, N., Buzdar, A. U., Asmar, L., Theriault, R. L., & Hortobagyi, G. N. (2000). Doxorubicin based adjuvant chemotherapy in elderly breast cancer patients:The M D Anderson Experience with long term follow-up. *Annals of Oncology, 11,* 1–5.

Izaks, G. J., Westendorp, R. G. J., & Knook, D. L. (1999). The definition of anemia in the older person. *Journal of the American Medical Association, 281,* 1714–1717.

Jacobson, S. D., Cha, S., & Sargent, D. J. (2001). Tolerability, dose intensity and benefit of 5FU based chemotherapy for advanced colorectal cancer (CRC) in the elderly. A North Central Cancer Treatment Group Study. *Proceedings of the American Society of Clinical Oncology, 20,* 384a, Abstr. 1534.

Jonasch, E., Kumar, U. N., Linette, E. P., Hodi, F. S., Soiffer, R. J., Ryan, B. F., Sober, A. J., Mihm, M. C., Tsao, H., Langley, R. G., Cosimi, B. A., Gadd, M. A., Tanabe, K. K., Souba, W., Haynes, H. A., Barnhill, R., Osteen, R., & Haluska, F. G. (2000). Adjuvant high dose interferon alfa 2b in patients with high risk melanoma. *Cancer Journal of Scientific American, 6,* 139–145.

Kim, Y. J., Rubenstein, E. B., & Rolston, K. V. (2000). Colony-stimulating factors (CSFs) may reduce complications and death in solid tumor patients with fever and neutropenia. *Proceedings of the American Society of Clinical Oncology, 19,* 612a, Abstr 2411.

Leith, C. P., Kopecky, K. J., Godwin, J., McConnell, T., Slovak, M. L., Chen, I. M., Head, D. R., Appelbaum, F. R., & Willman, C. L. (1997). Acute myelogenous leukemia in the elderly: assessment of multidrug resistance and cytogenetics distinguishes subgroup with markedly distinct responses to standard chemotherapy. *Blood, 89,* 3323–3329.

Marcantonio, E. R., Goldman, L., Orav, E. J., Cook, E. F., & Lee, T. H. (1998). The association of intraoperative factors with the development of postoperative delirium. *American Journal of Medicine, 105,* 380–384.

Petryk, M., & Grossbard, M. L. (2000). Rituximab therapy of B-Cell Neoplasms. *Clinics in Lymphoma, 1,* 186–194.

Raymond, E., Faivre, S., & Armand, J. P. (2000). Eidermal growth factor receptor tyrosine kinase as a target for anticancer therapy. *Drugs, 60,* Suppl1, 15–23.

Rudd, G. N., Hartley, G. A., & Souhani, R. L. (1995). Persistence of cisplatin-induced interstrand crosslinking in peripheral blood mononuclear cells from elderly and younger individuals. *Cancer Chemotherapy Pharmacology, 35,* 323–326.

Saltzman, J. R., & Russe, R. M. (1998). The aging gut. Nutritional issues. *Gastroenterology Clinics of North America, 27,* 305–324.

Santen, R. J., Yue, W., Naftolin, F., Mor, G., & Berstein, L. The potential of aromatase inhibitors in breast cancer prevention. *Endocrine Relations Cancer, 6,* 235–243.

Schagen, S. B., Van Dam, F. S., Muller, M. J., Boogerd, W., Lindeboom, J., & Bruning, P. F. (1999). Cognitive deficit after postoperative adjuvant chemotherapy for breast carcinoma. *Cancer, 85,* 640–650.

Schiffer, C. A. (1996). Hematopoietic growth factors as adjuncts to the treatment of acute myelogenous leukemia. *Blood, 88,* 3675–3685.

Sclaeppi, J. M., & Wood, J. M. (1999). Targeting vascular endothelial growth factor (VEGF) for anti-cancer therapy by anti-VEGF neutralizing monoclonal antibodies or VEGF receptor tyrosine-kinase inhibitors. *Cancer Metastases Review, 18,* 473–481.

Schrijvers, D., Highley, M., Du Bruyn, E., Van Oosterom, A. T., & Vermorken, J. B. (1999). Role of red blood cell in pharmakinetics of chemotherapeutic agents. *Anticancer Drugs, 10,* 147–153.

Seidman, A. D., Fornier, M. N., Esteva, F. J., Tan, L., Kaptain, S., Bach, A., Panageas, K. S., Arroyo, C., Valero, V., Currie, V., Gilewski, T., Theodoulou, M., Moyanhan, M. E., Moasser, M., Sklarin, N., Dickler, M., D'Andrea, G., Cristofanilli, M., Rivera, E., Hortobagyi, G. N., Norton, L., & Hudis, C. A. (2001). Weekly Trastuzumab and paclitaxel therapy for metastatic breast cancer with analysis of efficacy by HER2 immunophenotype and gene amplification. *Journal of Clinical Oncology, 19,* 2587–2595.

Sheehan, D. C., & Forman, W. B. (1997). Symptomatic management of the older person with cancer. *Clinical Geriatric Medicine, 13,* 203–219.

Short, K. R., & Nair, K. S. (2000). The effect of age on protein metabolism. *Current Opinions in Clinical Nutrition Metabolic Care, 3,* 39–44.

Sievers, E. L., Applebaum, F. R., & Spielberger, R. T. (1999). Selective ablation of acute myeloid leukemia using antibody targeted chemotherapy: a phase II study of an antiCD-33 calicheamicin immunoconjugate. *Blood, 93,* 3678–3684.

Sonneveld, P., de Ridder, M., van der Lelie, H., Nieuwenhuis, K., Schouten, H., Mulder, A., van Reijswoud, I., Hop, W., & Lowenberg, B. (1995). Comparison of doxorubicin and mitoxantrone in the treatment of elderly patients with advanced diffuse non-Hodgkin's lymphoma using CHOP vs CNOP chemotherapy. *Journal of Clinical Oncology, 13,* 2530–2539.

Spielberger, R. T., Stiff, P., Emmanouilides, C. (2001). Efficacy of recombinant human keratinocyte growth factor (rHuKGF) in reducing mucositis in patients with hematologic malignancies undergoing autologous peripheral blood progenito cell transplantation after radiation-based conditioning. Results of a phase 2 trial. *Proceedings of the American Society of Clinical Oncology, 20,* 7a, Abstr 25.

Stein, B. N., Petrelli, N. J., Douglass, H. O., Driscoll, D. L., Arcangeli, G., & Meropol, N. J. (1995). Age and sex are independent predictors of 5–fluorouracil toxicity. *Cancer, 75,* 11–17.

Stricker, H. J. (2001). Luteinizing Hormone Releasing Hormone antagonists in prostate cancer. *Urology, 58* (Suppl), 24–27.

Tirelli, U., Errante, D., Van Glabbeke, M., Teodorovic, I., Kluin-Nelemans, J. C., Thomas, J., Bron, D., Rosti, G., Somers, R., Zagonel, V., & Noordijk, E. M. (1998). CHOP is the standard regimen in patients ≥ 70 years of age with intermediate and high grade Non-Hodgkin's lymphoma: results of a randomized study of the European Organization for the Research and Treatment of Cancer Lymphoma Cooperative Study. *Journal of Clinical Oncology, 16,* 27–34.

Vestal, R. E. (1997). Aging and pharmacology. *Cancer, 80,* 1302–1310.

Witzig, T. E. (2001). Radioimmunotherapy for patients with relapsed B-cell non-Hodgkin's lymphoma. *Cancer Chemotherapy Pharmacology, 1,* S91–95.

Zinzani, P. G., Storti, S., Zaccaria, A., Noretti, L., Magagnoli, M., Pavone, E., Gentilini, P., Guardigni, L., Gobbi, M., Fattori, P. P., Falini, B., Lauta, V. M., Bendandi, M., Gherlinzoni, F., De Renzo, A., Zaja, F., Volpe, E., Bocchia, M., Aitini, E., Tabanelli, M., Leone, G., & Tura, S. (1999). Elderly aggressive histology non-Hodgkin's lymphoma: First line VNCOP-B regimen: experience on 350 patients. *Blood, 94,* 33–34.

Cancer Fatigue and Aging

Sandra Holley

Energy Crisis
At first I was energized
The diagnosis shocked me into action
The clutching fear galvanized me
The details demanded attention
The family's tears called for comfort
The decisions were made
The adrenaline flowed and I was energized
But one day all the energy was gone—
Physical, psychic, emotional—
The days turned into weeks
And the weeks into months
Now I search
Each cell of my body
Each corner of my mind
For one tiny spark . . . .(Hjelmstad, 1993)

Persons with cancer have identified fatigue as the major troubling symptom and the primary cause of distress in their lives as they contend with their illness and treatment (Dean, Spears, Ferrell, Quan, Groshon & Mitchell, 1995; Driever & McCorkle, 1984; Jamar, 1989; Kurtz, Kurtz, Given & Given, 1993; Nail & King, 1987; Piper, Rieger, Brophy, Haeuber, Hood, Lyver & Sharp, 1989; Rhodes, Watson & Hanson, 1988). An estimated 8,900,000 people live with cancer. As an individual ages, his or her risk for cancer occurrence increases. Nearly 80% of all cancers are diagnosed at age 55 or older, making cancer a disease of aging (ACS, 2001). Fatigue is a problem now, but one that will become an even greater problem as the cancer patient population increases in both absolute and relative numbers.

Distress is often associated with fatigue. Several researchers have examined symptom distress that has included fatigue (Cassileth, Lusk, Bodenheimer, Farber, Jochimsen & Morrin-Taylor, 1985; McCorkle & Young, 1978; McCorkle & Quint-Benoliel, 1986; Sarna, 1993; Strauman, 1986). Distress is the suffering that accompanies the experience of a phenomenon or symptom such as fatigue. Benoliel (1985) posits that "suffering is the inner experience of losing a part of the self" and Spross (1993) describes suffering as the evaluation of the significance or meaning of a phenomenon, not necessarily a perception or sensation. This distress or suffering is part of the cancer-related fatigue (CRF) experience.

Although we have systematically studied typical fatigue in various populations for more than 30 years, there is still no universal definition of fatigue. From the literature, typical fatigue has been identified as a phenomenon that is characterized by increased feelings of discomfort and decreased functional status related to decreased energy. Factors that may be involved are physical, mental, emotional, environmental, physiological, and pathological. There is also a voluntary component. This voluntary component means we are able to gather the energy to do something that we really want to do even though we are experiencing extreme typical fatigue (Aistars, 1987; Gordon, 1986; Hart & Freel, 1982; Pickard-Holley, 1991; Rhoten, 1982). The person with cancer experiences fatigue within the "wholeness" of his or her self. That is, the consequences of fatigue affect cognitive/attentional functions, alter one's expectations, have physical sequelae, and impact psychosocial and spiritual aspects, so that all realms of one's being suffer. Conceptually, fatigue is a subjective, multidimensional, unpleasant experience (Holley, 2000a).

The phenomenon of fatigue in persons with cancer has been pursued only in the past 25 years and continues to be a poorly understood and a distressing symptom. A burgeoning interest in the study of fatigue in persons with cancer is under way. A major funded project called *F.I.R.E.*® (Fatigue Initiative in Research and Education) is currently being sponsored by Ortho-Biotech through the Oncology Nursing Society. *F.I.R.E.*® provides funding to oncology nurses for research and education to improve and increase the understanding of fatigue in cancer patients.

Nurses are most frequently the health care providers responsible for helping persons with cancer to manage and adapt to the symptoms and side effects that are a part of the cancer experience. Thus, fatigue in persons with cancer is a significant issue for nursing. Although much attention is currently being paid to the symptom of fatigue in persons with cancer, it is still a poorly understood phenomenon. Fatigue can be discussed in its different aspects, but it is the impact on the whole person that constitutes the phenomenon of fatigue.

Patients often describe themselves as being healthy people who went to being people with cancer and suffering a *different* fatigue— cancer related fatigue (CRF). Since CRF is a *different* kind of fatigue, it is frequently unrecognized by patients, families, and health care providers. Because of the unfamiliarity with CRF, many patients misinterpret the experience of CRF as a negative consequence of their disease and a sign that a decline in their health is occurring. CRF is different from the transient tiredness and depletion of energy that everyone typically experiences and that accompanies physical exertion. Cancer patients report that they expected typical fatigue and CRF to be at least similar. The fact that they are different was confusing and disconcerting. Compared to typical fatigue, CRF was 1) more rapid in onset, 2) more intense, 3) more energy draining, 4) longer lasting, 5) often unexpected, and 6) frequently unrelenting (Holley, 2000a). CRF is a significant nursing concern because nurses are the major health care providers who assist persons with cancer to manage and adapt to the fatigue that is a part of the cancer experience. With an understanding of the phenomenon of fatigue, nurses can suggest interventions to help patients improve their quality of life and their ability to carry on their daily interactions.

PATHOPHYSIOLOGY OF FATIGUE

Exercise physiologists collaborating with physicians have studied healthy volunteer subjects regarding the effects of fatigue on muscle metabolism (Kent-Braun, Miller & Weiner, 1993; Miller, Boska, Moussavi, Carson & Weiner, 1988; Weiner, Mousavi, Baker, Boska & Miller, 1990). They found that significant decreases in the force from a maximal voluntary isometric contraction were associated with decreased phosphocreatine (Pcr), decreased pH, and increased inorganic phosphate (Pi). These studies used a noninvasive measurement protocol, which increases the appropriateness for use in ill individuals.

St. Pierre, Kasper and Lindsey (1992) examined the relationship of cancer and fatigue from a physiological framework. They explored the possible association of fatigue with the structural and biochemical changes in skeletal muscle that are produced by cancer or its treatment. The authors speculated that Tumor Necrosis Factor may be responsible in the mediation of skeletal muscle wasting, and the possibility that exercise may be inappropriate as an intervention for the fatigued cancer patient. Very little physiological research exists on cancer patients, so it is difficult to determine if what is appropriate for healthy subjects and animal models is also appropriate for persons with cancer.

CANCER TREATMENT AND FATIGUE

SURGERY

Surgery is the oldest form of cancer treatment. Fatigue has been recognized as a major debilitating symptom associated with surgery. Cimprich (1992) examined the relationship of attentional fatigue three days post-surgery for breast cancer surgery. She found no correlation with the use of narcotic pain medication, with mood-state, or with self-ratings of attentional functioning ability. She did find a decrease in attentional performance at return postoperative visits. Schroeder and Hill (1993) found no correlation with postoperative fatigue and anxiety, depression, hostility, and total body protein or fat. The best predictors of postoperative fatigue were preoperative fatigue, weight loss, a cancer diagnosis, and age.

The European medical community is active in studying fatigue in surgical patients. Physicians from Britain and New Zealand investigated factors related to postoperative fatigue (Christensen, Hjorts, Mortensen, Riis-Hansen & Kehlet, 1992; Christensen, Hougard & Kehlet, 1985; Christensen & Kehlet, 1989; Christensen, Kehlet, Vesterberg & Vinnars, 1987; Christensen, Nygaard & Kehlet, 1988; Christensen, Nygaard, Stage & Kehlet, 1990; Christensen, Stage, Galbo, Ghouri, Bodner & White, 1991; Zeiderman, Welchew & Clark, 1990). Unfortunately those studies did not indicate any relationship of fatigue to duration of surgery, gender, anxiety, weight loss, skeletal muscle fiber changes, nor extent of surgery. Increased heart rate, type of anesthetic, route of administration of analgesics, and weight loss were the only factors found that related to postoperative fatigue. From these studies, the researchers concluded that postoperative fatigue may be a symptom of cardiovascular deterioration, neuromuscular performance, and nutritional status. The findings acknowledge that fatigue is a problem after surgery, but the study findings leave the problem of postoperative fatigue poorly understood. Although well designed, none of these studies of surgical patients included patients with cancer. Patients with cancer may have a greater incidence of fatigue because of their disease process and treatments used in conjunction with surgery.

RADIATION THERAPY

At least 50% of cancer patients receive radiation therapy as a part of their treatment. Fatigue is recognized as a common side effect of this treatment modality (Faithfull, 1991; Greenberg, Sawicka, Eisenthal & Ross, 1992; Haylock & Hart, 1979; King, Nail, Kreamer, Strohl & Johnson, 1985; Kobashi-Schoot, Hanewald, Van Dam & Bruning, 1985). Haylock and Hart (1979) were the first oncology nurses to report their findings regarding fatigue in patients receiving radiation therapy. They found that fatigue increased from the onset of treatment throughout the course of radiation therapy. Fatigue decreased on the weekends and other times when patients were not undergoing treatment. Contrary to this study, Greenberg, Sawicka, Eisenthal and Ross (1992) found no reduction of fatigue on Sundays. Fatigue was the only symptom experienced by the majority of the subjects, and fatigue continued to be reported through the third post-treatment month. RT to the cranium is also associated with a somnolence syndrome (Faithfull, 1991), general malaise (Kobashi-Schoot, Hanewald, Van Dam & Bruning, 1985), and with rising Interleukin-I (Il_1) levels (Greenberg, Gray, Mannix et al., 1993).

Antineoplastic Chemotherapy

Studies of patients receiving chemotherapy have identified fatigue as the most frequently reported side effect, regardless of chemotherapy regimen (Greene, Nail, Fieler, Dudgeon & Jones, 1994; Musser, 1990; Piper, 1993). Jones (1994) found that the number of patient symptoms and level of fatigue before chemotherapy were significant predictors for the fatigue experienced during and after chemotherapy. Pickard-Holley (1991) found no significant relationship between fatigue and age, stage of disease, course of treatment, or depression. Weak-to-moderate relationships were found between fatigue and the ovarian tumor marker, CA 125. A much larger (N=451) study of outpatients receiving chemotherapy reported that psychological depression appeared related to fatigue (Morrow et al., 1992). Using a diary, the onset, pattern, duration, intensity, and distress of fatigue were described in 109 patients. Patterns of fatigue were related to timing and technique of treatment administration, particular types of cancer, and specific regimens. Maintaining a fatigue diary can help identify individual patterns of fatigue and assist nurses to help patients plan activities during treatment (Richardson, Ream & Wilson-Barnett, 1998).

All but one (Musser, 1990) of these studies are correlational. Seven standard instruments and one instrument designed for the study were used in the six studies analyzed. The multiplicity of instruments makes it very difficult to draw any consistent conclusions from the findings. Only two studies used theoretical frameworks (Musser, 1991 & Piper, 1993). Two of the studies (Musser, 1990; Pickard-Holley, 1991) had small sample sizes.

Biotherapy

Biological agents (Interleukins, interferons, and colony-stimulating factors) used for the treatment of cancer and cancer treatment sequelae have become the standard of care for certain cancers (Davis, 1984; Dean, Spears, Ferrell et al., 1995). Interferon alpha has been associated with cumulative dose-related fatigue. During treatment, fatigue impacted all of the domains of quality of life (Dean, Spears, Ferrell et al., 1995).

THE MEASUREMENT OF CANCER-RELATED FATIGUE

Tools have been developed specifically to assess and measure CRF. Some of the instruments in current use include the Piper Fatigue Scale, (PFS), the Multidimensional Fatigue Symptom Inventory (MFSI), the Schwartz Cancer Fatigue Scale and the Functional Assessment of Cancer Therapy-Anemia (FACT-A), and the Cancer Related Fatigue Distress Scale (CRFDS). These instruments provide a quantitative measure to CRF that can give the nurse a symptomatic baseline, an outcome measure, and a general overall assessment of treatment tolerance.

Piper Fatigue Scale

The revised Piper Fatigue Scale (PFS) is a 22-item self-report measure used to assess the subjective experience of fatigue. The four subscales consist of behavioral/severity, affective meaning, sensory, and cognitive/mood (Piper, Dibble, Dodd et al., 1998). The PFS also contains three open-ended items for assessment of any measures that subjects report as helping to relieve fatigue, causes of their fatigue, and symptoms associated with their fatigue. Cronbach's alpha measures for reliability of the PFS have been reported as ranging from .85 to .95. Face and content validity of the items were based on a literature review and 11 evaluations by fatigue experts. Concurrent validity was established with the subscales of the Profile of Mood States and the Fatigue Symptom Checklist (Piper, Dibble et al., 1998). The primary drawback to the PFS is that of measurement clarity. It is not clear what aspect of fatigue is being measured; therefore, it is difficult to interpret the meaning of the total score.

Multidimensional Fatigue Symptom Inventory

The Multidimensional Fatigue Symptom Inventory (MFSI) is an 83–item tool based on a review of the literature on fatigue and discussions with health care providers (Stein, Martin, Hann & Jacobsen, 1998). Five dimensions are included; global fatigue, somatic symptoms, affective symptoms, behavioral symptoms, and cognitive symptoms. The instrument was tested on 275 female subjects receiving treatment for breast cancer (n=184), women who were post treatment (n=92), and a group of apparently healthy women. Adequate validity and reliability data are reported. This instrument is very lengthy and not ideal for use with persons experiencing fatigue because of the response burden. Further testing is needed in other cancer patient populations, particularly men, given that the instrument was only used with female patients with breast cancer.

Schwartz Cancer Fatigue Scale. The Schwartz Cancer Fatigue Scale (SCFS) (Schwartz, 1998) is a 28-item scale with four subscales: physical, emotional, cognitive, and temporal. Reliability is reported between .82 and .93. Subscales and the item pool were derived from a literature review and "informal clinical interactions" (Swartz, 1998, p.714) of persons with cancer. Five oncology nurse experts and six patients assessed content validity. Reliability was assessed with a sample of 166 subjects with a ration of 6 subjects per item. The majority of the sample (n= 146) for testing this instrument were cancer patients who had completed treatment approximately four years previously. This tool reports good validity (at 0.05 level or higher) and reliability scores. The SCRS is somewhat burdensome with 28 items. It is also based on the literature and not on patients' experiences with CRF.

Functional Assessment of Cancer Therapy-Anemia. The Functional Assessment of Cancer Therapy-Anemia (FACT-An) (Cella, 1997) is a 40–item scale that was tested on a sample of fifty patients. Because of the limited testing, psychometric evaluation was not possible at that time. This instrument is a version of the FACT-G, which evaluates quality of life in cancer patients receiving treatment. This tool is also too cumbersome for the particular patient population for which it is intended. It focuses on only one aspect on CRF, functional status. Many of the other domains of well-being are not addressed. This tool is aimed at patients in treatment and does not accommodate patients with CRF who are not being treated or who are not anemic but are still experiencing fatigue.

Cancer Related Fatigue Distress Scale

The Cancer Related Fatigue Distress Scale (CRFDS) (Holley, 2000b) is a 20–item, single-factor scale on which patients rate the degree of distress they experience from their cancer related fatigue on a 0–10 numeric rating scale. All items for this scale are loaded on one factor with loadings > .80. Coefficient alpha was .98 for the measurement of CRF distress (Holley, 2000b). The CRFDS has strong content validity, high reliability, and very good construct validity. The CRFDS is a clinically useful and psychometrically sound tool for the measurement of CRF distress. This tool is clinically useful by virtue of being brief (20 items) but thorough, has clear instructions that required no training to use, and has a readability score at the third grade level.

Assessment of Cancer Related Fatigue

Any of the above instruments can be used to measure CRF in the clinical setting. Whatever tool is chosen, assessment of CRF must be on an ongoing basis. A simple list of questions can be used at the beginning of each encounter with a cancer patient. An example is:

How is your energy level? (if the response is "good," then there is no need to go further; if the response is " bad," then:)

Is fatigue a problem? (If yes, then. . . .)

On a scale of 0 to 10, with 0 being no fatigue and 10 being the worst fatigue imaginable, how would you rate your fatigue now?

On a scale of 0 to 10, what is the worst fatigue you have had in the past month?

On a scale of 0 to 10, what has been your usual level of fatigue this past week?

On a scale of 0 to 10, how much is fatigue interfering with yur normal activities?

These assessment questions are easy to remember, take very little time, and give a good deal of information. If the patient has a significant amount of fatigue, a referral may need to be made to other health care professionals such as a psychological consult to rule out depression.

Interventions for CRF

Journaling can help the nurse and the patient to see trends and triggers of fatigue and assist in a design of individually tailored interventions. Several drug companies have free patient journals created for this purpose. Also, patient education handouts are available for free on many health care and cancer websites such as the Oncology Nursing Society, American Cancer Society, and Cancersourcern, and from various pharmaceutical companies.

An occupational therapist (OT) can give instruction on energy conservation measures for the home. The OT may also be able to instruct in sleep hygiene. Napping is kept at a minimum of 30 minutes once or twice a day to prevent deconditioning.

A physical therapist consultant can instruct the patient in exercises that can be done in the sitting or lying positions. Mild exercise can help build stamina and correct or prevent de-conditioning due to inactivity.

Various psychoeducational groups are available both online and in the community. Knowing the available patient resources in a community is a must for oncology nurses in order to provide cancer patient support. Many hospitals, outpatient clinics, and other concerned health care providers offer groups. *I Can Cope* is sponsored by the American Cancer Society and is available in many communities. This program does not focus specifically on fatigue, but can put patients in contact with other patients and health care professionals who may be able to assist them with their concerns.

Energy for Living with Cancer: Managing Cancer Related Fatigue is an eight-week cancer rehabilitation program dealing specifically with cancer related fatigue and safety issues of cancer patients. The educational topics include risk factors, effects on daily life, barriers, and management strategies for cancer related fatigue. Reading and journaling homework assignments are a part of each session. Some examples of session topics include exercise instruction by a physical therapist, energy conservation instruction by an occupational therapist, and Tai Chi instruction by a Tai Chi master. There is also a sharing and support component to each session (Holley & Borger, 2001). This program is currently being offered in the central Florida area.

SUMMARY

The majority of literature on persons with CRF has focused on the prevalence, incidence, correlates, and dimensions of fatigue. Those studies have not addressed the morbidity of CRF or the suffering associated with CRF. The research on fatigue in persons with cancer is primarily descriptive and correlational, and frequently has had conflicting findings. A major limitation of studies has been the lack of a holistic approach to the measurement of the CRF experience on all aspects of the individual's life. In addition, little is heard from the individuals themselves who are experiencing fatigue associated with cancer. All of these studies suggest that fatigue has a tremendous impact on the individual with cancer.

The current oncology nursing literature and texts do not portray the morbidity of the CRF experience as it was described in previous work done by this author (Holley, 2000a). Clearly, the experience of CRF has an impact on the physical, social, spiritual, cognitive, and psychological dimensions of the patients' lives.

REFERENCES

American Cancer Society. (2001). *Cancer Facts and Figures—2001.* Atlanta, GA: American Cancer Society.

Aistars, J. (1987). Fatigue in the cancer patient: A conceptual approach to a clinical problem. *Oncology Nursing Forum, 14:* 25–30.

Benoliel, J. Q. (1985). Loss and adaptation: Circumstances, contingencies, and consequences. *Death Studies, 9,* 217–233.

Cassileth, B. R., Lusk, E. J., Bodenheimer, B. J., Farber, J. M., Jochimsen, P. & Morrin-Taylor, B. (1985). Chemotherapeutic toxicity—the relationship between patients' pretreatment expectations and post-treatment results. *American Journal of Clinical Oncology, 8,* 419–425.

Cella, D. (1997). The Functional Assessment of Cancer Therapy-Anemia (FACT-An Scale: A new tool for the assessment of outcomes in cancer anemia and fatigue. *Seminars in Hematology, 34*(3), Suppl, 13–19.

Christensen, T., Hjorts, N., Mortensen, E., Riis-Hansen, M., & Kehlet, H.(1992). Fatigue and anxiety in surgical patients. *British Journal of Surgery, 79,* 165–168.

Christensen, T., Hougard, F., & Kehlet, H. (1985). Influence of pre- and intraoperative factors on the occurrence of postoperative fatigue. *British Journal of Surgery, 72,* 63–65.

Christensen, T., Kehlet, H., Vertervberg, K., & Vinnars, E. (1987). Fatigue and muscle amino acids during surgical convalescence. *Acta Chirurgica Scandinavica, 153,* 567–570.

Christensen, T., Nygaard, E., & Kehlet, H. (1988). Skeletal muscle fiber composition, nutritional status and subjective fatigue during surgical convalescence. *Acta Chirurgica Scandinavica, 154,* 335–338.

Christensen, T., Nygaard, E., Stage, J. G., & Kehlet, H. (1990). Skeletal muscled enzyme activities and metabolic substrates during exercise in patients with postoperative fatigue. *British Journal of Surgery, 77,* 312–315.

Christensen, T., Stage, J., Galbo, H., Christensen, N., & Kehlet, H. (1991). Fatigue and cardiac and endocrine metabolic response to exercise after abdominal surgery. *Surgery, 105,* 46–50.

Cimprich, B. (1992). Attentional fatigue following breast cancer surgery. *Research in Nursing and Health, 15*(3), 199–207.

Davis, C. A.(1984). Interferon-induced fatigue (Abstract). *Oncology Nursing Forum, 11*(72), 67.

Dean, G., Spears, L., Ferrell, B. R., Quan, W. D. Y., Groshon, S. & Mitchell, M. S. (1995). Fatigue in patients with cancer receiving Interferon Alpha. *Cancer Practice, 3*(3), 164–172.

Driever, M. J. & McCorkle, R. (1984). Patient concerns at three and six months post-diagnosis. *Cancer Nursing, 4*(7), 235–241.

Faithfull, S. (1991). Patients' experiences following cranial radiotherapy: A study of the somnolence syndrome. *Journal of Advanced Nursing, 16*(8), 939–946.

Greene, D., Nail, L. M., Fieler, V. K., Dudgeon, D. & Jones, L. S. (1994). A comparison of patient-reported side effects among three chemotherapy regimens for breast cancer. *Cancer Practice, 2*(1), 57–62.

Greenberg, D., Sawicka, J., Eisenthal, S., & Ross, D. (1992). Fatigue syndrome due to localized radiation. *Journal of Pain and Symptom Management, 7*(1), 38–45.

Gordon, M. (1986). Differential diagnosis of weakness: a common geriatric symptom. *Geriatrics, 41:* 75–79.

Hart, L. K.& Freel, M. I.(1982). Fatigue. In C. M. Norris (Ed.), *Concept clarification in nursing.* Rockville, MD: Aspen.

Haylock, P., & Hart, L. (1979). Fatigue in Patients receiving localized radiation. *Cancer Nursing, 2,* 461–467.

Hjelmstad, L. (1993). *Fine black lines: Reflection on facing cancer, fear, and loneliness.* Englewood, CO: Mulberry Hill.

Holley, S. (2000a). Cancer related fatigue: Suffering a different fatigue. *Cancer Practice, 8*(2), 87–95.

Holley, S. (2000b). Evaluating patient distress from cancer-related fatigue: An instrument development study. *Oncology Nursing Forum, 27*(9), 1425–1431.

Holley, S., & Borger, D. (2001) Energy for living with cancer : Managing cancer related fatigue. A cancer rehabilitation group intervention study. Preliminary findings. *Oncology Nursing Forum, 28*(9), 1393–1396.

Jamar, S. (1989). Fatigue in women receiving chemotherapy for ovarian cancer. In S. Funk, E. Tornquist, M. Champagne, L. Copp, and R. Wiese (Eds.), *Key aspects of comfort.* New York: Springer.

Jones, L. (1994). Correlates of fatigue and related outcomes in individuals with cancer undergoing treatment with chemotherapy. *Dissertation Abstracts Int. (B), 54*(7), 3551.

Kent-Braun, J. A., Miller, R. G., & Weiner, M. W. (1993). Phases of metabolism during progressive exercise to fatigue in human skeletal muscle. *The Journal of Applied Physiology, 161,* 573–580.

King, K. B., Nail, L. M., Kreamer, K., Strohl, R., & Johnson, J. (1985). Patients descriptions of the experience of receiving radiation therapy. *Oncology Nursing Forum, 12,* 55–61.

Kobashi-Schoot, J., Hanewald, G., Van Dam, F., & Bruning, P. (1985). Assessment of malaise in cancer patients treated with radiotherapy. *Cancer Nursing, 8*(6), 306–313.

Kurtz, M., Kurtz, J., Given, C., & Given, B. (1993). Loss of physical functioning among patients with cancer. *Cancer Practice, 1*(4), 275–281.

McCorkle, R., & Quint-Benoliel, J. (1986). Symptom distress, current concerns and mood disturbance after diagnosis of life-threatening disease. *Social Science Medicine, 17*(7), 431–438.

McCorkle, R., & Young, L. (1978). Development of a symptom distress scale. *Cancer Nursing, 2*(3), 373–378.

Miller, R. G., Boska, M. D., Moussavi, R. S., Carson, P. J., & Weiner, M. W. (1988). 31P nuclear magnetic resonance studies of high energy phosphates and pH in human muscle fatigue. *Journal of Clinical Investigation, 81,* 1190–1196.

Morrow, G. R., Pandya, L., Barry, M., DiFino, S., Jennings, P., Flynn, P., Rosenbluth, R., & Dakhil, S. (1992). Chemotherapy-induced fatigue and patient-reported psychological depression (Meeting Abstract). *Proceedings of the Annual Meeting of the American Society of Clinical Oncology, 11,* A1329.

Musser, E. H. (1990). The self-reported needs of women with breast cancer who have recently completed treatment with chemotherapy (Meeting Abstract). *Oncology Nursing Forum, 17*(2 Suppl), 144.

Nail, L. M. & King, K. B. (1987). Fatigue. *Seminars in Oncology Nursing, 3,* 257–262.

Pickard-Holley, S. (1991). Fatigue in cancer patients: A descriptive study. *Cancer Nursing, 14*(1), 13–19.

Piper, B. F. (1993). Subjective fatigue in women receiving six cycles of adjuvant chemotherapy for breast cancer. *Dissertation Abstracts Int (B), 54*(1), 168.

Piper, B. F., Dibble, S. L., Dodd, M. J., Weiss, M. C., Slaughter, R. E., & Paul, S. M. (1998). The revised Piper Fatigue Scale: Psychometric evaluation in women with breast cancer. *Oncology Nursing Forum, 25*(4), 677–684.

Piper, B., Rieger, P., Brophy, L., Haeuber, D., Hood, L., Lyver, A., & Sharp, E. (1989). Recent advances in the management of bio-therapy-related side effects: fatigue. *Oncology Nursing Forum, 16*(supplement), 27–34.

Rhodes, V., Watson, P., & Hanson, B. (1988). Patients' descriptions of the influence of tiredness and weakness on self-care abilities. *Cancer Nursing, 11,* 188–194.

Rhoten, D. (1982). Fatigue and the postsurgical patient. In C. M. Norris (Ed.), *Concept clarification in nursing.* Rockville, MD: Aspen.

Richardson, A., Ream, E., & Wilson-Barnett, J. (1998). Fatigue in patients receiving chemotherapy: Patterns of change. *Cancer Nursing, 21*(1), 17–30.

St. Pierre, B., Kasper, C., & Lindsey, A. (1992). Fatigue mechanisms in patients with cancer: Effects of tumor necrosis factor and exercise on skeletal muscle. *Oncology Nursing Forum, 19*(3), 419–425.

Sarna, L. (1993). Correlates of symptom distress in women with lung cancer. *Cancer Practice, 1*(1), 21–28.

Schroeder, D., & Hill, G. (1993). Predicting postoperative fatigue: The importance of preoperative factors. *World Journal of Surgery, 17*(2), 226–231.

Spross, J. A. (1993). Pain, suffering and spiritual well-being: Assessment and interventions. *Quality of Life, 2,* 71–79.

Stein, K., Martin, S., Hann, D., & Jacobsen, P. (1998). A multidimensional measure of fatigue for use with cancer patients. *Cancer Practice, 6*(3), 143–152.

Strauman, J. J. (1986). Symptom distress in patients receiving phase I chemotherapy with Taxol. *Oncology Nursing Forum, 13*(5), 40–43.

Swartz, A. (1998). The Schwartz Cancer Fatigue Scale: Testing reliability and validity. *Oncology Nursing Forum, 25*(4), 711–717.

Weiner, M. W., Moussavi, R. S., Baker, A. J., Boska, M. D. & Miller, R.G. (1990). Constant relationships between force, phosphate concentration, and pH in muscles with differential fatigability. *Neurology, 40,* 1888–1893.

Zeiderman, M., Welchew, E., & Clark, R. (1990). Changes in cardio-respiratory and muscle function associated with the development of postoperative fatigue. *British Journal of Surgery, 77,* 576–580.

CHAPTER ELEVEN

Cancer-Related Anemia

Lodovico Balducci and Janine Overcash

A nemia and fatigue are often strictly interwoven (Cleeland et al., 1999; Demetri et al., 1998; Gabrilove et al., 1999; Gabrilove et al., 2000; Glaspy et al., 1998). Both conditions are relevant to the management of elderly cancer patients. This chapter is divided into two sections. The first concerns the prevalence, causes, consequences, and management of anemia in the older aged person, the second the causes, the consequences, and the management of fatigue in older cancer patients.

PREVALENCE AND CAUSES OF ANEMIA

Anemia has been defined by the World Health Organization (WHO) as hemoglobin concentration lower than 12 gm/dl in women and 13gm/dl in men (Ania et al., 1997). This definition has many merits in that it is based on large cross-sectional surveys of a population without known infirmity. It is consistent with the observation that the endogenous secretion of erythropoietin increases when hemoglobin values drop below 12 gm/dl (Goodnough et al., 1995). Clearly, the tissue oxygenation is sub-optimal for hemoglobin levels below 12 gm/dl, as the secretion of erythropoietin is stimulated by hypoxia. It is consistent with the observation that the risk of surgical complications increases below 12 gn/dl. It is consistent with the recent report that cardiac mortality in coronary care units was increased for patients with an hematocrit $\geq$ 33% (grossly equivalent to a hemoglobin of 11.5 gm/dl), if they did not receive blood transfusions (Wu et al.).

This definition is also problematic for two reasons. The first, a recent report from the Woman Health Study, showed that hemoglobin values lower than 13.4 gm/dl were an independent risk factor for death in healthy women aged 65 and older followed longitudinally (Chaves et al., 2001). The other reason is that two large studies (Gabrilove et al., 1999; Cleeland et al., 1999) showed that the highest incremental improvement in fatigue in cancer patients was obtained when the hemoglobin levels rose from 11 to 13 gm/dl. This observation suggests that the tissue oxygenation obtainable with hemoglobin levels over 12 gm/dl may be beneficial. For the purpose of this chapter we will entertain the WHO definition of anemia, with the understanding that this definition is still undergoing development.

Two epidemiological observations are of special interest in that they are opposite of each other. In a large cross-section of Italian patients (Imelmen et al., 1994), the average hemoglobin value did not change with age, at least until age 85. Conversely, in other studies both the prevalence (Ania, Suman, Fairbanks, Rademacher, & Melton, 1994; Smith, 2000) and the incidence (Ania, 1997) of anemia increased with age. The likely conclusions of these observations are that anemia is not a component of normal aging, at least until age 85, and that the prevalence and the incidence of conditions that cause anemia increase with the age of the population. Perhaps the best understanding of the causes of anemia in the elderly has been provided in a longitudinal study by Ania et al. (1997) (Table 11.1). From the examination of the records of the 98% of the population living in Olmstead County, Minnesota, these authors established that anemia of chronic disorders and iron deficiency accounted for more than 50% of the causes of anemia. Of special interest was the observation, reported also by other authors (Balducci & Hardy, 1998), that in approximately 20% of

TABLE 11.1 Causes of Chronic Anemias in Elderly Patients

Cause	Prevalence (%)
Post-hemorrhagic	7
Iron deficiency	15
Chronic disease	35
Unexplained causes	17
Renal failure, liver, and endocrine disease	6.5
Myelodysplasia or acute leukemia	5.5
Chronic leukemia or lymphoma	5.5
Vitamin B_{12} or folate deficiency	5.5
Other hematological disease	3

cases the cause of anemia was not apparent. A rationale for this occurrence could be that the number of cases reported actually represents early or undiagnosed myelodysplasia, whose incidence increases with age (Balducci & Hardy, 1998). Moreover, undiagnosed renal insufficiency may account for the majority of cases, despite a normal serum creatinine. The glomerular filtration rate declines in the majority of aging persons (Duthie, 1998), and this decline may be associated with a lower erythropoietin production. This type of anemia is reversible, thanks to the availability of recombinant erythropoietin (NIH Healthy People, 2000). Another possibility includes relative erythropoietin deficiency, which is production of erythropoietin that is inadequate for the degree of anemia (Goodnough, 1995; Hochberg, 1988). This possibility has been well documented, albeit not in the majority of older individuals (Balducci & Hardy, 1998; Balducci et al., 2001; Powers et al., 1991). This condition would be reversible with pharmacological doses of erythropoietin. Aging is associated with increased circulating concentrations of Tumor Necrosis Factor and Interleukin 6 (Hamerman et al., 1999), which are known to antagonize erythropoietin and cause anemia. In this situation, erythropoietin in pharmacological doses may help control the anemia (Figure 11.1). In this construct, anemia causes an accumulation of catabolic cytokines that in turn aggravate more anemia. In the meantime, the prevalence and severity of age-related organ dysfunction may increase as well due to catabolic cytokines. Erythropoietin might offset this self-aggrandizing process and in this way prevent the organ dysfunction of aging. A number of endocrine and nutritional effects may be responsible for anemia in older individuals. Of special interest are B12 deficiency and protein-calorie malnutrition, both reversible conditions (Balducci & Hardy, 1998).

DIFFERENTIAL DIAGNOSIS OF ANEMIA

The diagnostic workup of anemia is summarized in Figure 11.2. Essentially, anemia may be produced by one of two mechanisms—increased red blood cell loss and decreased red blood cell production. This distinction is easily made by measuring the reticulocyte count, which reflects the production of new red blood cell (RBC) in the bone marrow. If the reticulocyte count is low, the assessment of the RBC volume may help identifying the cause of the anemia. The diagnostic investigations for each type of anemia are listed in Table 11.2. It is imperative to understand the difference between iron deficiency anemia and anemia of chronic diseases. In iron deficiency the anemia is due to the fact that red blood cells cannot manufacture hemoglobin due to the scarcity of iron. In anemia of chronic diseases, instead, the

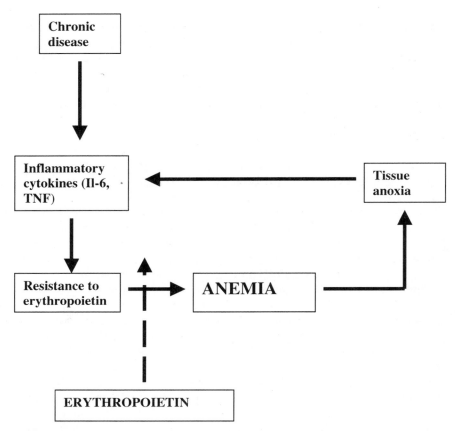

FIGURE 11.1 Hypothetical Activity of Erythropoietin in Reversing the Vicious Circle of Aging.

iron reserves are plentiful, but inaccessible, due to the effects of circulating cytokines that prevent iron utilization: it is a situation similar to that of an American having a checking account in a country hostile to the USA. The money is there, but cannot be withdrawn from the bank. The determination of the serum ferritin level, which reflects the iron reserves of the bone marrow, is essential to the differential diagnosis. The only situation in which this test is not reliable is in presence of an acute disease, in which case the level of free transferrin receptor concentration may establish the diagnosis.

Some important considerations related to elderly individuals are necessary when performing an assessment of anemia (Balducci & Hardy, 1998). First, the RBC volume should not be used as an absolute

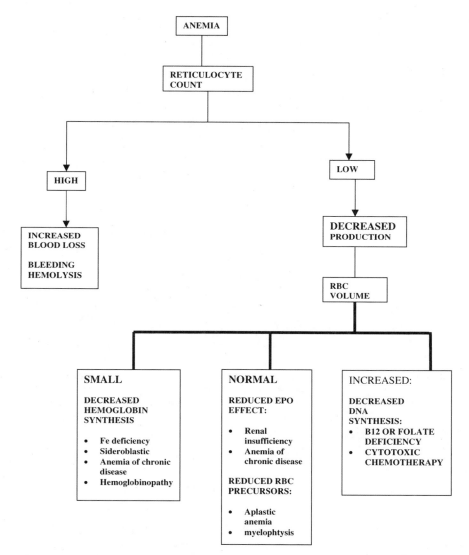

FIGURE 11.2 Algorithm for the Diagnostic Work-Up of Anemia.

guidance in the diagnostic workup, because multiple deficiencies with opposite effects on RBC volume are not uncommon with aging. For example, simultaneous iron and B12 deficiency may result in normocytic, rather than microcytic or megaloblastic anemia. B12 levels lower than 300 pg/dl should always be considered abnormal and treated

TABLE 11.2 Diagnostic Investigations of Anemia

Anemia suspected	Laboratory investigation	Clinical implications
Hemolytic anemia	Increased reticulocyte count, serum LDH and bilirubin	
Microvascular	Schystocytes in peripheral blood smear	Consider cancer Disseminated intravascular coagulation; thrombotic thrombocytopenic purpura, diabetes, hypertensive crisis, trauma
Autoimmune	Direct Coombs test Cold agglutinin RBC aggregates, microspherocytes, and ghost cell in peripheral blood	Lymphoproliferative disorders
FE Deficiency	Serum FE low, Fe Binding capacity increased and serum ferritin decreased; soluble transferrin receptors increased	Chronic blood loss (GI, genitourinary tract) Veganism (for 10 or more years)
Anemia of chronic disease	Serum Fe low Serum Iron binding capacity low Serum ferritin increased Free transferrin receptors: decreased Serum erytropoietin: may be inadequate to the degree of anemia	Chronic conditions (Cancer, arthritis, diabetes, chronic infections)
Anemia of renal insufficiency	GFR < 50 ml/minutes Serum erythropoietin low	Renal insufficiency
B12 or folate deficiency	B12 or folate levels low	Pernicious anemia; nutritional anemia

with B12 replacement. It should be remembered that B12 deficiency may also cause nervous disturbances, including dementia. The most common cause of B12 deficiency in older individuals is poor digestion of food B12 from gastric achylia (insufficient production of hydrochloric acid). These patients may receive oral, rather than parenteral, B12 replacement. Serum erythopoietin levels should always be obtained, in presence of hypo-proliferative anemia, due to the possibility of absolute or relative erythropoietin deficiency. Bone marrow aspiration and biopsy are mandatory in all cases in which there is pancytopenia, if one suspects myelophtysis (invasion of the bone marrow by neoplasia, infection or fibrosis), and whenever the cause of anemia is not clear.

The role of the nurse is pivotal in the diagnosis and management of anemia. On the forefront of the practice the nurse is the first to have access to the laboratory report in both primary care and specialistic clinic. It is not unusual for the nurse to initiate the work-up of abnormal values. In particular, in the geriatric patient, anemia has been all but ignored until recently, almost considered an expected consequence of age. This misconception may have had tragic consequences, including delayed diagnosis of a malignancy, such as cancer of the large bowel, at a stage when it was still curable. Progressive functional, cognitive, and medical deterioration of the older person, and increased mortality are issues associated with anemia and can be addressed by the nurse (Chavas et al., 2001; Izsak et al., 2001).

Despite the increased awareness of the problem, anemia in the elderly is still under-diagnosed and undertreated. As a patient advocate and as a health care educator, the nurse has unique opportunities for promoting this awareness. Finally, anemia is the main cause of fatigue, the most devastating chronic symptom of cancer, and an important realm of nursing intervention (Vailidres et al., 2001).

WHY ANEMIA SHOULD BE INVESTIGATED AND TREATED IN OLDER INDIVIDUALS

As mentioned before, anemia should not be considered a normal consequence of aging at least up to age 85; hence anemia, even mild anemia, may be an indicator of an underlying disease. While we cannot exhaust in this brief review all possible causes of anemia, some common pathologies will be identified.

Iron-deficiency anemia is always a sign of bleeding, generally chronic bleeding, unless a patient has been a vegan for ten or more years. Hence, iron deficiency should be worked up with investigation of the upper and lower gastrointestinal tract. In addition to cancer of the large bowel and of the stomach, diverticular disease of the large bowel, peptic ulcer, and angiodysplasia are common causes of chronic bleeding in older individuals. The diagnosis is important because it may provide a cure in some cases, and improvement of symptoms in most cases. Other cause of iron deficiency deserving to be investigated include chronic intravascual hemolysis, due to microvascular disease of red blood cell trauma (as it occurs in the presence of artificial cardiac valve).

B12 deficiency is associated with subtle neurological changes that may eventually lead to dementia. A megaloblastic anemia may reveal this deficiency and allow B12 replenishment, which will prevent the neurologic changes. Megaloblastic anemia may be a sign of underlying hypothyroidism, which in elderly individuals may be lethal unless treated in a timely manner.

Anemia may be an early sign of myelodysplasia, a preleukemic condition whose incidence and prevalence increase with age. In the early stages, myelodysplasia may be ameliorated by erythropoietin. In addition, a number of agents undergoing clinical trials may prevent the progression of myelodysplasia. Anemia and pancytopenia may be the first signs of a malignancy involving the bone marrow, especially a hematological malignancy. Anemia of chronic renal insufficiency and anemia of chronic diseases are reversible with erythopoietin treatment, and their diagnosis should be clearly documented.

In addition, anemia itself is a cause of severe morbidity and mortality and aggressive treatment is warranted. At least three studies (Chavas et al., 2001; Iszak et al., 1999; Kikuchi et al., 2001) showed anemia to be an independent risk factor for death in older individuals. The study of Chavas is very provocative because it showed that values of hemoglobin as high as 13.4 mg/dl may be associated with increased risk of death. Anemia may lead to fatigue, which in turn in older individuals may lead to functional dependence (Liao and Ferrell, 2000). Additionally, anemia may cause severe cardiovascular complications, including congestive heart failure, and death from coronary artery disease (Metivier et al., 2000; Silverberg et al., 2000; Wu et al., 2001). Cognitive decline in older individuals may also be the result of anemia (Brines et al., 2000; Pickett et al., 1999). Of special interest, erythropoietin seems to protect the brain in condition of injury. As already discussed and expressed in Figure 11.1, treatment of anemia may reverse or delay aging itself by preventing the accumulation of more catabolic cytokines in the circulation.

The management of anemia involves the treatment of the underlying disease, when that is possible. Initially, blood transfusions for an emergency (chest pain, symptoms of heart failure), or when the hemoglobin levels are below 8 gm/dl (10 gm/dl for patients with coronary artery disease) are vital. The nurse's first responsibility is to stabilize the patient. The use of erythropoietin in patients with renal insufficiency, cancer, rheumatoid arthritis, and other chronic diseases, when an absolute or relative erythropoietin deficit is present, is also a common component of the treatment plan (Chavas et al., 2001; Cleeland et al., 1999; Gabrilove et al., 1999).

ANEMIA-RELATED FATIGUE IN THE OLDER CANCER PATIENT

Fatigue is the most common chronic symptom of cancer and cancer treatment (Rieger 2001), and it is often caused by anemia. Fatigue in general is discussed in the prior chapter but its general relation to a remote will be discussed here. Fatigue involves a sensation of lack of energy that does not recover with rest, unlike normal tiredness, and that prevents the subject from having regular activity and conducting a normal life. (Cleeland CS, 2001). The social and emotional effects of fatigue cannot be overrated. Approximately 50% of the patients experiencing fatigue and 25% of their caregivers need to change jobs or quit their jobs altogether because of fatigue (Rieger et al., 2001). In older individuals, fatigue is associated with functional dependence (Liao and Ferrell), which may lead to a progressive functional decline, failure to thrive, and death. Even when functional dependence is reversible, rehabilitation may take several months, during which cancer treatment is aborted. Hence fatigue may result in undertreatment of cancer and worsening of its prognosis. Last but not least, functional dependence is the cause of major expenditure due to the employment of a full-time caregiver and to the nutritional, emotional, functional, and medical complications of reduced mobility. Clearly, fatigue needs to be addressed, prevented, and aggressively treated.

The main obstacle to the effective management of fatigue has been under-recognition and under-management of the symptoms. One of the major feathers in the hat of the nursing profession has been the original description of fatigue and the development of instrument capable to detect and quantify this devastating symptom. Of the most recent advances in medicine during the last twenty years, certainly symptom management has been one of the most significant in improving a person's outlook and quality of life, in translating the scary medical jargon into a familiar and friendly conversation. Of the several instruments available for the measurement of fatigue, two have been validated in older cancer patients: the functional assessment of cancer therapy general (FACT-G) (Overcash, 1998) and the Multidimensional Fatigue Symptom Inventory (MFSI) (Respini et al., 2002). Either instrument is very user-friendly and available for clinical practice.

As fatigue is multidimensional, the causes of this symptom are multiple; in general two groups of causes are recognized: energy imbalance and emotional distress, including pain, depression, anxiety, etc. (Gutstein, 2001). Major causes of energy imbalance include:

Anemia
Cachexia
Infection
Metabolic disorders

It is important to highlight the role of catabolic cytokines in each of these conditions, since the concentration of catabolic cytokines increases in the circulation with aging. In addition to TNF and IL-6, other cytokines of interest include Interleukin-1, interferons, leukemia inhibitory factor ciliary neurotrophic factor, and corticotrophin-releasing factor (Kurzrock, 2001). A number of agents, capable of antagonizing these substances, are undergoing clinical trials.

The management of fatigue requires an appreciation of the causes. The management of anemia, when this is present, is the mainstay of the treatment of fatigue. In this respect the use of erythropoietin has been invaluable. In multiple studies, summarized by Glaspy (2001), correction of anemia has been associated with improvement in fatigue. Since the highest incremental improvement in fatigue has been obtained when hemoglobin levels rose from 11 to 11 gm/dl, it is reasonable to recommend that the levels of HB be maintained at 12 gm/dl. In the meantime, the patient should be evaluated for depression and malnutrition: if depression is present it should be pharmacologically treated, while malnutrition should be reversed. Other treatments undergoing clinical trials include psychostimulants, such as methyphedinate, glucocorticoids, and the antidepressants inhibiting serotonine uptake (Burks, 2001). Nonpharmacological approaches, including regular exercise and support psychotherapy, are also desirable. Research in the management of fatigue should include:

- Prevention of anemia during chemotherapy, with erythropoietin;
- Role of exercise in randomized-controlled study;
- Role of psychostimulants in combination with erythropoietin;
- Role of medications that inhibit the action of catabolic cytokines, such as thalidomide.

REFERENCES

Anía, B. J., Suman, V. J., Fairbanks, V. F., & Melton, J. L. (1994). Prevalence of anemia in medical practice: Community versus referral patients. *Mayo Clinics Proceedings, 69,* 730–735.

Anía, B. J., Suman, V. J., Fairbanks, V. F., Rademacher, D. M., & Melton, J. L. (1997). Incidence of anemia in older people: an epidemiologic study in a well defined population. *Journal of the American Geriatrics Society, 45,* 825–831.

Balducci, L., & Hardy, C. S. (1998). Anemia of aging: a model of cancer-related anemia. *Cancer Control, 5,* Suppl. 17–21.

Balducci, L., Hardy, C. H., & Lyman, G. H. (2001). Hemopoietic growth factors and aging. *Current Opinions in Hematology, 12,* 125–132.

Brines, M. L., Ghezzi, P., Keenan, S., Agnello, D., de Lanerolle, N. C., Cerami, C. et al. Erythropoietin crosses the blood–brain barrier to protect against experimental brain injury. *PNAS, 97*(19):10526–10531.

Burks, T. F. (2001). New agents for the treatment of cancer-related fatigue. *Cancer, 92,* S6, 1714–1718.

Chaves, P. H., Volpato, S., & Fried, L. (2001). Challenging the world health organization criteria for anemia in the older woman. *Journal of the American Geriatrics Society, 49,* S3, A10.

Cleeland, C. S. (2001). Introduction, *Cancer, 92,* S6, 1657–1661.

Cleeland, C. S., Demetri, G. D., Glaspy, J. et al. Identifying hemoglobin levels for optimal quality of life: results of an incremental analysis. *Proceedings of the American Society of Clinical Oncology, 18,* 574a.

Demetri, G. D., Kris, M., Wade, J. et al: (1998). Quality of life benefits in chemotherapy patients treated with epoietin alfa is independent from disease response and tumor type. Result of a prospective community oncology study. The procrit study group. *Journal of Clinical Oncology, 16,* 3412–3420.

Duthie, E. (1998). Physiology of aging: relvance to symptom perceptions and treatment tolerance. In L. Balducci, G.H. Lyman, & W. B. Ershler (Eds.), *Comprehensive geriatric oncology* (pp. 247–326). London: Harwood Academic Publishers.

Gabrilove, J. (2000). Overview: erythropoiesis, anemia, and the impact of erythropoietin. *Seminars in Hematology, 37*(4 Suppl 6):1–3.

Gabrilove, J. L., Einhorn, L. H., Livingston, R. B., et al. Once weekly dosing of epoetin alfa is similar to three-times weekly dosing in increasing hemoglobin and quality of life. *Proceedings of the American Society of Clinical Oncology, 18,* 574a.

Glaspy, J. (2001). Anemia and fatigue in cancer patients. *Cancer, 92,* S6, 1719–1724.

Glaspy, J., Bukowski, R., Steinberg, C. et al. (1997). Impact of therapy with epoietin alfa on clinical outcomes in patients with non-myeloid malignancies during cancer chemotherapy in community oncology practices. *Journal of Clinical Oncology, 5,* 1218–1234.

Goodnough, L. T., Price, T. H., & Parvin, C. A. (1995). The endogenous erythropoietin response and the erythropoietic response to blood loss anemia: the effects of age and gender. *Journal of Laboratory Clinical Medicine, 126*(1), 57–64.

Gutstein, H. B. (2001). The biologic basis of fatigue. *Cancer, 92,* S6, 1678–1683.

Hamermann, D., Berman, J. W., Albers, G. W. et al. (1999). Emerging evidence for inflammation in conditions frequently affecting older adults: report of a symposium. *Journal of the American Geriatrics Society, 47,* 995–999.

Hochberg, M. C., Arnold, C. M., Hogans, B. B. et al: Serum immunoreactive erythropietin in Rheumatoid Arthritis impaired response to anemia. *Arthritis and Rheumatism, 31,* 1318–1321.

Kikuchi, M., Inagaki, T., & Shinagawa, N. (2001). Five-year survival of older people with anemia: variation with hemoglobin concentration. *Journal of the American Geriatrics Society, 49,* 1226–1228.

Kurzrock, R. (2001). The role of cytokines in cancer-related fatigue. *Cancer, 92,* S6, 1684–1688.

Inelmen, E. M., Alessio, M. D., Gatto, M. R. A., Baggio, M. B., Jimenez, G., Bizzotto, M. G., & Enzi, G. (1994). Descriptive analysis of the prevalence of anemia in a randomly selected sample of elderly people at home: some results of an Italian multicentric study. *Aging Clinical Experimental Research, 6,* 81–89.

Liao, S. & Ferrell, B. A. (2000). Fatigue in an older population. *Journal of the American Geriatrics Society, 48,* 426–430.

Metivier, F., Marchais, S. J., Guerin, A. P., Pannier, B., & London, G. M. (2000). Pathophysiology of anaemia: focus on the heart and blood vessels. *Nephrology and Dialysis Transplant, 15*(3):14–18.

NIH Healthy People 2000; Healthy people 2010: chronic kidney disease 2000; National Institute of Diabetes and Digestive and Kidney Diseases. Public Health Service. Healthy people 2000: national health promotion and disease prevention objectives. Washington, DC: US Department of Health and Human Services, Public Health Service, 1990; DHHS publication no. (PHS)90–50212.

Overcash, J. (1998). Symptom management in the geriatric patient. *Cancer Control, 5,* 46–47.

Pickett, J. L., Theberge, D. C., Brown, W. S., Schweitzer, S. U. , & Nissenson, A. R. (1999). Normalizing hematocrit in dialysis patients improves brain function. *American Journal of Kidney Disease, 33*(6), 1122–1130.

Powers, J. S., Kantz, S. B., Collins, J. C. et al. (1991). Erythropoietin response to anemia as a function of age. *Journal of the American Geriatrics Society, 39,* 30–32.

Rathore, S. S., Wang, Y. et al. (2001). Blood transfusions in elderly patients with acute myocardial infarction, *New England Journal of Medicine, 345,* 1230–1236.

Respini, D., Jacobsen, P. B., Thors, C. et al. (In Press). Issues of fatigue in the elderly. *European Journal of Cancer.*

Rieger, P. T. (2001). Assessment and epidemiologic issues related to fatigue. *Cancer, S6,* 1733–1736.

Silverberg, D. S., Wexler, D., Blum, M. et al. (2000). The use of subcutaneous erythropoietin and intravenous iron for the treatment of the anemia of severe, resistant congestive heart failure improves cardiac and renal function and functional cardiac class, and markedly reduces hospitalizations. *Journal of the American College of Cardiology, 35,* 1737–1744.

Smith, D. L. (2000). Anemia in the elderly. *American Family Physician, 62*(7):1565–1572.

Vailidres, R. U., Escalante, C., & Manzullo, E. (2001). Fatigue and debilitating symptoms. *Nursing Clinics of North America, 36,* 685–694.

CHAPTER TWELVE

Caring When Cure Is No Longer Possible

Ira Byock and Yvonne Corbeil

CARING WHEN CURE IS NO LONGER POSSIBLE

Care for persons who are dying is at once simple and complex. Comprehensive care for terminally ill patients is complex because dying is a multidimensional, multifactorial experience for the person whose life is ending. The evaluation and management of physical symptoms, such as neuropathic pain, intermittent bowel obstruction, or pruritus, are likely to require anatomic, physiologic, and pharmacologic considerations. Similarly, the psychological and medical evaluation and treatment of depression or of intermittent confusion in a patient with far-advanced disease may prove intricate and complex.

However, each of these clinical tasks is encompassed within a simple and straightforward orientation toward care for people who are dying and support for their families. As modeled by contemporary hospice/palliative care programs, care for people who are dying is organized around two major goals—alleviation of suffering and enhancement of the person's and family's ongoing quality of life. The concept of personhood and a model of lifelong human development can be applied to understand the nature of suffering, as well as quality of life of people living with progressive illness, disability, and the approach of death. This chapter is intended to provide the reader with an understanding of this care.

PERSONHOOD, SUFFERING, AND QUALITY OF LIFE

There are two poles of human experience associated with the last phase of life—suffering at one extreme, and a sense of well-being at the other. Suffering is the term that best describes the human experience of pervasive distress associated with dying. Cassell defines suffering as the state of severe distress that is associated with a perceived threat to the integrity of the individual.[1] Personhood in this model is conceived as a dynamic multidimensional matrix of spheres that collectively comprise one's experienced identity or sense of self. The dimensions include one's body (physical self), mind, past, family of origin, present family, culture, ethnicity, spiritual beliefs, political beliefs, roles in family (Mom/Dad, sibling, child), roles at work and organizations, preferences, aversions, habits, and so forth. (Figure 12.1)

A sense of meaning about who one is pervades a person's experience of self. A sense of meaning serves as a meshwork on and through which the process of personhood is woven.[2,3] Damage to this crucial dimension of self inevitably causes suffering, as if personhood were unraveling.

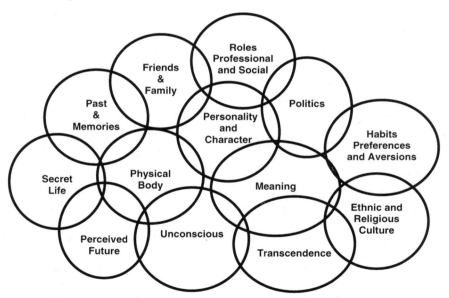

FIGURE 12.1 Cassell's Domains of Personhood
Adapted from Cassell, E. J. "The Nature of Suffering and the Goals of Medicine." *New England Journal of Medicine* 306, no. 11 (1982): 639–45.

If suffering occurs when a person experiences himself or herself to be coming apart and if the loss of meaning represents an *unraveling* of personhood, suffering among the dying could be expected to be universal and irremediable. Debilitated by illness, ultimately perhaps confined to bed, a person's sense of self is clearly assaulted. Empirically, however, we know that suffering is neither universal nor beyond our ability to affect through clinical interventions.

Interestingly, some people confronting the last phases of living report a new sense of wholeness and well-being despite progressive decline in function, the loss of roles, and the loss of relationships.[4,5,6,7] Herein lies the essence of the phrase *'healing versus curing.'* Seasoned clinicians working in palliative care recognize that people who have been hardened and made cynical by life frequently soften when illness forces them to accept kindness and caring from others. Anger that has kept one at odds with a family member or previous close friend commonly gives way to an attitude of openness to reconciliation. Those who have long felt isolated may once again, or for the first time, be able to feel loved. Such experiences are difficult to explain within the context of present-day health care, focused as it is on disease, medical treatment, and issues of service delivery and cost. Within hospitals and clinical settings, relief of suffering is the highest goal; however, it is too infrequently attained.[8-12] In these settings few dying persons experience an elevated quality of life and, when they do, these experiences go largely unrecognized.[13,14]

The phenomenology of positive experience in the phase of life called *dying* is of profound importance to developing a clinical approach to caring for people at the end of life. Instances of patients' and families' transitions from suffering to a sense of wellness and peacefulness are fundamental to understanding the human encounter with death. Patients and families have much to teach us about defining meaningful goals and emotional, spiritual, and social interventions that may provide support during this phase of life and through the process of dying.[15-22]

In examining the range of human experience associated with dying, one principle becomes clear. Although symptom management is the first priority for palliative care, it is not the ultimate goal. True person and family-centered care at the end of life strives not only to ensure comfort, but also to improve quality of life for people who are dying and for their families. This includes helping to preserve opportunities for them to grow through times of illness, caregiving, death, and grief.[23,24]

SYSTEMS ISSUES

INTEGRATING AND COMPLETING THE CONTINUUM OF CANCER CARE

Nurses working in oncology routinely encounter patients whose illness progresses despite aggressive efforts to extend life. While there have been important advances in cancer care over the past several decades, and recent remarkable progress in treating a few specific neoplasms, approximately half of all patients diagnosed with cancer will eventually die as a consequence of their illness or related complications. Caring for people as they die is, therefore, an integral part of oncology nursing practice.

In its statement on Cancer Care During the Last Phase of Life,[25] the American Society of Clinical Oncology has stated:

> "Cancer care optimizes quality of life throughout the course of an illness through meticulous attention to the myriad physical, spiritual, and psychosocial needs of the patient and family. ASCO believes that provision of optimal end-of-life care requires access to and availability of state-of-the-art palliative care rendered by skilled clinicians, buttressed when necessary, by palliative care experts."

Currently, comprehensive palliative care is often instituted only after life-prolonging care is no longer available, and effective treatment options have been exhausted, or have been rejected by the patient. (Figure 12.2a) However, the precepts of palliative care emphasize the importance of continuity of care, symptom management, skillful communication and psychosocial support throughout the course of illness[26,27] (Figure 12.2b). The continuity of palliative care in the management of patients with progressive cancer is well represented by the simple diagram in the World Health Organization monograph on palliative care.[28]

Correctly understood, palliative care represents a "both-and" model of care, enabling a seamless transition from mostly curative and life-prolonging treatments to therapeutic interventions for improving comfort and enhancing quality of life. As a patient's disease advances and there is proportionately less to offer in terms of life-prolongation, it is logical and natural for the goals of care to progress toward comfort and quality of remaining life. Thus, palliative and life-prolonging efforts complement one another and can properly proceed simultaneously.

The principle of proportionality, weighing the potential benefits of an available intervention against the risks, underlies the process of care planning and decision-making. The values and self-defined goals

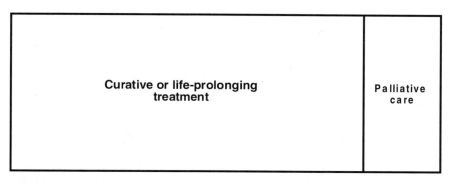

FIGURE 12.2a

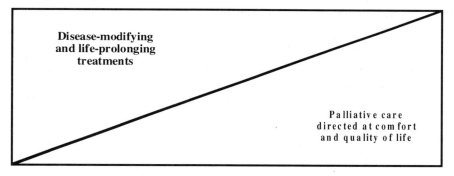

FIGURE 12.1b

Both figures adapted from Cancer Pain Relief and Palliative Care. Technical Report Series 804. Geneva: World Health Organization, 1990.

of the person, as well as the person's currently experienced quality of life, form the fulcrum for this ongoing decision-making process. At times, even as the end of life approaches, some life-prolonging measures may be warranted if they have potential for advancing the person's goals at a risk that is deemed acceptable. Such may be the case with yearly immunization against influenza, or oral antibiotic treatment for respiratory infection with fever in a debilitated, but stable patient.

This smooth progression of care requires excellent communication and coordination of a skilled interdisciplinary team. It also requires ongoing involvement of the patient and family actively participating in the care planning and decision making as partners in care delivery. The nurse's role is central to this interdisciplinary, patient-family centered approach.[29,30] The inherently intimate nurse/patient therapeutic relationship provides a privileged opportunity for the nurse to work closely with the patient and family in coordinating care and treatment with other members of the caregiving team.

Caring for the elderly dying patient presents particular challenges. Comorbid medical conditions and disabilities increase susceptibility to complications and add to the symptom burden. Skillful care requires oncology nurses to be knowledgeable about the physiological changes in the aging process, concomitant illness, such as diabetes, renal disease, and congestive heart failure, which may impact progressive illness and alter pharmacokinetics and response to treatment. Additionally, the social content frequently involves supporting and educating informal caregivers who may also be elderly.[31] The accumulated life experience of older adults inevitably contributes to preconceptions, of which they may be unaware, but which can impact the quality of their lives during illness, caregiving, and grief. Uncovering these expectations, hopes, and fears during early evaluation enables clinicians to be alert for particular values and concerns of a patient and family. This is often best accomplished by listening to people's stories of others they have known during illness and dying. This developed level of familiarity with patients and their families enables clinicians to prevent specific problems that people dread. It also allows clinicians to be reassuring and help people focus on realizing their own aspirations.

CASE MANAGEMENT AND CARE PLANNING

The process of ongoing care planning involving the patient with his or her family underpins this seamless model of life-prolonging and palliative care. At each point from diagnosis through death, the patient or surrogate retains the right to make informed choices among a full range of indicated and available options for care. Introducing the goals of comfort and quality of life and the concept of palliative interventions early in treatment establishes a foundation that extends continuity of care through the end of a patient's life, and extends support to the family during bereavement. Advance care planning often includes completion of documents, such as a living will conveying an individual's preferences for care and a durable power of attorney for health care formally appointing a proxy to make decisions if the person becomes unable to decide for himself or herself. Increasingly, the term advance care planning encompasses the iterative process of discussion that identifies patient and family values, assesses their needs, and weighs the risks and benefits of each therapeutic option in making decisions for the short and mid-term future.

Even at the time of diagnosis, professional caregivers err if they assume that every patient confronting a serious, life-threatening illness will choose aggressive life-prolonging care. It is particularly important in caring for the elderly patient to establish a context for medical decision-making that is rooted in the person's values, life goals, and general preferences. Some patients carefully consider all options and decide to forgo curative or remissive therapies despite a fair chance of disease-modifying efficacy. Inevitably there will be instances when clinicians disagree with the choices a patient or family makes. It can be intensely frustrating and emotionally painful for a nurse or doctor who feels that surgery, chemotherapy, or radiation therapy is indicated to support a patient who refuses a treatment.

Ultimately, clinicians can best serve patients and their families by providing the most current information available in words they can comprehend, and by offering clear recommendations throughout the course of illness and treatment. Within the ongoing process of care planning, it is the persons served who appropriately determine the proportion of life-prolonging to palliative treatments within the continuum of care at any point in time. In the end, it is the patient or appropriate surrogate whose lives are most affected and whose choices among available options must prevail.

CLINICAL ISSUES

PRINCIPLES AND PRACTICES

The essence of expert end-of-life care lies not merely in the technical competence of its components, but in the intention, vision, and synergism that permeate the whole. Within the current health care delivery system, excellence in care is best modeled by leading hospice programs.[32] A number of organizations have published definitions and precepts for hospice and palliative care.[33-35] The defining features of palliative care can be concisely conveyed by describing five basic principles of care.

Principle One: Symptom Management is the First Priority

This principle was introduced in the discussion of suffering and the notions of healing and curing. Pain and other types of physical distress commonly occur during the course of far-advanced illness. Fear of pain is among the most frequently expressed source of dread among patients and families who are facing a life-limiting illness. Symptoms of advanced illness have the power to destroy the quality of peoples' lives. Indeed, without effective control of severe pain and other sources of physical distress, the quality of life for the dying person predictably will be unacceptable. Witnessing a loved one live and die in physical agony impacts the lives of family members forever. For all these reasons, symptom management is the first priority for the palliative care team.

Regrettably, multiple studies have documented an astounding prevalence of unmet physical distress among people who are dying. Regulatory, financial and cultural barriers to appropriate prescribing and inadequate education relevant to symptom management contribute to problematic patterns in medical and nursing practice.[36-42]

Whatever resources are needed and the highest level of expertise available must be employed in service of controlling persistent symptoms. Symptom alleviating treatments can include analgesics and co-analgesics, chemotherapy, hormonal therapy, radiation therapy; neurosurgical, orthopedic, and oncologic surgical procedures; and behavioral therapy techniques. The commitment to alleviating suffering must be strong and the clinical approach must be organized, comprehensive, and ongoing. Palliative care teams, especially the physicians and nurses involved, must remain dedicated to do whatever is necessary to control physical discomfort.

A focused assessment of the patient's symptoms begins, quite simply, with a history and physical examination. Laboratory and radiologic evaluations are appropriate when they are needed in discerning the underlying pathophysiology of the person's discomfort. This information is processed by the clinician and the interdisciplinary team in developing a palliative plan of care. Implementation of the resulting care plan must be accompanied by ongoing evaluation of the person's subjective quality of life.

It is important to emphasize that there are no biologic or pharmacologic limits on the ability to control physical suffering in the context of far advanced illness, nor any legal or ethical reason for persons to be afforded less than whatever is required to achieve relative comfort as they die. Simply stated, no one need ever die in physical agony. In practice, even severe physical distress usually yields to fairly routine interventions. Adequate control of symptoms is not always easy and in unfortunate cases can prove to be very difficult. There are times when physical comfort can only be achieved at the cost of alertness. Infrequently, sedation is required to relieve otherwise intractable physical suffering.[43,44] But relative comfort is *always* possible.[45,46]

Principle Two: The Patient with His/Her Family is the Unit of Care

An important commonality in the human encounter with death is that people's lives remain interconnected—emotionally and physically— through the end of life and into grief. Palliative care recognizes the patient *with his or her family* as the unit of care. Families in this context are not defined solely by shared genetic endowment, marriage or adoption, but rather by the phrase "for whom it matters," encompassing the network of a person's relatives and close friends. Families have always and will always participate in this final transition from life and will always grieve for someone they love and have lost. The impending death of a loved one is as profound an experience in the lives of family members as is the coming birth of a new member. Each person in the patient's family, as well as the family as a whole, is inevitably, inescapably affected. As a corollary of this principle, extending support to a patient's family through the initial period of bereavement is an integral component of hospice and palliative care.[47]

Although each family is unique, there are common needs and opportunities that families tend to share. Each family wants to know that their loved one received the "best care possible," although they often only have a general sense of what this means. It almost always includes knowing that the person received, or had the chance to receive, the most current and effective treatments to cure illness and prolong life. It also extends to care that ensures that their loved one is as comfortable as possible. Whether it is stated, or simply assumed, the "best care possible" also extends to meeting the person's basic needs for hygiene, grooming, privacy, and dignity. Families need to know that their loved one's values and preferences for care were followed to the extent possible. It is not the details of an advance directive as much as the spirit of the person's and families' values that are important. Family members expect and need to know that the care extended will respect their loved one's inherent dignity. This is an important component of "the best care possible." A family that feels their loved one is treated in an undignified manner will be dissatisfied and at high risk for coming into conflict with clinicians.

Families who know that time with a loved one is limited value having an opportunity to say and do the things "that matter most." Expressing love for the person who is dying is a normal component of healthy family grieving which begins prior to death. In their time together and in their caring, loved ones value the opportunity to honor and celebrate the person dying. Lastly, many families feel a need to

TABLE 12.1 Family Needs and Family Opportunities

- To ensure the "best care possible"
- To be confident that preferences for care were respected
- To be confident that the person was treated in a dignified manner
- To say and do the things "that matter most"
- To honor and celebrate the person during his/her passing
- To grieve together

grieve together, honoring and celebrating the person who has died, and comforting one another in their shared loss (Table 12.1).

Principle Three: Palliative Care is an Interdisciplinary Team Approach and Process of Care

Care for people who are dying is optimally practiced as a team process and as a coordinated whole. Each member of the interdisciplinary clinical team represents a valuable resource during the procedure of devising and implementing a patient/family centered plan of care. Members of the team contribute through specific roles. The nurse case manager is the pivotal person coordinating care and serving as a conduit of information between members of the team and with the patient and family. The nurse regularly assesses physical and functional status, administers treatments, identifies new or impending problems, and drafts a plan of care. The patient's physician or the palliative care physician has responsibility for performing a medical evaluation, prescribing medications and symptom-alleviating treatments, and ensuring that an ethically sound process of decision making and informed consent has preceded significant treatment decisions. The social worker undertakes the financial and psychosocial evaluation and accesses sources of support for the patient and family. The chaplain explores spiritual or existential questions the patient might have, provides pastoral support, and helps the patient connect with his or her own local faith community and resources. Yet a reductionist approach to explaining a clinical palliative care team misses the essence of the model. In practice, the whole is more than the sum of its parts. Synergy is consciously recruited in the work of the team.[48,49]

Interdisciplinary care planning is the central dynamic—a genuinely creative process that invites input from all members of the clinical team. Thus the social worker or bath aide can lend their eyes and ears in gauging the impact that pain is having on the patient's activities and functional status. The nurse or physician may respond to a fearful patient's question about the future in a way that leads to a therapeutically valuable discussion of meaning and spiritual connection. In addition to providing respite to a patient's spouse, a volunteer may help the patient label pictures for an album or record spoken stories aiding the person in developing a sense of completion, or may assist in spiritual care by transporting and sitting with the patient for an hour in a cathedral or at the ocean or a riverside.

Principle Four: Dying is a Part of Living

The most fundamental feature of palliative care is a recognition of dying as a part of living—an important part.[50,51] Dying is characteristically hard, unwanted, and often tragic. Nevertheless, dying is a natural and normal human experience. While the symptoms and physical needs of dying persons require expert medical attention, dying is more than a set of medical problems to be solved. The fundamental nature of dying is as a *personal experience*. Viewed from the perspective of the life of the individual, even the multitude of medical problems is often dwarfed by the enormity of this final transition.

The philosophical stance of approaching dying as fundamentally personal and experiential distinguishes palliative care from even the most comprehensive problem-based medical care of people who are dying. The goal of improving quality of life and personal experience is a guiding principle in the design of each patient's palliative plan of care and is reflected in the subsequent interventions by members of the clinical team. Whether patients are at home, in a nursing home, or in an acute care hospital, medical testing and treatment should be as unobtrusive as possible, arranged whenever possible to accommodate the patient's and family's schedule and the sanctity of their time. The patient's and family's priorities dictate the priorities for the plan of care. Family visits; attendance at important family celebrations, such as weddings, graduations, and reunions; and participation in religious and cultural rituals often become important objectives for patients and, therefore, important objectives within a plan of care. Medical services may creatively utilize sophisticated home-based services and novel routes of medication administration in support of these goals. Psychosocial and spiritual support can focus on personal preparation and achieving comfort and a sense of completion and closure.

Principle Five: Palliative Care Represents Intensive Care

It is axiomatic that dying patients are among the very sickest in the health care system. While palliative care is often spoken of in terms of "supportive care," many patients seen by hospice and palliative care programs have multi-system failure and require many hours a week of skilled care and many more hours of supportive care. They may be taking 10 or more medications on any given day. Clearly, in meeting the needs of the patients and families, palliative care often represents *intensive care.*

It is a mistake to assume that hospice and palliative care must avoid sophisticated or expensive diagnostic workups and treatments. Issues of the cost or the "aggressive" nature of a proposed intervention do not obviate consideration of therapies of curative intention and must not limit consideration of treatments to relieve a patient's distress or improve quality of life in advanced illness. The intensive nature of some palliative interventions—such as neurolytic blocks for unrelenting neuropathic pain or sedation for management of severe terminal agitation—is properly limited only by patient-imposed restrictions.

INTERVENTION STRATEGIES

An important monograph from the Standards and Accreditation Committee of the National Hospice and Palliative Care Organization outlines a "treat, prevent, promote" intervention strategy.[52] It represents a systematic approach to comprehensive care planning throughout the terminal phase of illness. The Pathway assessment and intervention schema focuses on opportunities for clinical action. Consistent with the principles presented in this chapter, the Pathway assumes that the most pressing priority for patients and families is treatment of immediate sources of suffering—physical, emotional, social, or spiritual. The team then focuses on preventing symptoms and complications for which the patient is known to be at risk, and on early signs or foreseeable family conflicts or interpersonal discord. The interdisciplinary team plan of care also attends to promoting opportunities for a patient and family to grow, individually and together, through this final stage of life.[53-55]

When patients and families are supported at these levels, it is more likely that they will perceive that life retains value and offers treasured moments even as they face physical decline.[56]

DEVELOPMENTAL LANDMARKS AND TASKWORK

In approaching the apparent paradox of *'healing versus curing,'* it is worth emphasizing a fundamental tenet: Dying is a part of living. The period of time referred to as *dying* is a stage in the life of the individual and the family. Modern psychological theorists, among them Erik Erickson, Jean Piaget and Abraham Maslow, have recognized that human development is a lifelong process. Clinical experience in palliative care reveals that the end of life can be a time of remarkable opportunity and a time of profound richness and depth for the patients and families[57-64] The magnitude of the personal growth nurses witness is often surprising to both the patient and family. Furthermore, experienced nurses recognize that these developmental opportunities not only can be preserved, they also can be nurtured. People can be helped to identify the things that matter most to them now during this concluding phase of their life. Are there important things that they feel a need to say to another? Are there things that would be left undone if they were to die suddenly? Palliative care is practiced one patient and one family at a time. Through the skillful, effective management of symptoms, opportunity is preserved and through skillful, sensitive counseling, growth can be facilitated.

The specific characteristics of personal experience with advanced illness, dying, and grieving vary widely from person to person. The particular work that a person has need for, or interest in, doing as they confront life's end will vary. However, a person's individuality is not diminished by recognition of elemental commonalities within the human condition as life ends. Issues of life completion and life closure are available to each individual. One need not await serious, life-limiting illness for these issues to have relevance, but knowledge that time is limited lends urgency to these matters. The developmental landmarks and examples of end-of-life task work outlined here represent predictable personal challenges as well as important opportunities of persons as they die. Importantly, within a developmental model one need not sanitize nor glorify the experience of life's end to think of a person as having died well or, similarly, as having achieved a degree of wellness in their dying. Personal development is rarely easy. The touchstone of "dying well" is that the experience is of value and meaningful for the person and their family[65,66] (Table 12.2).

Empiric support for this developmental model is provided by a study conducted by Steinhauser and colleagues involving focus groups comprised of patients with advanced illness and their families. Qualitative content analysis of transcripts revealed that people assign importance to domains of preparation for death, a sense of completion, and feeling that they are or have contributed to others.[67] In a detailed ethnographic, participant-observer study of nine terminally ill individuals and their primary caregivers, Staton, Shy, and Byock demonstrated the relevance of this construct and of these develop-

TABLE 12.2 Byock's Working Set of Landmarks and Developmental Taskwork

Landmarks	Taskwork
Sense of completion with worldly affairs	Transfer of fiscal, legal and formal social responsibilities
Sense of completion in relationships with community	Closure of multiple social relationships (employment, commerce, organizational, congregational)
	Components include: expressions of regret, expressions of forgiveness, acceptance of gratitude and appreciation
	Leave taking; the saying of goodbye
Sense of meaning about ones' individual life	Life review
	The telling of "one's stories"
	Transmission of knowledge and wisdom
Experienced love of self	Self-acknowledgment
	Self-forgiveness
Experienced love of others	Acceptance of worthiness
Sense of completion in relationships with family and friends	Reconciliation, fullness of communication and closure in each of one's important relationships.
	Component tasks include: expressions of regret, expressions of forgiveness and acceptance, expressions of gratitude and appreciation, acceptance of gratitude and appreciation, expressions of affection
	Leave-taking; the saying of goodbye
Acceptance of the finality of life—of one's existence as an individual	Acknowledgment of the totality of personal loss represented by one's dying and experience of personal pain of existential loss
	Expression of the depth of personal tragedy that dying represents
	Decathexis (emotional withdrawal) from worldly affairs and cathexis (emotional connection) with an enduring construct
	Acceptance of dependency
Sense of a new self (personhood) beyond personal loss	Developing self-awareness in the present
Sense of meaning about life in general	Achieving a sense of awe
	Recognition of a transcendent realm
	Developing/achieving a sense of comfort with chaos
Surrender to the transcendent, to the unknown—"letting go"	*In pursuit of this landmark, the doer and "taskwork" are one. Here, little remains of the ego except the volition to surrender.*

Adapted from I. Byock. (1996). "The Nature of Suffering and the Nature of Opportunity at the End of Life." *Clinical Geriatrics Medicine, 12*(2): 237–52.

mental landmarks in the lives of people who are aware that they have only a few months to live.[68]

SAYING THE FIVE THINGS

The impending loss of relationships is emotionally painful for almost every person who is aware that death is near. Predictably, achieving a sense of completion in significant relationships is an important opportunity for ill persons and those who love them. The simple of exercise of saying "The Five Things"—"Forgive me. I forgive you. Thank you. I love you. Goodbye."—has helped many people develop a sense of having left nothing important unsaid. Relationships that become "complete" in this manner need not end. In acknowledging the inevitable loss that approaches, continued time together with friends and relatives often reflects a poignant, loving, solemn, and yet celebratory quality.

Sometimes relatively simple interventions can have profound clinical effect. The practice of eliciting stories can stimulate a process of life review that contributes to a patient's sense of meaning of their life. The clinician, family member, or trained volunteer who assists in the process can focus on highlights and major transitions in the person's life. Life review is not insight therapy and need not dwell on a person's history of loss and grief. Indeed, Kast recommends assisting patients in constructing "biographies of joy" as a way of balancing the grief that people facing the end of life often feel.[69] Stories also can be a gift that the ill person gives to others. People living with debilitating effects of illness may struggle with feelings of unworthiness and a sense of being a burden to others. The recording of family stories involving the marriage of matriarch and patriarch, seminal events, and the history of the family during war or natural disasters is a tangible way that people can contribute to their children, grandchildren, and the generations to come.

THE PROFESSIONAL CAREGIVER

THE THERAPEUTIC STANCE OF THE CLINICIAN

Training and experience are always valuable and while clinical competence is essential, also fundamental to providing superior care at the end of life is a *therapeutic stance* of the clinician from which team involvement and direct clinical interaction occur. Critical attributes of this caring orientation and attitude include the following:

RELIABILITY

Patients who are dying are in an inherently chaotic period of time and process. Health care providers must make preparations for predictable problems, but also develop contingency plans for the unpredictable problems that will arise. Doing so requires a systems approach. There must be enough resources and skillful, experienced personnel in the health care system to handle any emergency or contingency. Achieving this end requires broad and on-going education not only to staff and colleagues working on hospital floors or specialty units, nor only to hospice and palliative care staff, but also to the staff of area nursing homes, and the community's emergency medical services providers. Education and system planning should reflect the interdisciplinary and collaborative nature of the desired care.

HONESTY

Truth telling is a fundamental principle of clinical bioethics—and it is certainly applicable to palliative and end-of-life care. Patients have a clear right to be offered information about their condition and the treatment options available. Withholding bad news in an attempt to shield an ill person from the truth is virtually always a mistake and frequently arises from a misguided desire to protect the holders of the information, whether they are family members or professionals. Secrets tend to isolate people at the very time when closeness is most needed.[70]

In some cultures it is taboo or otherwise unacceptable to talk openly about dying with the ill person. Often the patient can be asked if he or she would like to discuss and make medical decisions. If not, the patient can indicate with whom clinicians can discuss care and who can make these decisions on his or her behalf.

NON-ATTACHMENT

Non-attachment is a component of the therapeutic stance that refers, firstly, to outcomes. While clinicians' commitment to alleviating suffering and enhancing the quality of life cannot be stressed too strongly, despite the very best of palliative care, sometimes, bad things happen. The world in which patients live, and therefore die, is imperfect. By contributing to reliability in their local health system and by ensuring that competent, caring attention is consistently provided, nurses model social responsibility one person to another. Professionals who choose to care for people who are dying do not deserve and must not accept guilt—including self-imposed guilt—when a patient or family's suffering persists despite concerted, good faith efforts to prevent and treat distress.

Non-attachment also refers to maintaining a nonjudgmental attitude toward our patients regarding their emotions and reactions. Even the most sensitive care during this trying time of life may provoke displaced anger toward professional caregivers. Alternately, expressions of love and devotion toward caregivers may be out of proportion to services rendered. The challenge for professionals is to absorb these emotions—somewhat like a sponge—while not reacting in overly personal ways to either.

AUTHENTICITY

In contemporary, colloquial shorthand, authenticity is referred to as *being real*. It refers to openness and emotional availability on the part of a clinician. This aspect of the therapeutic stance initially may seem antithetical to the quality of non-attachment. It is not. Instead, the willingness and ability to act with caring intention, while acknowledging the tension between the temptation to emotionally detach and flee on the one hand and the seductive draw of emotional involvement on the other, imbues a professional's practice with authenticity. The commitment and readiness to act out of genuine caring despite an acknowledged lack of complete clinical or philosophical clarity also contributes to the authentic quality of the clinician-patient relationship.

At its best, authenticity refers to a willingness to engage the patient in a personal, non-objectified manner. It is a willingness to extend friendship while maintaining professional standards of human interaction. This invites true compassion—which from its roots means not simply sympathy or kindness but a willingness to *suffer with* the other. To see the dying patient as a person to be met in friendship, shoulder to shoulder on a journey neither would choose, invites this meaning of compassion.

Additionally, authenticity implies willingness and the courage to say difficult things to patients when necessary—this may include an ability to set limits on inappropriate behaviors or demands. It may also extend to the clinician sharing with the patient his or her own feelings of frustration, disappointment, and sadness.

Authenticity is not merely an attribute that is valuable to the recipients of care. Within this personal investment lie the rewards for care providers. Clinicians who make home visits to hospice patients and their families have been known to remark on an ambience that often surrounds anticipated home deaths that is wonderful. It is notable how frequently the word "sacred" is used to describe these poignant scenes—even though the experience is stressful and always exhausting for the family. When friends and relatives gather to support one another in anticipation of their loved one's death, there is often a sense of solemnity; but sometimes, there is also a sense of celebration, accompanied by tears as well as interspersed moments of laughter. Participation in such experiences is an earned privilege of the caring professions. The clinician's commitment to service of others— investment in training and willingness to be present at difficult times— carries with it the opportunity to share in these most meaningful and intimate experiences in the lives of the person and family they serve.

IMAGINATION

Imagination is an essential element of the therapeutic relationship. One person cannot really know the intimate experience of another. Indeed, the assertion, "I know what you're going through," can sound callous. However, if the clinician has taken the time and invested the emotional energy to actually do so, the statement, "I can only imagine how difficult this must be for you," can communicate genuine empathy. This process involves what may be termed the *receptive imagination*. From within this stance the clinician listens to the patient's story as if he or she were the speaker and looks at the world *as if* through the patient's eyes.

The clinician can also draw upon the creative capacity of his or her *generative imagination* in helping a patient or family envision a satisfactory sense of completion and closure.[71] When working with a person who acknowledges that their life is limited, and after being confident of a therapeutic alliance, a clinician may invite a patient to look at the events of his or her illness as the middle portion of a poignant biographical novel. The person's imagination can be enlisted to address several questions: "What would be left undone if the hero/ heroine of the story died suddenly, today?" More provocative still, given what is known of the main character's history, values, and current terminally ill condition, "What would success look like, even now?" or "How might the story end in a way that was meaningful and valuable in the hero's or heroine's own terms?"

This use of generative imagination also gives rise to hope. Within the medical model, when there is no longer any realistic expectation of cure, hope is often spoken of as an expectation of comfort. This is tantamount to saying that all people who are living with a terminal illness can hope for is to avoid suffering. If human potential does exist at the end of life, our concept of hope can and must expand. The dictionary definition of hope specifies, "a desire for some good, accompanied with at least a slight expectation of obtaining it, or a belief that it is obtainable."[72] By sharing with the patient the knowledge that growth, at times, does occur in the context of terminal illness—that it is possible, and that the person can be supported in this process—the person is invited to have hope. He or she is presented with a goal that is both valuable and achievable.

CONCLUSION

Dying is more than a set of medical problems to be solved. Dying is fundamentally a profound personal experience for the person and family. Nurses and the other health professionals in oncology have essential roles to play in ensuring comfort and enhancing the quality of life for the dying person and the family. Pain and other sources of physical distress associated with far-advanced disease can be controlled. Even suffering that arises from deeply personal and spiritual or existential sources is clinically approachable. The first step is to acknowledge the person's suffering by listening in a skillful manner. Simply by doing what nurses do best—caring for the persons who are our patients—and by providing care without embarrassment about the inevitability of death, by caring within a team of committed providers, by keeping one's own commitment and that of the team strong, by preparation and education, and by acknowledging the lifelong human capacity for human development that exists within each dying person and his or her family, nurses can contribute to a healthy re-incorporation of the value of dying within the ongoing mystery of life.

REFERENCES

1. Cassell, E. J., (1982). The nature of suffering and the goals of medicine. *New England Journal of Medicine, 306,* 11.

2. Byock, I. and Merriman, M. P., (1998). Measuring quality of life for patients with terminal illness: The Missoula-Vitas Quality of Life Index. *Palliative Medicine, 12,* 231–244. [Byock, 1998 #46].

3. Byock, I., (1997). *Dying well: The prospect for growth at the end of life.* New York: Riverhead, Putnam.

4. Cleeland, C. S. et al., (1994). Pain and its treatment in outpatients with metastatic cancer. *New England Journal of Medicine, 330,* 9.

5. Byock, I. (1996). The nature of suffering and the nature of opportunity at the end of life. *Clinics in Geriatric Medicine, 12,* 2.

6. Byock, I. *Dying Well: The Prospect for Growth at the End of Life.*

7. Steinhauser, K. E. et al. (2000). In search of a good death: observations of patients, families, and providers. *Annals of Internal Medicine, 132,* 10.

8. Byock, I. The nature of suffering and the nature of opportunity at the end of life.

9. Kearney, M. (1992). Palliative medicine—Just another specialty? *Palliative Medicine 6,* 93–95.

10. Byock, I. Growth: A paradigm for hospice care. (paper presented at the IXth International Congress on Care of the Terminally Ill, Montreal, November 3, 1992).

11. Byock, I. The nature of suffering and the nature of opportunity at the end of life.

12. Steinhauser et al. In search of a good death: Observations of patients, families, and providers.

13. Staton, J., Shuy, R. & Byock, I. (2001). *A few months to leave.* Washington, DC: Georgetown University Press.

14. Peschel, R. & Peschel, E. (1989). Sisyphus and the triumphs of medicine. *Psychological Reports 64,* 891–5.

15. McSkimming, S. A., et al. (1997). *Living and healing during life-threatening illness.* St. Louis: Catholic Health Association of the United States.

16. Byock, I. *Dying well: The prospect for growth at the end of life.*

17. Byock, I. (1996). Notes of a Hospice physician. *Western Journal of Medicine 164,* 4.

18. Broyard, A. (1992). *Intoxicated by my illness and other writings on life and death.* New York: Ballantine Books.

19. Bernardin, J. (1997). *Gift of peace: Personal reflections.* Chicago: Loyola Press.

20. Albom, M. (1997). *Tuesdays with Morrie.* New York: Doubleday.

21. de Hennezel, M. (1997). *Intimate death.* New York: Alfred A. Knopf Inc.

22. Staton, J., Shuy, R. & Byock, I. (2001). *A few months to leave.* Washington, DC: Georgetown University Press.

23. Steinhauser, K. E. et al. (2000). In search of a good death: Observations of patients, families, and providers. *Annals of Internal Medicine, 132,* 10.

24. Byock, I. (1996). The nature of suffering and the nature of opportunity at the end of life. *Clinics in Geriatric Medicine, 12,* 2.

25. ASCO, (1998). Cancer care during the last phase of life. *Journal of Clinical Oncology, 16,* 5.

26. The Robert Wood Johnson Foundation Last Acts Task Force. (1998). Precepts of palliative care. *Journal of Palliative Medicine 1,* 2.

27. ASCO. Cancer care during the last phase of life.

28. Cancer pain relief and palliative care. *Technical Report Series 804.* Geneva: World Health Organization, 1990.

29. Coyle, N. (2001). Introduction to palliative care nursing. *Textbook of Palliative Care Nursing,* Ed. B. R. Ferrell and N. Coyle. New York: Oxford University Press.

30. Vachon, M. L. S. (2001). The nurse's role: The world of palliative care nursing. *The Textbook of Palliative Care Nursing.* Ed. B. R. Ferrell and N. Coyle. New York: Oxford University Press.

31. Dery, S. and O'Mahony, S. (2001). Elderly patients. *Textbook of Palliative Care Nursing.* Ed. B. Rollings and N. Coyle. New York: Oxford Unversity Press.

32. ASCO. Cancer care during the last phase of life.

33. Last Acts Task Force. Precepts of palliative care.

34. Standards and Accreditation Committee National Hospice Organization. (1997). *A pathway for patients and families facing terminal disease.* Arlington, VA: National Hospice Organization.

35. CPCA. (1995). Palliative care: Towards standardized principles of practice. Canadian Palliative Care Association.

36. White, K. R., Coyne, P. T. & Patel, U. B. (2001). Are nurses adequately prepared for end-of-life care? *Journal of Nursing Scholarship, 33,* 2.

37. Last Acts Task Force. Precepts of palliative care.

38. Cleeland, C. S. & Chapman, C. R. (1993). *Documenting barriers to cancer pain management in current and emerging issues in cancer pain: Research and practice.* Ed. K. M. Foley. New York: Raven Press Ltd.

39. Wallace, K. G. et al. (1995). Staff nurses' perceptions of barriers to effective pain management. *Journal of Pain and Symptom Management, 10,* 3.

40. Cleeland, C. S., Von Roenn, J. H. & Gonin, R. (1993). Physician attitudes and practice in cancer pain management: A survey from the Eastern Cooperative Oncology Group. *Annals of Internal Medicine, 119,* 121–6.

41. McCormack, J. et al. (1993). Inadequate treatment of pain in ambulatory HIV patients. *The Clinical Journal of Pain, 9,* 4.

42. Cleeland, C. S. et al. Pain and its treatment in outpatients with metastatic cancer.

43. Byock, I. (1993). Consciously walking the fine line: Thoughts on a hospice response to assisted suicide and euthanasia. *Journal of Palliative Care, 9,* 3.

44. Quill, T. E., and Byock, I. (2000). Responding to intractable terminal suffering. *Annals of Internal Medicine, 133,* 7.

45. Twycross, R. G., and S. A. Lack. (1986). *Therapeutics in terminal care.* New York: Churchill Livingstone.

46. Levy, M. H. (1996). Pharmacologic treatment of cancer pain. *New England Journal of Medicine, 335,* 15.

47. Egan, K. (1998). A patient-family value based end-of-life care model. Largo, FL: Hospice Institute of Florida Suncoast.

48. Cummings, I. (1997). The interdisciplinary team." In *Oxford Textbook of Palliative Medicine, 2d Edition.* Ed. G. W. C. Hanks, D. Doyle, & N. MacDonald. New York: Oxford University Press.

49. Lattanzi-Licht, M., Mahoney, J. J., & Miller, G. W. (1998). *The Hospice choice.* New York: Simon and Schuster.

50. National Hospice Organization Standards and Accreditation Committee. Standards of a Hospice program of care. *The Hospice Journal, 9,* 4.

51. Last Acts Task Force. Precepts of palliative care.

52. National Hospice Organization. *A Pathway for Patients and Families Facing Terminal Disease.*

53. Byock, I. The nature of suffering and the nature of opportunity at the end of life.

54. Byock, I. *Dying well: The prospect for growth at the end of life.*

55. Steinhauser, K. et al., In search of a good death: Observations of patients, families, and providers.

56. Mount, B. M., & Scott, J. (1983). Wither hospice evaluation. *Journal of Chronic Disease, 36,* 11.

57. Ibid.

58. Bartholome, W. Living in the light of death. *Bulletin of the University of Kansas Medical Center.*

59. Byock, I. Growth: A paradigm for hospice care. Paper presented at the IXth International Congress on Care of the Terminally Ill, Montreal, November 3, 1992.

60. Byock, I. The nature of suffering and the nature of opportunity at the end of life.

61. Kearney, M. Palliative medicine—Just another specialty?

62. Egan, K. A., & Labyak, M. J. (2001). Hospice care: A model for quality end-of-life care. In *Textbook of palliative nursing,* Ed. B. R. Ferrell and N. Coyle. New York: Oxford University Press.

63. Jaffe, C., & Ehrlich, C. (1997). *All Kinds of Love.* Amityville: Baywood Publishing.

64. Kelley, P., & Callanan, M. (1992). *Final gifts.* New York: Poseidon Press.

65. Byock, I. Growth: A paradigm for hospice care.

66. Byock, I. The nature of suffering and the nature of opportunity at the end of life.

67. Steinhauser, K. et al. In search of a good death: Observations of patients, families, and providers.

68. Staton, J., Shuy, I., & Byock, I. *A few months to leave.*

69. Kast, V. (1991). *Joy, inspiration and hope.* Trans. D. Whitcher. Texas A&M University Press.

70. Saunders, C. (1984). On dying well. *The Cambridge Review, 80,* 16–8.

71. Byock, I. (1994). When suffering persists. *Journal of Palliative Care 10,* 2.

72. *Webster's New Universal Unabridged Dictionary,* (1983), second ed. New York: Simon & Schuster.

SECTION THREE

Related Issues

Mr. Brown's Story

"Why did you let him do it? Why did you not tell him that he might have lived six more months with treatment, that he might even have seen the birth of his grandchild?"

This was the first and only time Dr. Oren saw Tammy cry. Out of grief or out of anger, the Nurse Practitioner broke down for the first time in four years. Full-time professional, full-time mom, full-time graduate student, Tammy single-handedly organized and directed the hospital's Geriatric Oncology Program. Mr. Brown had made Tammy cry: a 78-year-old bank lawyer with metastatic prostate cancer who attended the clinic every six weeks in a dark suit. After hearing the report of the latest tests, Mr. Brown went back to his office to conclude a twelve-hour day of work. Lately the news related to his health had gone from bad to worse, but we never could notice a grimace of disappointment in his face or a wrinkle of frustration in his suit, or a shadow of neglect on his white shirt and his dark tie. One more time, cancer was closing in on another victim. Mr. Brown had elected to look the enemy in the face, unlike the majority of his peers who would have tried a desperate and useless escape in the treacherous land of experimental treatment. His bravery disconcerted Tammy, used, like the other members of the health care team, to offering the patients a temporary refuge during their impossible flight from death, to medicate the expanding wounds, to provide a berth for a few hours of restless sleep.

"I did not try to dissuade him because I admire him and envy him," was Dr. Oren's somber answer to Tammy. *Like most of the cancer stories, Mr. Brown's story had been a story of hope and desperation in alternance, a story started 10 years earlier, in a doctor's office, with an abnormal blood test.*

As part of the yearly checkup to which Mr. Brown submitted religiously, a measurement of the blood concentration of the Prostate Specific

Antigen (PSA) was performed. The PSA was found mildly elevated to 6.8 ng/ml, which prompted the exam of the prostate with an ultrasound that revealed a small cancer sitting in the middle of the prostate, a cancer that never could have been detected by an exploring finger. His wife and his two daughters still remembered the relief experienced as the surgeon emerged from the OR with a triumphant expression, the sterile mask hanging around the neck and dark spots of blood and betadine on the scrub-suit. He looked like a crusader back from a bloody and victorious battle, with the armor stained with dust and blood. "Mr. Brown had tolerated the surgery very well: in two hours he will be awake and out of the recovery room. And the margins were free of tumor, not even one small cell had migrated outside the capsule. For all practical purposes he was cured. Once more, health maintenance had paid off; Mr. Brown should be proud of himself for complying with prostate cancer screening that allowed the diagnosis of cancer at an early stage, when it was fully curable."

Intensely private, the Browns had made no fuss about the impotence that complicates prostate surgery almost universally, after age 60. From half words, involuntary facial expressions, mute questions, I had a hint that the inability to achieve full intercourse saddened the last 10 years of this close couple. In my experience, the unusual couples that become closer with aging are those that learn to appreciate the advantages of growing old. One of these advantages is intimacy free of the risks of pregnancy and of the constraints of limited time. Like a favored vacation spot, which becomes every year richer of memories and more varied in sensations, intimacy turns more predictable and more fulfilling with age, for people able to look into the quality of their lives more than into the quality of their bed performance.. Never would the Browns have considered to begrudge an operation that had saved Mr. Brown's life and returned him whole to his family, to his clients, to his world. With the same stern determination with which they had endured the heat of a cheap apartment without air conditioning during law school, with which they had endured seven weekly days of work, fourteen hours a day, throughout the school years of their children, they endured now deprivation of intimacy. It never occurred to the Browns that being alive at the cost of intimacy was anything less than a privilege offered by the prodigious advances of medical research; it never occurred to the Browns that their personal disappointment might have tainted the joy of being alive, independent, and loved.

After surgery, every six months, Mr. Brown had driven his blue Mercedes to the doctor's office to check the PSA levels. In the waiting room he used to go through a number of briefs and computer prints he carried in a heavy briefcase of dark leather, waiting his turn without impatience over the frequent delays. He reserved four hours of his time for the doctor appointment, not to make his own customers wait. After the doctor visit, Mr. Brown would meet his wife in a small Mexican restaurant on Howard and celebrate with a Marguerita the good news that his PSA was still below 0.1 ng/ml. This ritual came to a brisk end after three years of joyful celebrations. Mrs. Brown has a chilly recollection of that day:

"When Bill did not reach out of the car window for me with a smile, I realized something had gone sour, I just hoped it was his job. After parking he joined me on the driveway, kissed me on the cheek and we walked together in silence. We took place at our usual table, by the window, ordered our meals, and when the Margueritas arrived Bill attempted a smile and said only one word: "one.one." Suddenly I realized the honeymoon with cancer was over."

The doctor asked Mr. Brown to come back in two weeks, hoping for a mistake, but two weeks later the PSA had climbed further from 1.1 to 1.4. There were no mistakes, the cancer had come back. . . . A thorough workup, including a bone scan, and a CAT scan of the abdomen and the pelvis failed to reveal any signs of cancer, but the message of the PSA could not be clearer; somewhere, somehow, in the body of Mr. Brown, a little seed of cancer was budding and was getting ready to suffocate his life. With the same stern determination that had directed his life through most critical conjunctures, Mr. Brown underwent an orchiectomy, that is the removal of both testicles, the time-honored treatment of testicular cancer since 1941. He disdained the alternative treatment by chemical castration with subcutaneous injections of hormones every three months. He knew very well that the injections would have cost his Medicare $5000.00 a year, while an operation costing less than $1000.00 would have eliminated his testicles for good. An old-fashioned sense of social responsibility kept him from charging a costly pretense of manhood to an overburdened system unable to take care of life-and-death issues for lack of funds. The PSA disappeared eight weeks after the orchiectomy and stayed put for more than five years, then, a new, gnawing pain in his left hip announced the final phase of the disease.

"Bill did not mention the pain for a few months, but I noticed he was not sleeping well,"

recollects Mrs. Brown, and the level of aspirin tablets in our medicine cabinet kept going down. He tried to joke that at our age arthritis is just normal, but I insisted taking him to the doctor. This time the PSA was 33 and worse, a bone scan showed that the cancer had invaded most of his back bones." Dr. Oren sat down with the Browns for more than an hour to explore together the options for the management of hormone-refractory prostate cancer, that is, prostate cancer that cannot be controlled anymore with standard treatment:

> "We can relieve the pain in your bone with a few sessions of radiation therapy; we can give you a medicine called strontium that will control for five or six months all cancer in your bone, but may lower your white-blood cells and your platelets in the blood, with increased risk of severe infections or bleeding; or we may try some chemotherapy to slow down the progression of your disease . . ."

The goals of Mr. Brown were crystal clear: he wanted to keep enjoying a life that had been so rich and generous as much as possible and thereafter to go as quickly as he could. He was not interested in any treatment with debilitating side effects. He came as close as humanly possible to obtaining his wishes.

Three times we had to administer radiation to painful sites of his bones, over one year, as his PSA climbed to more than 200 ng/ml. Finally one day his serum creatinine, which had been well in the normal range at less than 1 mg/ml, jumped to 7 mg/ml; his kidneys were becoming obstructed by the growing tumor; in a few days he would have become unable to urinate, to eliminate all poisons that his body produced daily in the chemical reactions that support a normal life. We could have restored the patency of the kidneys with a stent, and given him six more months of life, or let the disease follow its course and let him die over the next couple of weeks. Mr. Brown had no doubts: consistent with his staunch beliefs expressed throughout his disease, he decided it was time for him to go. He knew the additional six months of life would have been complicated by continuous infections, growing bone pain, ingravescing disability; he knew that death by renal failure was a virtually painless death, as close as you can get to a peaceful death. Surrounded by his wife and his daughters, who held his hands crying, he asked to see the hospice nurse. Two weeks later Dr. Oren signed his death certificate. He had died in his sleep after five days of coma, in the bed he had shared with his wife for more than half a century. He had lost almost one third of his body weight, in his fight against death, but none of the dignity that had been the backbone of his countenance. Death could deprive him of his flesh, not of the leadership of his life. As much as possible by human means, he had conquered death. Simplicity made Mr. Brown's death so exemplary. Somehow, the majority of us, human beings, would like to carry through death the same serenity of Mr. Brown and at the same time we would like to see his bravery rewarded by a happy end. Like Tammy, we had hoped that he had opted for a temporary relief of his kidney, to gain some time for some new miraculous cure to emerge. This but too human ambivalence is the main obstacle to an unperturbed discussion of death, including our own death. "How much time, Doctor, six months, like they always say in television?" really means for the majority of patients "how much time I have for my appeal before the death sentence is carried out?"

The composure of Mr. Brown's death stemmed from the way he had lived. His death has been the culminating event of a life conducted under the banner of self-reliance expressed in a series of realistic choices. More than Mr. Brown's equanimity in the face of death, we envy the ownership he exercised on his life. Equanimity had been just the expression of that ownership. We envy his ability to let life go when it had become too burdensome, we envy the intimate satisfaction with his previous life that allowed him to give up the last crumble of life, the way a well-fed diner gives up without second thoughts an attractive dessert at the end of a meal. More simply, we envy Mr. Brown's success in exploiting the present, free of regrets and grief, unfettered by hopes and expectations in a hypothetical future. Ultimately, we envy the way Mr. Brown had learned to wield his power of choice throughout his life.

CHAPTER THIRTEEN

Social Support Networks of the Older Cancer Patient

Janine Overcash and Lodovico Balducci

This chapter will address some definitions of social support and contrast them with the concept of social networks. The following question will be addressed:

- Who are the people that most often become caregivers to older people?
- What are some of the issues that can arise for many caregivers, as well as the person receiving the care?
- What are some of the nursing interventions that can be offered to accommodate both the patient and the caregiver?

This chapter will include a review of recent published literature and will act as a nursing reference for addressing social support of the older cancer patient.

BACKGROUND INFORMATION

Increasing numbers of people are living longer and more healthy lives. The Census Bureau in 1994 reported that people aged 85 and over are the fastest-growing segment of the United States population. Despite the increasing number of older people reaching the age of 85, the National Cancer Institute 1994 SEER data suggests that 50% of all cancers are diagnosed in patients 65 and over and 60% of all cancer deaths occur in this segment of the population. When confronted with such a diagnosis, surgery, chemotherapy, and/or radiation therapy are generally recommended. Frequently these treatments leave the patient in need of emotional support and with the inability to perform the activities that promote self-care. The gerontological literature suggests that as people age it is not uncommon to have a decrease in the available social support systems that provide assistance with instrumental tasks (bathing, dressing) and emotional support (Auslander & Litwin, 1990). Without a person to assist with the above supports, a patient may not be as able to tolerate cancer therapy and therefore may experience a less positive cancer treatment outcome (Balducci, 1994). Adequate social support systems have been linked with less depression, better adjustment to illness, less probability of nursing home placement, and even lower risk of mortality (Cohen & Syme, 1985; Funch & Marshall, 1983).

DEFINITIONS

Social support can be described as an "exchange of resources between at least two individuals perceived by the provider or the recipient to be intended to enhance the well-being of the recipient" (Shumaker & Brownell, 1984, p. 13) (Table 13.1). The resources exchanged within social support can be tangible help, which involves providing material aid, or service, or emotional support, which can be empathy, love, caring, trust, and the information with which to solve

TABLE 13.1 Definitions of Social Support as Compared to Social Network

Social Support	Social Networks
When two individuals are in the role of provider and recipient of care that will enhance the well-being of the recipient (Shumaker & Brown, 1884). Tangible help that includes material help or aid.	Links between people (Mitchell, 1974).
	Social network may be an acquaintance who does not have a reciprocal relationship that may enhance the well-being of one of the participants.
Emotional support including love, empathy, caring, and trust which can solve a problem (Krause & Markides, 1990).	
A positive act from one person to another (Lackner et al., 1994).	

a problem (Krause & Markides, 1990). Social support tends to be a positive act offered from one person to another person in need and does not have to be reciprocal (especially for frail elderly). A diagnosis of cancer can reduce the ability of a person to reciprocate support and increase the amount of social support required (Lackner, Goldenburg, Arrizza & Tjosvold, 1994).

In contrast to social support, a social network can be described simply as the links between people (Mitchell, 1974). Occasionally "social networks" and "social support" are used synonymously in the literature and it is important to understand that these terms have different meanings. Individuals who make up social networks are not necessarily people who exchange resources. Some members of a network are simply acquaintances and do not provide anything that can be called "support" (Wellman, Carrington & Hall, 1988). Individuals who may be included in a social network may only have brief contact with a person on a superficial level that is typically less than intimate.

Social support can be conceptualized as a type of coping assistance offered in response to a need (Thoits, 1985). Social support has been described in the social science literature to mean a pool of individuals who provide "emotional support, material aids and services, information, and new social contacts" (Walker, MacBride & Vachon, 1977). Social support can be explained in two ways; functionally and structurally (Cohen & Syme, 1985). A structural definition can be explained in terms of interpersonal relationships or the construction and preservation of social bonds. A structural theorist would assess the existence of the social ties and the connection between individuals. A functional approach to social support would focus on social contacts and the functions they serve, such as transportation and/or emotional support.

Two types of social support are recognized: formal and informal support (Table 13.2). Formal support refers to social workers, nurses, home health aides, etc. Informal support usually refers to kin, friends, and neighbors (Cantor, Brennan & Sainz, 1994). Both formal and informal support systems act to meet the needs of an individual by provid-

TABLE 13.2 Two Types of Social Support

Formal Social Support	Informal Social Support
Nurses	Kin
Social Workers	Friends
Home Health Aide	Neighbors
Hired Caregivers	Partner

ing emotional support, daily activities, and personal assistance during times of need. The persons who make up an individual's informal support system may not always act in the role as "supporter" and often these roles change depending on the situation. The "provider" to a person in need may encounter a stressful occasion and become a "recipient" of social support. The individual contacts that make up the informal support network can become "activated" in times of "crisis, conflict, and stress" (Peters-Gordon, 1982). Social support is a multidimensional concept that varies from situation to situation, with ever-changing roles and responsibilities. Social support necessary for one person in a particular situation can be very different than for another individual in a similar situation. The support needs of an older person with a cancer diagnosis can be very different from the support needs of an older person without a malignancy. People living with a diagnosis of cancer may require and seek out reassurance and acceptance from others who have also encountered a cancer diagnosis and have survived. For this reason, the use of support groups is a very important entity in the lives of many cancer patients. Coping strategies, community resources, and reassurance are offered and obtained within the arena of a formal support group for many who face the long road of cancer therapy.

DOMAINS OF SOCIAL SUPPORT

Social support can include many different tasks and functions that are necessary to fulfill the needs of a recipient (Table 13.3). For older people with cancer, social support may present itself as much-needed instrumental support during chemotherapy or as a friendly discussion about issues far removed from the language of cancer. The domains of social support were identified by the foremost supportive needs often required by older cancer patients (emotional and instrumental support) (Rose, 1990; Cohen and McKay, 1984). Emotional support is the domain of social support most frequently utilized by cancer patients (Rose, 1990). This may be due in part to a sense of fatalism and acute fear of dying often associated with a diagnosis of cancer (Powe, 1996). Emotional support is vital to the patient encountering such fears, and helps patients cope with cancer and cancer treatment. The five concepts that make up the emotional support domain are reassurance, esteem support, intimacy, the need to ventilate, and the need for open communication (Rose, 1990).

Instrumental support (bathing, dressing, transportation) is also vital to the well being of an older cancer patient. Without someone to

TABLE 13.3 Domains of Social Support

Emotional Support	Reassurance
	Esteem Support (Encouragement)
	Intimacy
	Communication
Instrumental Support	Tangible Aid
	Advocacy
	Directive Guidance

provide transportation and assistance in activities of self-care, a person could be unable to receive cancer treatment (Goodwin, Hunt & Samet, 1991). Often cancer therapies are indicated to be administered everyday, and without reliable transportation it can be very difficult to undergo necessary treatments. Tangible aid, advocacy, directive guidance, and social diversion are concepts found to describe the notion of instrumental support (Rose, 1990).

The concepts identified as components of social support can be incorporated into clinical instruments useful to identify deficiencies in available support. It is important, however, to culturally adjust these instruments with respect to the individuals being assessed. The needs of older adults cannot be pigeonholed into specific domains and made to fit universally. Older people are a heterogeneous population even within the United States. Assessments and interventions pertaining to social support must be customized to the individual before formal services are obtained.

SOCIAL SUPPORT AND THE CANCER PATIENT

An adequate social support environment has been associated with enhanced post-mastectomy self-esteem and reduced mortality in people with breast cancer (Reynolds & Kaplan, 1990; Wortman & Dunkel-Schetter, 1979). Social support has been suggested to be useful to the cancer patient by acting as a buffer during diagnosis and treatment and by moderating distress throughout rehabilitation (Irwin & Kramer, 1988). A model is provided that helps illustrate how social support factors into the life of an older cancer patient (Figure 13.1).

The benefits of social support can be different depending on the site and stage of the cancer diagnosis. In a study by Ell et al. (1992), the relationship between social support and the site of cancer (breast,

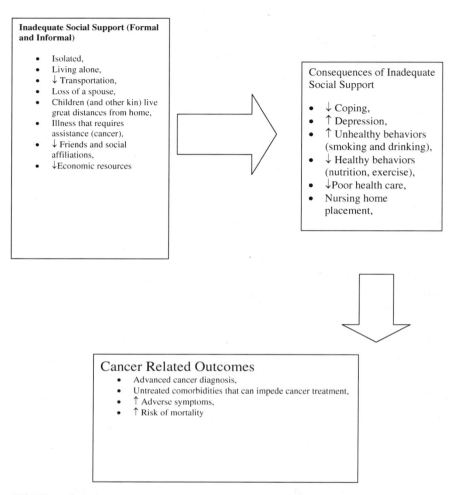

FIGURE 13.1 A Model of Social Support in the Older Cancer Patient

lung, or colon) found that for women with breast cancer, adequate social support was significantly associated with survival. For colon or lung cancer patients, the only predictor of survival was stage of illness and not social support. It should be mentioned that 10 years ago, when the study was performed, colon and lung cancer were rather acute diseases with a much shorter survival. Hence, social support might have played a minor role, because social support is mainly important in chronic situations, requiring multiple doctor visits, changes of living conditions, changes in function. Nowadays the situation is quite different: the majority of patients with colorectal cancer present with an early stage of their disease and they also tend to live longer. Chemotherapy has become more effective both in metastatic colorectal and lung cancer, and then the role of social support may become more prominent.

In older patients with breast, lung, and colorectal cancer who had low levels of social support functional impairment, pain, comorbidities (multiple diagnosis), and advanced malignancy (regardless of site) were recognized as part of their health assessment (Willey & Silliman, 1990). Based on these findings, an important component of the nursing assessment would be to determine if there was a lack of social support, or if disease-related demands were so extensive that the existing social support could not manage. It is possible that patients with more advanced disease and multiple health problems had the same amount of support, but this support was simply inadequate to match more pervasive needs. If instead these people had indeed lower resources, then an important correlation may exist between inadequate social support, development of advanced cancer, and multiple comorbidities that would call for a "preventive" institution and adjustment of social support.

Several current research articles have been published on the matter of actual support versus assumed social support. One interesting element in the literature is that the perceived availability of support is frequently not available for cancer patients due to the negative stigma cancer often produces. Those who do not have a diagnosis of cancer commonly direct avoidance behaviors toward cancer patients. Additionally, 56% of healthy people would avoid someone with a diagnosis of cancer (Peters-Golden, 1982). When subjects were asked if they would expect to be treated differently in the event of a cancer diagnosis, 81% stated they would. Of those, 32% felt they would be pitied, 29% felt people would be nicer to them, and 15% felt they would be avoided. For subjects diagnosed with breast cancer, 52% felt they actually were avoided or even feared by those without a diagnosis of cancer. Only 3% felt people were nicer to them. A detrimental aspect is that cancer patients, and the medical community, are often optimistic regarding cancer prognosis due to new cancer treatment therapies. When patients are avoided, it can be unsettling to have this optimism dashed by family, friends and social support that fail to materialize.

One study contradicts the previous information on the avoidance of cancer patients. Tempelaar et al. (1989) reported that cancer patients who have undergone surgery or chemotherapy have more positive and less negative social support experiences than people without a diagnosis of cancer. The study revealed that the more advanced the cancer diagnosis, the more positive the social support. It was also noted that older cancer patients had less social support than younger cancer patients. The fact that older people have fewer people involved in their social support system than younger people is widely represented in the literature (Willey & Silliman, 1990; Matt & Dean, 1993).

In terms of the older cancer patient, Goodwin, Hunt, and Samet (1991, 1993, 1996) have published several studies on aspects of survival in the older cancer patient. It has been shown that social support and access to transportation are two very important provisions supplied by social support that can have a positive outcome in cancer treatment. Factors that may construct a barrier to cancer treatment were found to be advanced age, poor social support, impairment in functional status, and decreased mental status (Goodwin, Hunt & Samet, 1993). Lack of these components can mean a delay in diagnosis and treatment and a diminished probability of survival. Access barriers have been shown to be greatest for older women, minorities, and individuals with a low socioeconomic status (Guidry et al., 1996).

Because of the importance of adequate social support, a routine psychosocial assessment including social support is conducted on every new patient who enters the Senior Adult Oncology Program at the H. Lee Moffitt Cancer Center at University of South Florida. The assessment is comprised of several open-ended questions that assess patient need and level of comfort with having, or not having, a social support network (Table 13.4). Patients who do not have an informal support (friends, family) system (and would like to have one) are connected to formal support systems such as cancer support groups, home health care agencies, and transportation organizations. Patients who report available social support yet perceive negative interactions are then referred for psychosocial counseling (if desired). Patients

TABLE 13.4 Senior Adult Oncology Program Current Life Situation Questionnaire

1. List those people living in the home with you.
2. Which relatives live near you?
3. Do you have children living in other places?
4. So you have a "best friend"? If so, where does this person live?
5. How many times per week do you socialize with friends/family?
6. What activities do you enjoy when you are feeling well?
7. Do you have a specific religious affiliation?
8. Are you active with a specific religious group?
9. How many hours of television do you watch per day?
10. Do you attend a cancer support group?

and families can be instructed on how to maximize their relationships to provide positive, supporting behaviors to aid the cancer patient in adapting to the disease. "Support systems must become part of the solution rather than the problem" (Irwin & Kramer, 1988).

ADVANTAGES OF SOCIAL SUPPORT

People with an adequate social support system enjoy a higher health status than those who do not have ample support (Ell et al., 1992; Pilisuk et al., 1993). Weak social support bonds can promote pessimism with regard to health and wellness related behaviors. Older people with a poor social support system often have a reduced health status and a higher mortality when compared to those who have an adequate social support system. A "consistent pattern of an increased mortality rate associated with each decrease in social connection" tends to be explained by the unhealthy behaviors such as smoking, alcohol consumption, and decreased physical activity more prevalent in people with reduced support (Berkman & Syme, 1979, p. 190).

Being married has been shown to have a positive effect on health status and mortality. Gliksman et al. (1995) found that being unmarried was a risk factor for cardiovascular disease among men, but not for women. The lack of social support is associated with a significant increase in the prevalence of smoking and other behaviors that can cause cardiovascular problems. Men may benefit from healthy behaviors (diet and exercise) that may be initiated and established by their wives. Bryant and Rakowski (1992) found that elderly women with frequent social contact have a lower risk of death than men who do not have these social contacts.

Social support patterns are different for the aged (65 and over) when compared to those of younger people. Many elders have survived spouses, family, and friends and thus have a limited or inadequate support network. This is unfortunate because the social support of friends and family is very important in the fulfillment of many of the everyday needs of the elderly cancer patient. Furthermore, the available support may be comprised of old spouses and old family members, all of whom have health problems and limited function on their own. One of the foremost reasons why a frail, older person can remain living in the community is the level of informal support they receive (Bowling & Brown, 1991). For many older Americans, especially within the African-American community, the church can be a major source of informal support. The level and extent of support offered by the church is often connected to the size of the church (as measured by membership) and affiliation with other churches throughout the nation (Morrison, 1991). Small churches with limited membership tend to only "fill in" when family is not available. The more active seniors within a church membership (people who participate in choir, women's organizations, classes, etc.) are often the recipients of more social support. It is widely recognized that the African-American church has provided both formal and informal social support to its members throughout American history. Morrison (1991) writes, "The importance of social supports such as churches in sustaining elderly in their communities and preventing more costly institutionalization cannot be overlooked" (p. 107).

When family and friends are not available to care for frail or seriously ill elderly, formal support services are sought to subsidize the needs of the older person. Unfortunately, those elderly that do not have adequate informal support may live in areas that are without a highly developed system of formal support services and often have no or little support supplementation. At this point, many turn to formal support systems such as nursing home placement (Auslander & Litwin, 1990; Cantor, 1980). The social support of family members is important in preventing institutionalization of an older person, and more precisely the absence of a spouse nearly triples the risk of nursing home placement (Freedman et al., 1993). Most elders receive the supportive care they need, which is reflected in that older Americans (people 70 and over) live very independent lives and only 5% of the nation's elders are placed in nursing homes (Havlik et al., 1994). A profile of institutionalized elderly is illustrated in Table 13.5.

In areas of the world that have traditionally relied on younger generations taking care of the older generations, increasing industrialization and urbanization along with more men and women in the workforce has made the family's responsibility for caring for elderly members

TABLE 13.5 Profile of People in Nursing Homes

Age Range	Sex	Race	Place of Residence Prior to Nsg Home Placement
14%			
36%			
85+ 51%			
	3:1 women to men	89% white	
Living at home with family			18%
Living at home alone			13%
Hospital or other nursing home			58%

difficult. In Korea, Choi (1996:8) states that, "the values of familism and communalism (the author uses familism to indicate that the family takes care of the person in need and communalism to refer to living as a group and contributing to the needs of the whole) are withering away and, instead individualism and a nuclear-family orientation is developing and expanding." Changes in informal support provided by family members to elders are diminishing before the government of Korea can put in place formal support facilities. The elderly are the people most often hurt by these sociological changes, as their primary supports are less able to help.

Reduction in adverse symptomatology association with a diagnosis of cancer is another advantage of adequate social support. Researchers found a decrease in depression and stress in the presence of a social support system. Stressors that occur as a result of a past cancer diagnosis have a tremendous psychosocial impact on many cancer patients, and especially the elderly. Fear of recurrence, social reorientation, adjustment of physical compromise, and depression are related to adequate support (Halstead & Fersler, 1994). Larger social networks and greater support systems reported less stress and depression in older white respondents (Beigel, Magaziner & Baum, 1991). However, black respondents with a larger social support system had more stress and depressive symptoms. The rationale for this finding is presumed to be that caregivers of black elders may have more responsibilities and greater levels of stress that is transferred to the older person (Beigel, Magaziner & Baum, 1991).

In the case of cancer survivorship, coping strategies are useful in modifying stress and feelings of depression. The effects of social support by source on depressive symptoms are that spouse, friends, and adult children were found to rank in descending order regarding the extent to which the lack of interaction and support caused depression (Dean, Kolody & Wood, 1990). Older people in need of social support often look to friends before adult children. This may be due to the potentially great geographic distances adult children may live from their aging parents in the United States (this will be discussed later in the paper). It is helpful for the medical community to assess for predictors of depression in elderly, as depression can interfere with the willingness of a person to seek cancer screening and even treatment.

Predictors of depression among elderly Chinese immigrants were found to be poor health status, living alone, and dissatisfaction with family support (Mui, 1996). Chinese elder immigrants do not often seek formal support and often rely on family members. Nurses should "facilitate shared living arrangements with family members or others" before entertaining other formal support interventions when working with the Chinese community (Mui, 1996: 643).

SOURCES OF SOCIAL SUPPORT

Many of the individuals who make up the social support systems of the older person may not be in a position to offer support. Often older people outlive family members, a spouse, and friends. Children are usually the only family members available to provide support and often children do not live with, or even near an aging parent. Three generations living under the same roof are becoming more and more rare in industrialized societies. Urbanization and industrialization have created a "push" toward the cities for the youth, which often leaves the extended family living in rural areas without adequate social support (Shanas, 1979). As parents grow older and/or encounter a diagnosis of cancer, it may be difficult for the children to act as caregivers over large geographic distances. Adams and Blieszner (1995, p. 214) report that "increased geographic mobility have led to smaller households, with more elders living alone and more dispersed family networks." Personal assistance and support are difficult to provide when large distances separate families. Shi (1994) discusses this problem in China. As the birth rate declines and fewer multigenerational families share the same residence, family support systems are threatened. The government of China provides little formal support to the elderly, thus the family must make arrangements to provide the necessary support systems, even over great distances.

With the demographic changes in the world, the family has taken on a new appearance called the "beanpole" family (Adams & Blieszner, 1995). Increased longevity, and a decrease in birth rates mean fewer members of each generational cohort (five generations may exist, each with fewer members). In years past, often families had many children who were responsible to care for a few aging family members. Today fewer children are available to care for an increasing number of family members who are growing older. So instead of a "pyramid" family, a "beanpole" family now exists.

Within the United States, the job of providing support to aging parents often falls on daughters (Beigel, Magaziner & Baum, 1991). As women continue to make up a large portion of the labor force around the world, they find themselves acting in the role of career woman, mother, housekeeper, wife, and caregiver to aging family members (Brody, 1981). Not only are adult daughters the people most often responsible for caring for aging parents within the United States, but also daughters suffer more stress in the role of caregiver when compared to the spouse of the aging parent (Jones & Vetter, 1984). When the primary social support person has the same residence as the person in need, then often family and friends withdraw support, which typically leaves the caregiver isolated and lonely. The member of the support system who lives with the person in need bears the brunt of the obligations. Formal support services should proactively target the caregivers who share the residence of the care-receiver for stress management and respite services (Rose, 1990). Extending help to the primary support person before they become entirely overwhelmed with daily caregiving responsibilities may prevent the caregiver from becoming ill themselves or resigning from the support role completely. Respite services are very important for the mental wellness of the primary support person (Brawell, Mackenzie, Larschinger & Cameron, 1995).

Having a family support system helps the older person cope with bereavement issues and live with the loss of a spouse, close relatives, and friends. Families provide much-needed companionship and understanding to the older person through illness (Silverstein & Bengston, 1994). When the older person becomes in need of instrumental support then the children are often expected to help, more so than friends and/or neighbors. Antonucci (1985) writes that older people who require instrumental assistance are most comfortable with their families providing these services. This may result from the expectation that family members will meet the needs of other family members out of the sense of familial obligation. As stated previously, Cantor, Brennan and Sainz (1994, p. 106) report "children are the most crucial element in the social support of older people."

Not all adult children are motivated by the same reasons to take on the role as the primary support person of an aging, ill relative. Silverstein, Parrott and Bengston (1995, p. 473) assessed the factors that motivate sons and daughters to provide support to aging parents. The study concluded that sons provide support based on obligation, familiarity, and self-interest, "implying that they contribute to the support of parents more out of service and selfishness than out of sentiment." Daughters were found to be influenced by "intimacy and altruism" (p. 473).

For all the benefits of having the support of family, there are also some challenges (Krause, 1995). Negative interactions are likely to occur between family members more so than between friends, and elderly kin are usually the recipients of these negative interactions. Krause (1995: 71) states, " . . . it is likely that negative interactions will exert a more noxious effect on the elderly because older adults may

be less able to extricate themselves from problematic encounters."
Lack of a confidante and sense of objectification (treating the care-
receiver like a object or thing) were found to be major causes of
conflict and negative social interaction (Johnson, 1996). Support from
adult children can be beneficial emotionally in moderate levels and
distressful at higher levels (Silverstein & Chien, 1996). In other words,
at a certain point the amount of support can be detrimental and cause
a decrease in the well being of the older parent. It would be unwise of
a researcher to assume that all relationships, friend and kin, are positive and the source of mainly pleasurable interactions. Thoroughly
examining the quality of social support as part of the nursing history
before assuming that actual positive support is the yield is crucial in
understanding how the patient is able to have their emotional, physical, functional, and social needs met while enduring a diagnosis of
cancer and cancer treatment (Kaufman, 1990).

The persons offering support can also experience distress from
negative interactions perpetrated by the care-receiver. Adverse social
support contributes to the amount of strain experienced by the caregiver. Caregiver strain may result from the stress of adjusting to the
deterioration of a family member (often a parent), which often spurs
feelings of helplessness and anger that can result in negative interactions. Caregiver strain may lead to a decline in health, reduced social
contacts, and a reduction in self-esteem (Spaid & Barusch, 1991).

Friends also play an important role in the support systems and
social networks of older persons suffering from diagnoses such as
cancer. Patients who have suffered a cancer diagnosis look for esteem, directed guidance, and reassurance from many different sources
(friends, family, and health professionals) due to "the importance of
restoring self-esteem in coping with a life-threatening illness such as
cancer" (Rose, 1995, p. 459). Friends are frequently utilized at higher
rates then have been generally reported, especially in areas of bereavement (Adams, 1986). Friends who are older themselves may have
experienced loss and are better able to provide advice and assistance
in coping with such issues. The social support of friends is often
called upon when someone experienced in matters of aging is needed,
when elderly have no family, or when the need for help is unpredictable (Adams & Blieszner, 1995).

For the people 85 and older, it has been found that lack of friend
support leads to higher psychological distress (Matt & Dean, 1993).
Older people often feel greater importance toward the support they
receive from friends. As people grow older they are less likely to have
a spouse, be employed, or even live close to family members. The

importance placed on the support of friends is crucial to good psychological health and possibly physical health.

The role of sibling relationships to the support has been evaluated. Unfortunately, sibling relationships were rather infrequent and generally nonsupportive, even if the older person and the sibling lived nearby (Wilson, Calsyn & Orlofsky, 1994). Nurses should not assume that siblings living nearby will necessarily provide adequate support to the person in need, and other plans for support, either formal or informal, should be formulated.

NURSING RECOMMENDATIONS DIRECTED TOWARD SOCIAL SUPPORT ISSUES

This review is not complete without a section focused on nursing interventions. No matter what social support situation is in place for the older cancer person, it is important to define: Is anyone providing support? Who are the people providing support? To what extent are people providing support? How do the people providing supports, and the people receiving the support, feel about their situation? These questions can establish a starting point to determine whether further interventions such as transportation, caregiver respite, furnished meals, and/or home care are necessary.

Older people undergoing cancer care not only may require someone to provide assistance and support, but they may also be the support to an ill spouse or another person who requires care (Overcash, 2001b). In a study of older women with breast cancer, 6 of the 12 participants were also caregivers to another person while they themselves were undergoing cancer treatment. Assessments specifically geared to determine the patient's roles and responsibilities can reveal some potential problems that should be addressed before an acute situation occurs.

Nursing in conjunction with social work can provide a comprehensive assessment to make the journey through cancer diagnosis and treatment as functional as possible. It is hard to make suggestions of specific assessment and intervention components because every situation is different, with varied individual needs and limitations. Asking the "right" questions and listening to the responses (as common sensical as it sounds) is the best skill to determine what a patient needs as social support.

As referred to in Table 13.3, even asking the right questions may not render a clear, simplistic solution for solving social support problems such as a lack of caregiver, but it will define the need so a plan can be formulated. Accessing community agencies (possibility in conjunction with social work) may help resolve outstanding social support problems. Limited economic resources may qualify the patient for services offered through Medicaid; however, these services are often limited. There is no easy solution to the myriad of problems associated with a lack of social support, but knowing the available options helps to develop realistic plans that may help the patient receive the cancer care they need.

CONCLUSION

This chapter has addressed only some of the issues related to the social support networks of the older cancer patient. Malnutrition, increased medication use, and comorbidities (multiple diagnosis) are health concerns that may also play a part in the concept of social support networks, and should be explored in further research. There is no lack of available social support literature, nor experts who have dedicated their professional work to this topic in the disciplines of psychology, nursing, anthropology and medicine. New information is added to this body of knowledge monthly as noted by the growing citations in the medical and psychosocial databases.

REFERENCES

Adamchak, D. J., Wilson, Adrian, A., Nyanguru, A., & Hampson, J. (1991). Elderly support and intergenerational transfer in Zimbabwe: An analysis by gender, marital status, and place of residence. *The Gerontologist, 31*(4): 505–513.

Adams, R. (1986). Friendship and aging. *Generations, 10*: 40–43.

Adams, R. G. & Blieszner, R. (1995). Aging well with friends and family. *American Behavioral Scientist, 39*(2): 209–224.

Antonucci, T. (1985). Social support: Theoretical advances, recent findings and pressing issues. In Social support: Theory, research and applications. I. G. Sarason & B. Sarason, Eds. pp. 21–37. The Hague, Holland: Martinus Nijhoff.

Auslander, G. K., & Litwin, H. 1990). Social support networks and formal help seeking: Differences between applicants to social services and a nonapplicant sample. *Journal of Gerontology, 45*(3): S112–119.

Balducci, L. (1994). Do we need geriatric oncology? *Cancer Control, 1:* 91–93.

Berkman, L. F., & Syme, L. (1979). Social networks, host resistance, and mortality: A nine-year follow-up study of Alameda County residents. *American Journal of Epidemiology, 109*(2): 186–203.

Biegel, D. E., Magaziner, J., & Baum, M. (1991). Social support networks of white and black elderly people at risk for institutionalization. *Health and Social Work, 16*(4): 245–255.

Bramwell, L., MacKenzie, J., Laschinger, H., & Cameron, N. (1995). Need for overnight respite for primary caregivers of hospice clients. *Cancer Nursing, 18*(5), 337–343.

Brody, E. M., (1981). Women in the middle and family help and older people. *The Gerontologist, 21*(5): 471–481.

Bowling, A., & Brown, P. D. (1991). Social networks, health and emotional well-being among the oldest old in London. *Journal of Gerontology, 46*(1): S20–32.

Bryant, S., & Rakowski, W. (1992). Predictors of mortality among elderly African-Americans. *Research on Aging, 14*(1): 50–67.

Bucquet, C., & Colvez, A. (1992). Sources of instrumental support for dependent elderly people in three parts of France. *Aging and Society, 12*: 329–354.

Cantor, M. H. (1980). The informal support system: Its relevance in the lives of the elderly. In *Aging and Society.* E. Boratta & N. McClusky, Eds. Beverly Hills, CA: Sage.

Cantor, M. J., Brennan, M., & Sainz, A. (1994). The Importance of ethnicity in the social support systems of older New Yorkers: A longitudinal perspective (1970 to 1990). *Journal of Gerontological Social Work, 22*(3/4): 95–127.

Chio, S. J. (1996). The family and ageing in Korea: A new concern and challenge. *Aging and Society, 16*: 1–25.

Cohen, S., & MaKay, G. (1984). Social support, stress and the buffering hypothesis: A theoretical analysis. In *Handbook of Psychological Health.* (pp. 253–267). Baum, A., Taylor, S. E., & Singer, J. E., Eds. Hillsdale, NJ: Erbaum.

Cohen, S., & Syme, A. (1985). *Social support and health.* New York: Academic Press Inc.

Dean, A., Kolody, B., & Wood, P. (1990). Effects of social support from various sources on depression in elderly persons. *Journal of Health and Social Behavior, 31*: 148–161.

Ell, K., Nishimoto, R., Mediansky, L., Mantell, J., & Hamovitch, M. (1992). Social relations, social support and survival among patients with cancer. *Journal of Psychosomatic Research, 36*(6): 531–541.

Freedman, V. A., Berkman, L., Rapp, S. R., & Ostfield, A. M. (1994). Family networks: Predictors of nursing home entry. *American Journal Of Public Health, 8*: 843–845.

Funch, D., & Marshall, J. (1983). The role of stress, social support and age in survival from breast cancer. *Journal of Psychosomatic Research, 27*(1): 77–83.

Goodwin, J. S., Samet, J. M., & Hunt, W. C. (1996). Determinants of survival in older cancer patients. *Journal of the National Cancer Institute, 88*(15): 1031–1838.

240

Gliksman, M. D., Lazarus, R., & Leeder, S. R. (1995). Social support, marital status and living arrangement correlates of cardiovascular disease risk factors in the elderly. *Social Science and Medicine, 40*(6): 811–814.

Guidey, J. J., Greisinger, A., Aday, L. A., Winn, R. J., Vernon, S., & Throckmarton, T. A. (1996). Barriers to cancer treatment: A review of published research. *Oncology Nursing Forum, 23*(9): 1393–1398.

Halstead, M. T., & Fernsler, J. I. (1994). Coping strategies of long-term cancer survivors. *Cancer Nursing, 17*(2): 94–100.

Hannum, R. J. (1990) Social support and cancer: Adult patients' desire for support from family, friends and health professionals. *American Journal of Community Psychology, 18*(3): 439–461.

Havil, R. J., Yancik, R., Long, S., Ries, L., & Edwards, B. (1994). The National Institute on Aging and the National Cancer Center Institute SEER Collaborative study on comorbidity and early diagnosis of cancer in the elderly. *Cancer, 77*:2101–2106.

Irwin, P. H., & Kramer, S. (1988). Social support and cancer: Sustained emotional support and successful adaptation. *Journal of Psychosocial Oncology, 6*(1/2): 53–71.

Johnson, R. J. (1996). Risk factors associated with negative interactions between family caregivers and elderly care receivers. *International Journal of Aging and Human Development, 43*(1): 7–20.

Jones, D., & Vetter, N. J. (1984). A survey of those who care For the elderly at home: Their problems and their needs. *Social Science and Medicine, 19*(5): 511–514

Jow-Ching Tu, E., Freedman, V. A., & Wolf, D. A. (1992). Kinship and family support in Taiwan. *Research on Aging, 15*(4): 465–486.

Kaufman, A. V. (1990). Social network assessment: A critical component in case management for functionally impaired older persons. *International Journal of Aging and Human Development, 30*(1): 63–75.

Krause, N. (1995). Negative interaction and satisfaction with social support among older adults. *Journal of Gerontology, 50B*(2): P59–P73.

Krause, N., & Markides, K. (1990). Measuring social support among older adults. *International Journal of Aging and Human Development, 30*(1): 37–53.

Lackner, S., Goldenberg, S., Arrizza, G., & Tjosvold, I. (1994). The contingency of social support. *Qualitative Health Research, 4*(2): 224–243.

Matt, G. E., & Dean, A. (1993). Social support from friends and psychological distress among elderly persons: Moderator effects of age. *Journal of Health and Social Behavior, 34*: 187–200.

Mitchell, J. C. (1974). Social networks. *Annual Review of Anthropology, 3*: 279–299.

Morrison, J. D. (1991). The Black church as a support system for black elderly. *Journal of Gerontological Social Work, 17*(1/2): 105–119.

Mui, A. (1996). Depression among elderly Chinese immigrants: An exploratory study. *Social Work, 41*(6): 634–643.

Ogawa, N., & Retherford, R. D. (1993). Care of the elderly in Japan: Changing norms and expectations. *Journal of Marriage and the Family, 55*: 585–597.

Peters-Golden, H. (1982) Breast cancer: Varied perceptions of social support in the illness experience. *Social Science Medicine, 16*: 483–491.

Pilisuk, M., Montgomery, M. B., Oarks, S. H., & Acredo, C. (1993). Locus of control, life stress, and social networks: Gender differences in the health status of the elderly. *Sex Roles, 28*(3/4): 147–165.

Powe, B. D. (1996). Fatalism and participation in colorectal cancer screening among poor, elderly, black individuals. Ph.D. Dissertation, School of Nursing, University of South Carolina.

Reynolds, P. & Kaplan, G. (1990). Social connections and risk for cancer: Prospective evidence from the Alameda County study. *Behavioral Medicine, 16*(3): 101–110.

Shanas, E. (1979). The family as a social support system in old age. *The Gerontologist, 19*(2): 169–174.

Shi, L. (1994). Elderly support in rural and suburban villages: Implications for future support system in China. *Social Sciences and Medicine, 39*(2): 265–277.

Shumaker, A. S. & Brownell, A. (1984). Toward a theory of social support: Closing conceptual gaps. *Journal of Social Issues, 40*:11–13.

Silverstein, M. & Bengtson, V. L. (1994). Does intergenerational social support influence the psychological well-being of older parents? The contingencies of declining health and widowhood. *Social Science and Medicine, 38*(7): 943–953.

Silverstein, M. & Chen, X. (1996). Too much of a good thing? Intergenational social support and the psychological well-being of the older parents. *Journal of Marriage and the Family, 58*: 970–982.

Silverstein, M., Parrott, T. M., & Bengtson, V. (1995). Factors and predispose middle-aged sons and daughters to provide social support to older parents. *Journal of Marriage and Family, 57*: 465–475.

Spaid, W. & Barush, A. (1991). Social support and caregiver strain: Types and sources of social contacts of elderly caregivers. *Journal of Gerontological Social Work, 18*(1/2): 151–159.

Tempelaar, R., De Haes, J. C. J. M., De Ruitter, J. H., Bakker, D., Van den Heuvel, W. J. A., & Van Nieuwenhuijzen, M. G. (1989). The social experiences of cancer patients under treatment: A comparative study. *Social Science and Medicine, 29*(5): 635–642.

Thoits, P. A. (1985). Social support and psychological wellbeing: Theoretical possibilities. In *Social support: Theory, research and applications.* I. G. Sarason & R. B. Sarason Eds. Den Haag, Holland: Martinus Nijhoff.

Walker, K. N., MacBirde, A., & Vachon, M. L. (1977). Social support networks and the crisis of bereavement. *Social Science and Medicine, 11*(1): 35–41.

Wellman, B., Carrington, P. J., & Hall, A. (1988). Networks as Personal Communities. In B. Wellman, S. D. Berkowitz (Eds.), *Social structures: A network approach to structural analysis in the social sciences,* Vol. 2 (pp. 130–184). New York: Cambridge University Press.

Willey, C., & Silliman, R. A. (1990). The impact of disease on the social support experiences of cancer patients. *Journal of Psychosocial Oncology, 8*(1): 79–95.

Wilson, J. G., Calsyn, R., & Orlofsky, J. L. (1994). Impact of sibling relationships on social support and morale in the elderly. *Journal of Gerontological Social Work, 22*(3/4): 157– 950.

Wortman C., & Dunkel-Schetter, C. (1979). Interpersonal relationships and cancer. *Journal of Social Issues, 35*: 120–128.

CHAPTER FOURTEEN

Helping Family Caregivers of Elderly Cancer Patients: The CARE Model

John J. Barrett, William E. Haley, and Leah Sisler

Nursing's role in the care of elderly cancer patients and their family members is profound. Because of the aging of our population, the close association of age and cancer prevalence, and pressures to keep patients at home whenever possible, families will likely assume increasing responsibility for older relatives with cancer (Schonwetter, 1992). Increasingly, family members care for their elders at home after initial diagnosis and treatment due to the shift from inpatient to community cancer treatment. With little, if any, preparation, many family caregivers face new care demands, which vary depending upon the stage of the illness and phase of treatment (Given & Given, 1996) and compete with already existing demands. Many family caregivers are threatened with exhaustion from the ongoing daily stress of taking care of a loved one with cancer. Caregivers look to nurses for direction and assistance with the management of their elder's cancer care (Given & Given, 1996; Hileman, Lackey & Hassanein, 1992; Reuben, 1997; Siegel, Raveis, Houts & Mor, 1991).

However, nurses often find older patients with cancer a formidable challenge for several reasons. The traditional medical evaluation of the older patient with cancer often falls short in assessment and treatment of comorbid problems, and on the effects of cancer and other disabilities on the family. Because cancer and its treatment are associated with medical and functional impairments as well as psychological sequelae such as depression, elderly patients with cancer require careful symptom management and thorough psychosocial support, and their families have parallel needs. Nurses face another challenge in their management of elderly cancer patients, namely, cognitive impairment, with delirium a common problem in cancer patients (Lawlor, Fainsinger & Bruera, 2000), and nearly half of those over age 85 having Alzheimer's disease. Many assessment tools rely upon the patient's active and accurate participation and self-report. Impaired memory along with depression and sensory impairment (e.g., hearing) can hinder assessment and treatment of such symptoms as pain. Nurses can expect to see increasing numbers of elderly cancer patients with complex comorbid problems given the increasing incidence rates, longer survival, and the aging of the population (Ferrel, Rhiner, Cohen & Grant, 1991; Nijboer, Triemstra, Tempelaar, Sanderman & Van Den Bos, 1999; Reuben, 1997; Yancik, 1997).

Family caregivers are central to the nurse's assessment and care of the older patient with cancer. Given the trend toward outpatient care, a major portion of the responsibility for caring for these patients frequently lies with a family member, or in some cases a significant other, friend, or neighbor (Harrington, Lackey, & Gates, 1996; Hileman & Lackey, 1990; McMillan, 1996). They often provide emotional support, assist with activities of daily living, administer and monitor medications and side effects, ensure proper nutrition, and help with other physical aspects of care (Hileman & Lackey, 1990; McMillan, 1996). Any regimen prescribed by the physician will often be implemented with the assistance of these caregivers. The nurse depends on these caregivers to report relevant information, especially when the elder's comorbid conditions such as dementia, depression, or hearing impairment threaten the accuracy of the patient's self-report. These caregivers provide vital assistance to the nurse in assessment and care of their loved one with cancer. Nurses and caregivers must work collaboratively to provide care to the elderly cancer patient.

However, caregivers are at risk for adverse outcomes such as depression, anxiety, sleep disruptions, psychosomatic symptoms, disruption in family relationships, and diminished physical health (Miaskowski, Kragness, Dibble & Wallhagen, 1997; Toseland, Blanchard & McCallion, 1995). Succumbing to these negative consequences seems related to characteristics of the caregiver, the patient, and the care situation (Nijboer et al., 1999). Influential caregiver factors include their age, gender, living situation, socioeconomic status, health, type and quality of the relationship between elder and caregiver, and caregiver's perceptions. For example, caregiver's perception of caregiving is associated with their mental health (Nijboer et al., 1999). Caregiver's optimism has been found to be an influential predictor of caregiver burden and depression (Given & Given, 1996). Patient characteristics such as dependency seem to negatively affect the caregiver (Given & Given, 1996). Finally, the caregiver's vulnerability to negative consequences may also be influenced by characteristics of the care situation including duration, intensity, and type of care. For example, some personal tasks such as feeding and bathing the patient seem to be perceived as more difficult and burdensome than nonpersonal tasks (grocery shopping) (Given & Given, 1996). While many experience increased levels of strain upon assuming this new role, some caregivers experience much satisfaction associated with successfully providing care to their elder.

Nurses must attend to family caregivers to assure that the elderly cancer patient receives the best possible care. With little, if any instruction, these family caregivers assume this major responsibility for patient care. They need:

1. support (e.g., psychological and spiritual),
2. information about the disease (e.g., prognosis, treatment, and "how to" physically care for their elder), medications (administration guidelines, common side effects), and community resources (e.g., delivery of home care, hospice, respite, legal and financial advice); and
3. assistance with problem solving (Blanchard, Albrecht & Ruckdeschel, 1997; Bucher, Houts, Nezu & Nezu, 1999; Ferrel et al., 1991; Harrington et al., 1996; Hileman et al., 1992; McMillan, 1996; Yates, 1999).

The family caregiver becomes a vital member of the health care team working collaboratively with other health care professionals to provide quality care for the elderly cancer patient. Many caregivers are not familiar or comfortable with this role. It is important to acknowledge their value, listen to their concerns, and identify their goals. When caregivers are under acute stress (newly admitted to hospice, new diagnosis, newly discharged from hospital to home), information and direct assistance are particularly vital.

The relative importance of caregivers' needs changes over the course of their elder's illness. If these caregivers are uninformed or lack adequate support, elderly cancer patients' physical well-being may be compromised. These caregivers can benefit from nurses' expertise and support.

While nurses cannot directly provide all services at various stages of the disease, they can enlist the support of family caregivers and allied health professionals to accomplish a four-step approach to patient assessment and care. This approach allows the family caregiver to benefit from the nurse's expertise and enhances the nurse's success in assessment and care of the cancer patient, given the many competing demands on the nurse's time. Nurses can improve the quality of life for patients and their caregivers across all stages of the disease by following this simple, cost-effective, four-step strategy summarized in the acronym CARE: (C) conceptualize the caregiving situation, (A) assess the caregiving situation, (R) respond to assessed needs, and (E) evaluate response and situation. Caregivers want a thorough evaluation and explanation of their relative's condition, and they need the facts. Family caregivers depend on nurses' informed responses to questions about patient care or referrals to community support. The basic goal of cost-efficient management strategies is to maximize the independence and dignity of the patient while minimizing the negative impact on the family caregiver. Nurses should not underestimate the benefits of these steps in helping family members care for their elders with cancer.

C: CONCEPTUALIZE THE CAREGIVING SITUATION

Nurses working with older cancer patients and their family caregivers encounter numerous complex problems that may be difficult to understand. In working with family caregivers, it is useful for the clinician to have a clear conceptual model to guide assessment and intervention. For example, a nurse observes that an elderly man is not providing adequate care for his wife with breast cancer. Without a theoretical approach in understanding this circumstance, the nurse may conclude that the husband does not care, or is unwilling to provide care. The stress process model of caregiving, described below, provides nurses with a conceptual framework for understanding the dynamics of the caregiving situation and guiding their assessment and interventions. In the example given, it may be that the husband is overwhelmed by the stressors he is facing; that he has poor understanding of the cancer and has very low self-efficacy for his ability to provide the care; that he has cognitive impairment or other limitations; or that he is depressed and has too little energy to provide the needed care.

The stress process model assumes that multiple factors and processes account for the individual differences in caregiver outcome (i.e., physical and psychological health). This conceptual model consists of four components:

1. stressors,
2. caregiver appraisals,
3. psychosocial resources, and
4. mental and physical well-being.

Stressors refer to the cancer patient's ill health (i.e., physical and psychological) and associated care tasks (Haley et al., 1996; Nijboer et al., 1999). Stressors are classified as primary and secondary. Primary stressors are direct consequences of the elder's cancer and disability. They include stressors that directly related to caregiving tasks, such as assisting the patient with self-care tasks, managing patient symptoms and treatment regime, and witnessing the suffering of the relative with cancer (Blank, Longman & Atwood, 1989; Hinds, 1985; Stetz, 1987; Zarit & Zarit, 1998). Secondary stressors refer to the consequences of the primary stressors on the caregiver's life, such as role strain including strains on finances and employment, changes in family structure due to providing care to the patient, and changes in the caregiver's self-concept (Zarit & Zarit, 1998). Research suggests that the severity of patient self-care impairments alone has relatively little direct relationship to caregiver well-being, but that patient behavioral problems, pain, and mood disturbances are more likely to be related to caregiver depression and burden (Miaskowski et al., 1997; Schultz, O'Brien, Bookwala & Fleissner, 1995). However, taken together, these stressors account for a surprisingly small portion of the variance of caregiver well-being and strain (Zarit & Zarit, 1998). Nevertheless, cancer in the elderly with its accompanying stressors is a context ripe for caregiver distress. Whether caregivers succumb to this distress depends upon additional factors in the stress process model (Zarit & Zarit, 1998).

Caregivers can respond differently to similar stressors due in part to caregivers' differential appraisals of their elder's problems, changes in their lives due to the demands of caregiving, and their resources. Carey, Oberst, McCubbin and Hughs (1991) reported that a negative appraisal of the caregiving situation mediated the relationship between caregiver burden and patient dependency. Subjective appraisals of caregiving stressors have been found to be more predictive of caregiver burden and depression than objective severity of patient illness. Caregiving events become stressful through their interface with caregiver's appraisal along with other factors.

Available psychosocial resources can buffer the effects of stressful events. These resources include formal and informal support and cop-

ing skills. Spouses with lower levels of social support have more difficulty adjusting than those with a higher level of social support (Northhouse, 1988). A recent study found that cancer caregivers with a low
level of daily emotional support became more depressed over time (Nijboer, Tempelaar, Triemstra, Van Den Bos & Sanderman, 2001). However,
research suggests that the caregivers' perception of social support, not
the sheer amount, is crucial. A longitudinal study (Ell, Nichimoto, Mantel
& Hamovitch, 1988) found that low levels of perceived social support
predicted poor functioning in the caregiver. Patterns of social support
established during caregiving may have important implications for subsequent adjustment of the caregiver during bereavement in the case of
terminally ill patients (Bodnar & Kiecolt-Glaser, 1994).

Coping skills can also serve as an effective stress buffer. Approach
coping involves directly facing the stress through such means as seeking out information or problem solving. On the other hand, avoidance
coping attempts to ignore problems or engage in wishful thinking
(Moos, Cronkite, Billings & Finney, 1984). While avoidance coping may
be effective in reducing distress in the short run, research finds that
caregivers who use approach coping more extensively have better
psychological adjustment.

One adaptive personality trait to note is the caregiver's level of
optimism. More optimistic caregivers appear less depressed and appraise the caregiving situation as having less of an impact upon their
health and schedule than caregivers who scored low on optimism
(Kurtz, Given & Given, 1995). Given et al. (1993) also reported that the
caregiver's disposition of optimism predicted the caregiver's mental
health status and their reactions to caregiving.

In sum, caregivers' mental and physical health depends upon multiple factors and processes. Caregiver outcome is not determined solely
by the demands of the situation or available resources, but in part by
the caregivers' appraisal of the relationship between these demands
and available resources (Zarit & Zarit, 1998). These dynamics of the
stress process model can focus the nurse's assessment and response.

A: ASSESS THE CAREGIVING SITUATION

Nurses usually meet family caregivers while they are caring for the
elderly cancer patient. In addition to evaluating the patient, nurses
must assess the family caregiver, given their essential role in patient
care. The stress process model can guide nurses' assessment, and
should include assessments of stressors, appraisals, psychosocial resources, and caregiver mental and physical well-being.

First, nurses must evaluate caregivers' understanding of their elder's illness, symptoms, treatment, prognosis, and the important role they play in patient care. These caregivers often lack understanding about various aspects of the illness and desire more information to enhance their care for their elder (Yates, 1999). Next, nurses need to identify the stressors (i.e., primary and secondary) and determine which stressors the caregivers appraise to be stressful or problematic. Their ratings may change as stressors emerge and recede in importance during the course of the disease. The Memorial Symptom Assessment Scale (MSAS) is an outstanding instrument in this area (Portenoy et al., 1994). In addition, nurses should assess caregivers' emotional distress. Although a rare occurrence, despondent caregivers have killed their terminally ill spouses and then themselves. Nurses can assess for depression and suicidal thoughts by administering a brief self-report rating scale, such as a caregiver strain measure or a depression inventory (e.g., Beck Depression Inventory) (Zarit & Zarit, 1998).

Given caregivers' vulnerability to exhaustion and frustration, nurses must also assess for elder abuse. Estimates indicate that 800,000 to 2 million adults are victims of abuse or neglect each year. Risk factors include stressful lifestyle of the abuser and/or victim, limited social support network, behavioral problems, incontinence, the need to be fed, alcohol or drug abuse, a family history of violence, isolation of the victim, and a history of mental illness (Ebersole & Hess, 1998). For further assessment and treatment strategies for elder abuse, readers may find Quinn and Tomita's (1997) classic text a helpful reference.

Next, nurses need to explore the effectiveness of the caregivers' past and present strategies to manage patient care and problems. As nurses gather this information, they can evaluate whether these coping strategies reflect more an approach or avoidant style. Nurses should pay attention to the caregivers' level of optimism, and caregivers' perceived adequacy of support (i.e., informal and formal) and their awareness of available community resources.

If nurses suspect that an elderly caregiver has memory problems that could jeopardize patient care, then they may assess the caregiver's awareness of any memory lapses and may administer a brief cognitive screen, such as the Mini-Mental State Examination (Folstein, Folstein & McHugh, 1975). An outside referral to a neurologist or neuropsychologist may be warranted for a definitive diagnosis. Based upon a thorough assessment, nurses can tailor their responses to the needs of the caregiver and the elderly cancer patient, which can change relative to the type of cancer, the stage of the disease, and phase of treatment (Given & Given, 1996).

R: RESPOND

Nurses can respond to problems caregivers find distressing by using a combination of emotional support, information, and problem solving. Although nurses' training tends to emphasize solving problems and providing information, emotional support is as essential to caregiving as their efforts in problem solving, education, and referrals. An essential early step that is often assumed but is critical is the development of rapport, and a sense in the family that the nurse is a caring and empathic person. This is key to any helping relationship. Caregivers also appreciate the emotional support nurses can provide. These caregivers experience a range of feelings throughout the course of their elder's illness. They may be ashamed of some feelings. When nurses acknowledge, accept, and normalize the range of feelings that caregivers often experience, they create a "safe" environment for these caregivers to discuss difficult issues. If the nurse believes the caregiver could benefit from more in-depth psychological support, she can refer the caregiver to a mental health professional. Nurses' encouragement and praise of caregivers' appropriate responses can promote the well-being of their elders. Because these caregivers may at times feel underappreciated, nurses can empathize with them and underscore the valuable service they are providing for their loved one.

Nurses must educate caregivers about their elders' illness, symptoms, treatment, treatment side effects, prognosis, and the need to take care of their own health. Some family caregivers are aware of their need for further education. For example, family caregivers of patients facing bone marrow transplantation reported the need for information about preparing for caregiving, managing the care, facing challenges, and developing supportive strategies (Stetz, McDonald & Compton, 1996). Other caregivers may be misinformed and need to be educated. For example, some caregivers may believe that their elder will become addicted to pain medication. Consequently, they may under-medicate their elder, which can worsen their elder's problems. Research has shown that education about cancer pain improves family caregivers' knowledge about pain and their experience caring for the elderly patient in pain (Ferrel, Grant, Chan, Ahn & Ferrel, 1995).

Nurses can also inform caregivers about available community resources that can benefit their elders and themselves. Nurses can refer caregivers to community agencies. Appropriate referrals afford caregivers access to available support systems such as Hospice, chore services, respite care, support groups, individual counseling, and Meals on Wheels. In a recent survey assessing primary caregivers' needs for overnight respite, nearly 60% of primary caregivers reported the amount of sleep they are getting is inadequate and 70% of all respondents indicated that they would use overnight respite services (Bramwell, MacKenzie & Laschinger, 1995). Nurses' referrals afford caregivers access to available support systems. For example, one recent study found that a short length of stay by a cancer patient in an inpatient hospice, less than eight days, was associated with better psychological well-being for spousal caregivers (Gilbar, 1998). Names of local support groups and other helpful information can be obtained through the National Cancer Institute (1–800–422–6237) and the American Cancer Society (1–800–227–2345). Appropriate and timely referrals benefit the caregiver and the elderly cancer patient.

To work successfully on problem solving, nurses collaborate with the caregiver to identify, prioritize, and describe the problems related to caregiving. Successful interventions depend upon an accurate assessment of the problematic patient behavior, circumstances before the behavior occurs (i.e., antecedents), and consequences of the behavior. The nurse should investigate the problem behavior and determine such basics as: when did it first occur?; when does it occur (i.e., time of day)?; who is present?; and how often does it occur? Determining these factors can further refine nurses' assessment of the problem, and provides baseline data to evaluate the effects of future intervention(s). The nurse can ask the caregiver about the antecedents and consequences of the problematic behavior, which may inadvertently reinforce the problematic behavior (Zarit & Zarit, 1998).

Next, nurses must collaborate with elderly cancer patients and their caregivers to find appropriate solutions, including pharmacologic or behavioral interventions. Pharmacologic interventions may lessen such symptoms as pain, though not without the risk of adverse side effects and complications. Because elderly cancer patients are at risk for complications resulting from polypharmacy, it is important to gather a comprehensive medication history including past experience with medications prescribed for symptom management (especially pain, dyspnea, or constipation), over-the-counter medication (including herbal/alternative remedies), current medication, allergies, and sensitivities. Current medications should always be reviewed when new therapies are prescribed, to avoid negative drug interactions. Possible side effects underscore the need for close monitoring by nurses. Nurses value the caregiver's feedback regarding the patient's compliance with a drug regimen and response to the drug. It is helpful to instruct the caregiver to keep a log of medications given with the time and response noted. The nurse should ask the caregiver to observe possible side effects (e.g., nausea, vomiting, sedation, dizziness, constipation, diarrhea, hallucinations, urinary retention, increased agitation).

However, many problems may not respond to pharmacological interventions.

Sometimes behavioral strategies are a more effective response to modify the environment, patient, or caregiver. Nurses can reduce caregiver distress through teaching caregivers new coping skills, such as cognitive strategy of "reframing." The stressfulness of the caregiving situation can be reduced by helping caregivers view the situation from a different perspective. For example, by explaining to caregivers about the appropriate use of pain medication for cancer patients, nurses can help change a caregiver's perspective that their elder will become addicted. Nurses may also recommend modifying the environment by utilizing formal and informal supports for patient care. In collaboration with caregivers, nurses might have to identify the pros and cons of proposed solutions and agree upon trying one solution (Zarit & Zarit, 1998). After agreeing to implement one, the nurse might encourage the caregiver to rehearse the steps involved in carrying out the proposed solution. This "dry run" can address and speak to overcoming possible obstacles. Then, the nurse encourages the caregiver to implement the solution and monitor the problem for reduced frequency. Finally, the nurse in collaboration with the caregiver evaluates the success of the response. If nurses are not familiar with these procedures, they may refer caregivers to an appropriate allied health professional who is (e.g., psychologist, nurse, social worker) (Zarit & Zarit, 1998).

E: EVALUATE THE RESPONSES AND SITUATION

Ongoing evaluations are indicated for elderly cancer patients and their caregivers. Periodic evaluations are needed to monitor the patient's physical changes, medication regimen, and the caregiver's management of coping with patient behaviors. Thus, the nurse focuses not only on the patient's changes over time but also on the caregiver's coping with these changes. Family caregivers rely on the nurse to provide advice and support regarding management of their elder. In turn, nurses can receive valuable feedback from the caregiver about the relative's compliance with a prescribed regimen, as well as the patient's physical, emotional, and behavioral changes. The cancer symptoms can vary over time. Ongoing management of functional loss and behavior problems can prevent the caregiver from reaching a crisis point. Caregiver burnout may lead to premature institutionalization of their elder or to serious physical and mental health problems in the caregiver.

One important element to consider in ongoing evaluation is to consider the need for discussion of end of life issues. Medicine, in particular oncology, can be highly focused on finding a cure, but when curative approaches have reached their limits, patients and families need to consider palliative care, hospice, advance directives, and preparation for bereavement. Since there can be an unspoken agreement among the patient, family, and health care providers to avoid addressing the reality of death, many patients do not receive appropriate hospice and palliative care. Family members are often key to such discussions and decisions.

CASE EXAMPLE

M.G. is a 75-year-old married African-American male diagnosed with stage four prostate cancer with bony metastasis two weeks ago. He is experiencing severe low back and leg pain which he currently rates as a "9" on a 10 point scale. He reports that the best his pain has been in the past 24 hours is an "8" and the worst is a "10." He states that it is worse when he moves and it is better when he sits or lies very still. Mr. G. lives in his home with his wife of 55 years. Mrs. G. (71 years old) has been identified as Mr. G.'s primary caregiver in the home. Mrs. G. has been reluctant to give Mr. G. his pain medication because she doesn't want him to become addicted. Mr. G. was referred by his primary care physician to hospice for pain and symptom management.

Use of the stress process model of caregiving as a conceptual framework (C) allows the nurse to assess (A) Mrs. G.'s stressors and psychosocial resources as she provides care for Mr. G. at home. Because of Mr. G.'s deteriorating physical condition (progressive disease resulting in increased debility and pain), Mrs. G. provides for his physical care including bathing and dressing. She is also experiencing secondary stressors related to role reversal and strain because as Mr. G. was once responsible for the financial dealings of the household, Mrs. G. finds that now she must manage the household finances—a role that she is not accustomed to. Mrs. G. reports that this is "very stressful" for her and that her only son is not able to help because he has a family to take care of himself, and she has a relative absence of social support. She reports that she is tired and feels "worn out" because Mr. G. is not sleeping well at night because of the pain. She does have a number of assets in coping, including an optimistic personality, strong religious faith, and excellent problem-solving abilities. It is determined that she has particular needs for more information about cancer and its treatments, and problem-solving aimed at getting more help from her son and learning to manage the family's finances.

The nurse, in response (R), provides emotional support and information and assists the caregiver with problem-solving. The nurse listens to Mrs. G.'s concerns regarding her husband's condition. He/she acknowledges that Mrs. G. is an active participant on the health care team and explains to Mrs. G. the principles of good pain management, including the difference between physical dependence on and addiction to pain medications. Together, they develop a plan to help Mr. G. achieve maximum pain control, including giving him his medications around the clock as prescribed, assessing for side effects of the pain medication, and reporting emergency symptoms of pain to the health care team. Mrs. G. and the nurse discuss ways to let her son know how much he is needed at this time. In addition, Mrs. G. makes a plan to get help in managing her finances from a neighbor and member of her church who is an accountant.

Together, Mrs. G. and the nurse evaluate (E) the plan during follow-up telephone calls and visits. Mr. G. now rates his pain as a 2/10 and is able to enjoy conversations with his wife. He is also sleeping better at night—and so is Mrs. G. This greatly improves her sense of well-being. Mrs. G. has asked her son to spend two nights a week, giving her a 'break' from the intensive care that her husband requires. She has successfully learned to manage the checkbook, but needs additional help to understand her husband's pension plan and insurance. Continuing assessment, response, and evaluation are key to successful outcomes in caring for elderly cancer patients and their caregivers.

CONCLUSIONS

The nurse is pivotal in the care of elderly cancer patients and their caregivers throughout all stages of the disease. A comprehensive approach involves the four steps summarized in the acronym CARE: (C) conceptualize the caregiving situation, (A) assess patient and caregiver, (R) respond to their needs and problems, and (E) evaluate on an ongoing basis patient management. This approach emphasizes a close working relationship between the nurse and family caregivers. The caregiver can benefit from nurses' conceptualization of his or her situation, accurate assessment, appropriate and timely responses in the form of education, problem solving, referrals, and emotional support, and periodic evaluations of patient care. Furthermore, patient care can be enhanced when nurses elicit caregivers' input throughout this four-step process. Finally, through this approach, nurses can monitor the caregiver's physical, mental, and emotional well-being and can recommend that the caregiver take appropriate steps to safeguard his or her own health. The increasing numbers of elders with cancer will make care of these patients and their families a substantial part of the practice of many nurses in the years ahead.

REFERENCES

Blanchard, C. G., Albrecht, T. L., & Ruckdeschel, J. C. (1997). The crisis of cancer: Psychological impact on family caregivers. *Oncology, 11*(2), 189–194.

Blank, J. J., Longman, A. J., & Atwood, J. R. (1989). Perceived home care needs of cancer patients and their caregivers. *Cancer Nursing, 12,* 78–84.

Bodnar, J. C., & Kiecolt-Glaser, J. K. (1994). Caregiver depression after bereavement: Chronic stress isn't over when it's over. *Psychology of Aging, 9,* 372–380.

Bramwell, L., MacKenzie, J., & Laschinger,H. (1995). Need for overnight respite for primary caregivers of hospice clients. *Cancer Nursing, 18,* 337–343.

Bucher, J. A., Houts, P., Nezu, C. M., & Nezu, A. (1999). Improving problem-solving skills of family caregivers through group education. *The Application of Problem-Solving Therapy to Psychosocial Oncology Care, 16,* 73–84.

Carey, P. J., Oberst, M. T., McCubbin, M. A., & Hughs, S. H. (1991). Appraisal and caregiving burden in family members caring for patients receiving chemotherapy. *Oncology Nursing Forum, 18,* 1341–1348.

Ebersole, P., & Hess, P. (1998). *Toward healthy aging: Human needs and nursing response.* (5th ed.). St. Louis, MO: Mosby-Year Book, Inc.

Ell, K., Nichimoto, R., Mantel, J., & Hamovitch, M. B. (1988). Longitudinal analysis of psychosocial adaptation among family members of patients with cancer. *Journal of Psychosomatic Research, 32,* 429–438.

Ferrel, B., Rhiner, M., Cohen, M. Z., & Grant, M. (1991). Pain as a metaphor for illness Part I: Impact of cancer pain on family caregivers. *Oncology Nursing Forum, 18*(8), 1303–1309.

Ferrel, B. R., Grant, M., Chan, J., Ahn, C., & Ferrel, B. A. (1995). The impact of cancer pain education on family caregivers of elderly patients. *Oncology Nursing Forum, 47,* 1211–1218.

Folstein, M. G., Folstein, S. E., & McHugh, P. R. (1975). Mini-Mental State—A practical method for grading the cognitive state of patients for the clinician. *Journal of Psychiatric Research, 12,* 189–198.

Gilbar, O. (1998). Does length of stay at a hospice affect psychological adjustment to the loss of the spouse? *Journal of Palliative Care, 14,* 16–20.

Given, B., & Given, C. W. (1996). Family caregiver burden from cancer care. In R. McCorkle, M. Grant, M. Frank-Stromborg, & S. Baird (Eds.), *Cancer nursing: A comprehensive textbook* (pp. 93–109). Philadelphia: W.B. Saunders.

Given, C. W., Stommel, M., Given, B., Osuch, J., Kurtz, M. E., & Kurtz, J. C. (1993). The influence of cancer patients' symptoms and functional states on patients' depression and family caregivers' reaction and depression. *Health Psychology, 12*(4), 277–285.

Haley, W. E., Roth, D. L., Coleton, M. I., Ford, G. R., West, C. A. C., Collings, R. P., & Isobe, T. L. (1996). Appraisal, coping, and social support as mediators of well-being in Black and White Alzheimer's family caregivers. *Journal of Consulting Clinical Psychology, 64,* 121–129.

Harrington, V., Lackey, N. & Gates, M. (1996). Needs of caregivers of clinic and hospice cancer patients. *Cancer Nursing, 19,* 118–125.

Hileman, J., & Lackey, N. (1990). Self-identified needs of patients with cancer at home and their home caregivers: A descriptive study. *Oncology Nursing Forum, 17*(6), 907–913.

Hileman, J., Lackey, N., & Hassanein, R. (1992). Identifying the needs of home caregivers of patients with cancer. *Oncology Nursing Forum, 19*(5), 771–777.

Hinds, C. (1985). The needs of families who care for patients with cancer at home. *Journal of Advanced Nursing, 10,* 575–581.

Kurtz, J. C., Given, C. W., & Given, B. (1995). Relationship of caregiver reactions and depression to cancer patients' symptoms, functional status and depression- a longitudinal view. *Social Science and Medicine, 40,* 837–846.

Lawlor, P. G., Fainsinger, R. L., & Bruera, E. D. (2000). Delirium at the end-of-life: Critical issues in clinical practice and research. *Journal of the American Medical Association, 284*(19), 2427–2429.

McMillan, S. C. (1996). Quality of life of primary caregivers of hospice patients with cancer. *Cancer Practice, 4*(4), 191–198.

Miaskowski, C., Kragness, L., Dibble, S., & Wallhagen, M. (1997). Differences in mood states, health status, and caregiver strain between family caregivers of oncology outpatients with and without cancer related pain. *Journal of Pain and Symptom Management, 13,* 138–147.

Moos, R. H., Cronkite, R., Billings, A., & Finney, J. (1984). *Health and Daily Living Form Manual.* Palo Alto: Social Ecology Laboratory, Stanford University and Department of Veteran's Affairs Medical Centers.

Nijboer, C., Tempelaar, R., Triemstra, M., Van Den Bos, G., & Sanderman, R. (2001). The role of social and psychological resources in caregiving of cancer patients. *Cancer, 91,* 1029–1039.

Nijboer, C., Triemstra, M., Tempelaar, R., Sanderman, R., & Van Den Bos, G. (1999). Determinants of caregiving experiences and mental health of partners of cancer patients. *Cancer, 86,* 577–588.

Northhouse, L. L. (1988). Social support in patients' and husbands' adjustment to breast cancer. *Nursing Research, 37,* 91–95.

Portenoy, R. K., Thaler, H. T., Kornblith, A. B., et al. (1994). The Memorial Symptom Assessment Scale: An instrument for the evaluation of symptom prevalence, characteristics and distress. *European Journal of Cancer, 30A,* 1326–1336.

Quinn, M., & Tomita, S. (1997). *Elder abuse and neglect: Causes, diagnosis, and intervention strategies.* (2nd ed.) New York: Springer.

Reuben, D. (1997). Geriatric assessment in oncology. *Cancer, 80,* 1311–1316.

Schonwetter, R. S. (1992). Primary Care: Clinics in office practice. *Geriatric Oncology, 19,* 451–463.

Schulz, R., O'Brien, A. T., Bookwala, J., & Fleissner, K. (1995). Psychiatric and physical morbidity effects of dementia caregiving: Prevalence, correlates, and causes. *Gerontologist, 35,* 771–791.

Siegel, K., Raveis, V., Houts, P., & Mor, V. (1991). Caregiver burden and unmet patient needs. *Cancer, 68,* 1131–1140.

Stetz, K. M. (1987). Caregiving demands during advanced cancer. *Cancer Nursing, 10,* 260–268.

Stetz, K. M., McDonald, J. C., & Compton, K. (1996). Needs and experiences of family caregivers during marrow transplantation. *Oncology Nursing Forum, 23,* 1422–1427.

Toseland, R. W., Blanchard, C. G., & McCallion, P. (1995). A problem solving intervention for caregivers of cancer patients. *Social Science and Medicine, 40,* 517–528.

Yancik, R. (1997). Cancer burden in the aged. *Cancer, 80,* 1273–1283.

Yates, P. (1999). Family coping: Issues and challenges for cancer nursing. *Cancer Nursing, 22*(1), 63–71.

Zarit, S. H., & Zarit, J. M. (1998). *Mental disorders in older adults: Fundamentals of assessment and treatment.* New York and London: The Guilford Press.

CHAPTER FIFTEEN

Nursing Research and Quality of Life

Janine Overcash and Lodovico Balducci

I mprovement and maintenance of Quality of Life (QOL) are a major goal of medical care, especially in conditions in which the improvement of survival is limited and is paid at the price of significant complications. This issue is particularly relevant to the older aged person with cancer, who has a limited life expectancy and increased risk of complications from cancer treatment. While there is almost universal agreement on the principles, the first attempt to measure QOL was performed in 1973. In 1973 a literature review rendered only five articles using the term "quality of life" in the abstract (Testa & Siminson, 1996). In 1993, a MEDLINE search revealed 1252 cites, and that figure does not include a PsyLit or General Academic database search. Oncologists have used the construct of QOL in research as early as the 1940s to help understand some of the effects of cancer treatment (Bowling & Brazier, 1995). This wide body of research has provided important results, but has also revealed serious pitfalls in the measurements of QOL, including the lack of a comprehensive assessment capable to encompass all the aspects of an individual life. This assessment is particularly desirable for older individuals, given the high degree of diversity in this patient population (Overcash & Balducci, 2002a). The extensive amount of literature reviewed for this chapter reflects varying definitions of QOL and the need for clarity of the construct in research projects. This chapter will be a review for nurses using both quantitative and qualitative QOL measures.

TABLE 15.1 Definitions of Quality of Life

General Definition of Quality of Life (QOL)	Health-Related Quality of Life Definition (HRQOL)
A general definition of QOL considers a very holistic set of domains that exist beyond health and physical being. Domains such as economics, housing, independence (both physical and politically), general life satisfaction, relationships, and occupation.	As implied in the title, health-related quality of life tends to look at factors associated with immediate health. Domains of physical, functional, emotional and social well-being are common to HRQOL.

DEFINITIONS OF QUALITY OF LIFE

QOL can be defined in essentially two ways—a general definition of QOL and health-related quality of life (HRQOL) (Table 15.1). The former integrates the notion of all the very different elements and experiences that tend to figure into QOL (Bowling, 1995). Finances, housing, independence, general life satisfaction, relationships, and occupational issues are some of the elements that can determine how someone may rate their QOL at any given time (Farquhar, 1995; Marshall, 1990; Rogerson, 1995; Rosenberg, 1995). Rosenberg (1995) writes that typically health is not an issue of QOL unless it is in some way compromised. The saying about taking health for granted may be true for many when considering QOL. Another way of considering QOL is that of a continuum of pleasure and displeasure, with satisfaction somewhere in the middle. The perception of where QOL should be marked on the continuum is dynamic, changing with respect to situations that arise as part of daily life (Andrews, 1974). The definition of QOL varies then with the perspective of the student. In this chapter we are particularly interested in HRQOL, and then we'll refer to this construct when mentioning QOL. In the meantime we will try to highlight all aspects of life that may influence the perception of QOL in the older person and that must be taken into account both in the practice of oncology and in clinical trials.

Within the wide body of knowledge of "health," many disciplines use the notion of QOL as an endpoint on which to base interventions. Clinicians working with people experiencing mental and/or physical disabilities, aging, cancer, and AIDS/HIV have used QOL in research or clinical practice (Cella et al., 1993; Cella et al., 1998; Farquhar, 1995;

Felce, 1997; Moore, 1999; Testa & Lenderking, 1999). Cella and Tulsky (1990) focus on the effects of disease on physical function. These authors postulate that function deterioration is associated with poorer QOL and function improvement with better QOL. This definition has the merit of assessing the most likely consequence of diseases, but may be age-weighted, to some extent. Perceptions of QOL can be variable between individuals, as we age, and specific to individual health histories. An adolescent who requires bed rest may be more concerned with a reduced social life than is someone who is older and has had a history of health problems and limited activities.

Another assessment of QOL may focus on personal relationship. In this case QOL can be a multilevel, complex construct evaluable at three levels: *intrapersonal,* which means that people consider QOL on how they might, would, or could envision themselves; *interpersonal,* which are comparisons between people and *sociocultural,* in which the person's condition is compared with societal expectations (Sartorius, 1987). Skevington (1994) performed a study to further assess Sartorius's (1987) theories and found that interpersonal comparisons were the most common in clinical research. Again, this type of assessment may be problematic in older individuals, whose function and health may be highly variable even in a short age range (Overcash & Balducci, 2002b).

Others consider QOL to be a multifaceted construct involving physical, social, and emotional dimensions and the way health and health care are perceived. These QOL measures tend to have the merit to assess the patient's feelings toward health and treatment, thus shifting some power toward the patient in terms of rating how their personal needs are being met (Smart & Yates, 1987). Empowering the patient to rate QOL dependent on health care, or tell their perceptions of the cancer experience, highlights the personal aspects of QOL, including the influence of symptom management, the individual perception of remission, disease progression, and cancer diagnosis. This approach also highlights the limitations of quantitative measurements of QOL in encompassing all aspects of a person's existential experience. In general, quantitative measurements have a "low ceiling," meaning that they can differentiate very well bad and very bad QOL, but less well bad, good, and very good. Hence the need of a qualitative, more comprehensive approach.

In addition to providing important end points in interventional and descriptive research, and providing a measure of treatment outcome, qualitative or quantitative definitions of QOL can be a patient quality assurance measure of nursing care, or health care in general, apart from the research component. Nursing can have the option to utilize the construct as an evaluation of care or as a research outcome measure, which makes QOL an applicable research component.

Aside from all the formal, multidimensional definitions, QOL may simply be an entity that is assessed by asking the patient, "So, how is your QOL today?" The term "assessed" is used here because this way of determining QOL is not typically considered an empirical measure as science considers a measure, but it is a way, simplistic as it is, to gather everything that a person feels encompasses their own personal QOL. This question can trigger a quick personal assessment of all health issues, symptomatology, social relations and every other element influencing QOL at that particular time point (Allison, Locker & Feine, 1997; Rosenberg, 1995). This simple question may be more of a component of a nursing assessment as compared to empirical research data, but nevertheless it may be a valuable way of understanding how patients are coping with cancer and cancer treatment (Farquhar, 1995). This method of QOL assessment is considered a "global" assessment. Global assessments are attractive due to their simplicity, but lack sensitivity for detecting issues often associated with cancer (Balducci, 1994).

Opposite to simply assessing QOL by a one-question survey, a formula has been developed that considers how objective and subjective dimensions together translate the complete assessment into the actual QOL experienced ("quality of life" = (L) $\times$ (Σ(qol)$_n$ I) $\times$ M) (Testa & Simonson, 1996). Buchholz (1996, p. 520) writes that "the overall quality of life depends on the length of life (L), the sum of the quality of life (qol) in "n" different areas multiplied by the importance (I) of each area, and the transpersonal meaning (M) of that area." This sort of way of defining QOL is highly empirical, but may not fit with all types of nursing research. This type of data may not reflect some of the patient's experiences that may contribute to a more personal account of QOL.

As seen in this discussion of definitions of QOL, there are many diverse ways in which this construct is conceptualized. Some researchers feel that QOL is whatever the individual feels is important to their life at a particular time and other researchers develop an empirical formula that is suggested to represent and measure QOL. However, if the construct of QOL is used in research and practice, it is important to provide a definition that relates to the specific project and uniform validated measurements. A review of research projects that used QOL in 1994 found that only 15% of the articles concerning QOL in the MEDLINE database offered a conceptual definition of the construct (Gill & Feinstein, 1994). Less than half (35%) identified domains of QOL measured. Well constructed research should consist of a clear

TABLE 15.2 Semi-Structured Interview Questionnaire

1. List those people living in the home with you.
1. Tell me some aspects that you feel are important to your life.
2. Tell me about some of the roles for which you are, and have been, responsible.
3. How has breast cancer changed your life?
4. What are some concerns and worries that are associated with breast cancer?
5. What are some positive aspects associated with breast cancer?
6. Describe a "good" day since your breast cancer.
7. Describe a "bad" day since your breast cancer.
8. How has chemotherapy affected your life?
9. What does QOL mean to you?
10. How would you define QOL?
11. How has breast cancer influenced your QOL?
12. Would you like to share any stories related to your life before and/or after your breast cancer?

definition of the construct, followed by measurement instruments that address the domains reflected in the definition. In using the term "instruments" it is important to consider that obtaining a patient narrative is also an appropriate method for assessing patient/family perceptions of QOL. Asking a patient/family a series of open-ended questions concerning how QOL is personally defined and rated will provide an understanding of the extent that medical and nursing care are meeting needs and expectations (Table 15.2).

CULTURAL CONCERNS OF EVALUATING QUALITY OF LIFE

It is important to note that perceptions of what constitutes QOL may vary among cultures (Marshall, 1990). Lawton (1991) writes that definitions of life quality are largely a matter of personal or group preferences, and different people typically value different things. Several indicators of QOL have been found to vary between the United States and Western Europe (Scitovsky, 1976). Issues such as the availability of fresh produce, gardening, and time spent playing outdoors were all found to be indicators of enhanced general QOL (as opposed to Health Related Quality of Life) in Europe and not within the United States. With these types of differences in mind, Marshall (1990) warns that the multicultural integration of a single QOL instrument should be approached cautiously.

Several QOL instruments have been developed for use in different languages and cultures (Aaronson, Cull, Kaasa & Sprangers, 1994; Bullinger, 1995; Cella et al., 1998; Sullivan, Karlsson & Ware, 1995; Uki, Mendoza, Cleelad, Nakamura & Takeda, 1998; The WHOQOL Group, 1995). A certain degree of cultural relativism should be employed when developing a cross-cultural instrument. Using a culturally relative approach may require a new instrument to be developed specific to each culture being explored. Instead of constructing new instruments, many QOL measures are translated and validated to fit various cultures using methods of iterative translation-back translation, focus group work, panel review, and testing (Kuyken, Orley, Hudelson & Sartorius, 1994).

A Spanish-language version of the Functional Assessment of Cancer Therapy General (FACT-G) scale was developed for use in Spanish-speaking oncology patients living in the central United States and Puerto Rico (Cella et al., 1998). Items were translated using iterative translation-back translation and "decentering." Cella et al., (1998) report that *decentering* refers to "treating the original document as subject to improvement/modification based on input received in cross-cultural review. A spirituality domain is being added to the Spanish translation measure as recommended by Spanish committee reviewing the FACT-G.

Items were converted for use in several European cultures for the European Organization for Research and Treatment of Cancer (EORTC) QOL questionnaire (Aaronson, Cull, Kaasa & Sprangers, 1994). Several biomedical, sociodemographic and cultural factors using multivariate regression analysis were assessed and it was found that culture did have a statistically significant effect on QOL. The motivation for these types of uniformed QOL translations is to have an instrument useful for evaluating the impact of medical treatment in patients of many cultures, which can provide a baseline for interventions that potentially can help families cope and live with a serious illness (Bernhard et al., 1998).

A study by European and United States investigators aimed at trends in current directions of QOL research found that researchers in the UK were active in pursuing methods for assessing QOL, integration of measures into clinical trials, coping, rehabilitation, and supportive care. American researchers were more involved in the psychosocial sequelae of a cancer diagnosis (Ganz, Bernard, & Hurny, 1991). Findings suggest that the US scientists may be interested in simply treating the cancer and UK researchers may be interested in helping patients cope with the cancer.

The message from understanding the cultural relevancy of any clinical measure is to consider that because a measure is translated from one language to another does not mean that it makes sense to peoples of different backgrounds. Researchers such as Cella et al. (1998) make a point of modifying their instruments so that elements determined to be important to one group of people are reflected in that particular instrument. Comparisons of groups across cultural boundaries may not be as easy as evaluating summary scores of QOL instruments. Nursing researchers performing QOL research projects must determine what methods and instruments are relevant to their research and consistent between the survey groups. Considerations in narrative research methodologies may be prudent to gain cultural reflections not sensitive to QOL measures.Why is Quality of Life a Useful Measure?

To what extent is this type of quantitative instrument or qualitative methodology actually beneficial? If QOL is a highly dynamic and personal construct, is it even reasonable to consider that a measure would accurately represent such a complex concept? It has been suggested that QOL is something that has to be rated by the individual and not assessed simply by observing a person. Oncologists and caregivers were surveyed as to how their patient or family member would rate their own QOL. The researchers found that the oncologist's perceptions of QOL were worse than those of the patients. This study suggests that it is important to assess, and not assume, the quality of a patient's life.

As mentioned earlier in the chapter, empirical QOL measures are beneficial to provide an additional assessment of treatment outcome (Cella et al., 1997; Gill & Feinstein, 1994; Martin & Stockler, 1998; Moinpour & Hayden, 1990). Having a QOL instrument that is able to reflect some of the effects of toxicity related to cancer treatment can be helpful in orchestrating proactive interventions (Gotay & Wilson, 1998). A QOL instrument can be a predictor of treatment status and survival for many cancer patients (Osoba, 1994).

The evaluation of hospital stays and health care management can also be determined and measured by using a QOL scale. Bulstein and Mackowiak (1997) have integrated the concept of QOL with the development of a point-of-service outcome instrument to assess asthma. The project is being piloted currently and has been implemented as a real-time desktop software program. QOL as an outcome measure was found to be useful in understanding that patients experienced an enhanced QOL while undergoing palliative care at home as compared to in a hospital (Payne, 1992). This type of study may help clinicians be more accommodating to provide care in a setting in which the patient feels most comfortable.

In the area of oncology, QOL measures have been found to be useful in understanding patient perceptions of breast preservation surgical options (Kiebert, de Hayes & de Velde, 1991) and prediction of survival and survival duration (Coates, Gebski, Murray, McNeil, Byrne & Forbes, 1992; Fleishman et al., 1994; Hurny, Bernhard, Coates, Castiglione-Gertsch, Peterson & Gelber, 1996). QOL measurement outcomes have also been shown to be beneficial in formulating treatment procedures for localized prostate cancer (Litwin et al., 1995). QOL measures have also been shown to contribute positively in the treatment of metastatic prostate cancer for palliating some of the pain associated with the disease (Tannock, Gosposarowics, Meakin, Panzarella, Stewart & Rider, 1989).

A word of warning is necessary when a very complex, subjective construct such as QOL acts as a basis for medical decisions, resource allocation, and policy interventions. Meran (1996) illustrated a situation in which a person without brain activity was deemed to be without QOL, even though death was not imminent. Meran (1996, p. 521) states, "It is only a short step from regarding someone as having no quality of life (absent brain function) to making a judgment about which lives are worth sustaining and which are not."

MEASURING QOL

A review of the numerous instruments is an overwhelming, however necessary, precursor task to a well-constructed QOL research project results. An understanding of the domains incorporated into each instrument and how they can address the questions identified in the nursing research project. While it is difficult for any one instrument to reflect all aspects of a particular population, many measures have been developed for specific disease sites and age groups (Cella et al., 1993; Overcash, Extermann, Parr et al., 2001). An extensive review will familiarize the researcher with many of the concepts repetitive in the QOL data. Issues like the common domains of physical, emotional, social, functional and spiritual well-being developed as the foundations of a great many of the QOL instruments will become apparent. Table 15.3 addresses some of the many QOL instruments and provides a cursory understanding of what domains are reflected in each.

Often researchers may use two methodologies (qualitative and quantitative methods) to address a specific research question. This type of project construction is often the proverbial "best of both worlds." As will be discussed in a later portion of this chapter, narrative methods tend to identify elements that an individual may feel are incorporated into their personal QOL that are not identified on a particular instrument. An instrument coupled with open-ended questions may yield

TABLE 15.3 Some Commonly Used QOL

Name of Instrument	Authors	Description	Domains
MOS 36–Item Short-Form (SF-36)	Ware & Sherbourne 1992	Designed to measure health status and QOL. Can be administered over the phone in 15 minutes and is translated into several languages. It has age-related norms.	Physical Functioning, Social Functioning, Bodily Pain, General Health Perceptions, Vitality, Role Limitations due to Emotional Problems, Mental Health
Sickness Impact Profile (SIP)	Bergner, Bobbitt, Kressel, Pollard, Gilson & Morris, 1976	136-item self-report scale	Physical, Emotional, Psychosocial, Functional
Geratric Quality of Life Questionnaire (GQLQ)	Guyatt, Eagle, Sacket, Willan, Griffen, & McIlroy 1993	Allows for an individual approach that allows participants to identify items relevant to their own personal health.	Activities of Daily Living, Symptoms, Emotional Function
The World Health Organization Quality of Life Assessment (WHO-QOL)	WHOQOL Group, 1993	100 questions assess QOL in the perceptions culturally relevant to the participant. Four open-ended questions concerning individual perceptions of QOL are included.	Physical Health, Psychological Concerns, Levels of Independence, Social Relationships, Environment, Spirituality/Religion, and Personal Beliefs.
Icelandic Quality of Life Questionnaire	Bjoernsson, Tomasson, Ingimarsson & Hellgason, 1997	30-item measure with qualitative and quantitative components.	Physical, Emotional, Functional
Japanese Questionnaire for Quality of Life	Yamaoka, Ogoshi, Haruyama, Kobayashi, Takeda, Hayashi, 1998	20-item instrument shown to be valid in cancer and non-cancer patients and people without health concerns	Psychological, Physiological, and Environmental

(continued)

TABLE 15.3 *(continued)*

Name of Instrument	Authors	Description	Domains
McGill Quality of Life Questionnaire (MQOL)	Cohen, Bruera, Provost, Rowe & Tong, 1997	Is a general measure used for all diagnoses	Physical and Existential Well-Being
Assessment of Quality of Life at the End of Life (AQEL)	Axelsson & Sjoden, 1999	Swedish measure shown to be valid and reliable in palliative care patients	Physical, Emotional and Social Well-Being
Functional Assessment in Cancer Therapy Scale (FACT-G)	Cella, Tulsky, Linn, Bonomi, Silberman, 1993	This is a series of 28 items for cancer and non-cancer diagnosis that has been shown to be valid and reliable in older cancer patients.	Physical Well-Being, Social/Family Well-Being, Emotional Well-Being, Functional Well-Being, and Relationship with Doctor
Functional Living Index-Cancer (FLIC)	Schipper, Clinch, McMurray & Levitt, 1984	22-item measure which uses visual analogue scales in which the participant places a mark on a continuum to indicate response.	Functionality, Pain, Emotional Stress, Day-to-Day Life
European Organization for Research and Treatment of Cancer QLQ-30	Hjermstad, Fossa, Bjordal & Kaasa, 1995; Aasonson et al., 1993	30-item measure, with disease-specific sites shown to be valid and reliable to English and non-English speaking countries. It also consists of a global QOL question.	Physical, Role, Emotional, Social, and Cognitive Functioning
Comprehensive Quality of Life Measurement Tool (CARES)	Schag & Heinrich, 1990	Consists of 139 problems that affect cancer patients routinely.	Physical, Psychosocial, Medical, Marital, and Sexual
Quality of Life-Radiation Therapy Instrument (QOL-RTI)	Gwede, Friedland, Johnson, Casey, Cantor & Sauder, 1996	24-Item visual analogue scale developed specifically for people undergoing radiation therapy.	Function, Emotion, Family, Socioeconomic, and General QOL

*Generic (G) or Disease Specific (DS)

empirical data that at the same time provide personal account, narrative data, which can be analyzed and used in tandem with the quantitative data. A narrative research component can yield issues that may be identified as key personal QOL issues not addressed using a survey instrument. Using narrative methods in conjunction with a QOL instrument revealed (with the use of narrative data collection) that epilepsy patients did not like being labeled as an "epileptic," which was a QOL issue for many of the people surveyed (Scambler & Hopkins, 1990). Cummins, McCabe, Romeno and Gullone (1994) suggest that subjective and objective data are both highly relevant variables in QOL research, but the correlation between them is relatively low. Subjective narrative data are typically an individual's perspective, and objective questionnaire data are usually associated with norms. Not all research projects call for the same standardized QOL methods (Felce, 1997). Often subjective, narrative methods will be particularly relevant and other situations may warrant objective instruments; "no one approach is better than the other, but they are different, with different strengths and weaknesses to illuminate aspects of peoples' quality of life" (Felce, 1997, p. 134).

When embarking on any study, it is important to select data collection methods that are most able to answer the questions identified in the research. There certainly is no shortage of options when selecting a QOL instrument. A consideration when performing research specific to older people is the length or the data collection methods. Not to assume all older people have difficulty with long, complicated questionnaires or interviews, but for some a long involved data collection process when enduring cancer treatment can be taxing to the point that neither the participant nor the researcher has a good experience. If targeting people over 75 with comorbidities in association with a cancer diagnosis and cancer treatment, a short QOL questionnaire such as the FACT-G (Cella et al., 1993) may be more appropriate than a longer, more involved questionnaire. The timing of when the data is collected is also of great importance. Participants symptomatic with nausea or flu-like symptoms may not want to be questioned at a time when they are feeling poorly. These are common sense statements but they do need to be addressed when conducting geriatric/oncology research. For its convenience, the FACT-G was validated in older cancer patients, by comparing this test and the most commonly used general instrument of QOL in older individuals HR-36 (Overcash et al., 2001). As a result of this validation, the FACT-G was adopted as standard assessment of QOL in the SAOP of the H. Lee Moffitt Cancer Center.

As discussed earlier in the chapter, determining a patient's QOL by simply asking the general question of, "So how is your QOL?" may be a good general nursing assessment item, but difficult to measure consistently among research participants (Balducci, 1994; Gill & Feinstein, 1994). In contrast, there are researchers who feel this global question is a valid research measure as compared to the often-lengthy QOL instruments common to clinical research. For older people a general, global QOL question may be an appropriate way of determining QOL (Butler, 1994). Farquhar (1995) found that not only are people, specifically older people, capable of rating their own QOL, but were found to frequently mention the term "quality of life" in response to a general satisfaction question even before the interviewer introduced the QOL term.

THE ROLE OF NARRATIVE RESEARCH IN IMPROVING UNDERSTANDING OF QUALITY OF LIFE

A considerable amount of QOL literature supports the need for more qualitative, personal accounts when measuring QOL (Bowling, 1995; Gill & Feinstein, 1994; Leplege & Hunt, 1997; Rosenberg, 1995). A hermeneutical approach to QOL by encompassing a comprehensive dimension of an individual must be derived by the self-expression of concepts, such as interpretation of life events, analysis or morals, and other notions that are difficult to capture with standardized questionnaires (Rosenberg, 1995).

A narrative interview approach may help detect concerns that are apart from the well-defined domains of QOL and will be culturally relevant in that the individual is providing their own account of how QOL is experienced. With a highly complex, culturally relative notion such as QOL it may be reasonable to be skeptical of a single quantitative measure translated in many languages. Subtle issues of cultural diversity are unlikely to be detected, and the scores obtained may not be entirely reflective of QOL (Leplege & Hunt, 1997). Marshall (1990) calls for more ethnographic methods to insure adequate representation of individual, culturally diverse perceptions of QOL.

Narrative methods can be used synergistically with QOL questionnaires by allowing for personal discussion. Ebrahim (1995, p. 1391) writes that the "Routine use of QOL measures may highlight the need for deeper inquiry about mood, cognition or pain relief." Narrative interviews may help facilitate patient communication about problems not identified in a questionnaire. Plans could then be put into place to help deal with issues defined as problematic by the patient and the nurse. Narrative measures can transcend the "analytical conventions" set by quantitative measures by motivating boundless, unrestricted communication about individual factors which affect QOL at a particular time in a person's life (Rogerson, 1995).

Narrative methods are seemingly familiar to nursing. We use narrative methods to some extent when we take a health history or assess social/family interactions. Narrative data collection allows the nurse to perform skills intrinsic to nursing. Combining narrative methods with empirical instrument also provides a good balance of data collection that can enhance understanding of patient and family QOL concerns.

CONCLUSIONS

The amount of literature available over the last ten years on the topic of QOL is overwhelming. After spending time considering the topic and assessing the current ways in which QOL is used, consistencies appeared in the literature. Commonalities in QOL involving the physical, emotional, functional, spiritual, and psychosocial well-being are well cited in the published lierature. The intent of this chapter is to provide a cursory review of a very extensive topic and to illustrate the various methodologies that are available to measure QOL in a clinical setting. Understanding all the options that are available to measure QOL can be an important step in developing a sound, well-constructed nursing research project. From a practical standpoint, in clinical practice as well as in treatment research, the FACT-G seems to provide useful additional information and should be incorporated in all clinical trials involving older individuals with cancer.

Urgent issues of nursing research include:

• Use of narrative methods in addition to or in lieu of quantitative instruments. These methods are time-consuming and unlikely to benefit all patients, yet they may be essential to gather information in a particular situation, including patients with some complex personal history and specific goals in life. For example, we had as a patient a tribal Indian chief having as a goal to complete the writing of the history of his tribe before dying of prostate cancer. Clearly, the achievement of this goal influenced his perception of QOL, but could not be obtained from quantitative instruments;

• Use of global questions, that are time-saving, to screen patients in whom a more complete assessment of QOL is indicated;

• Comparison of the prognostic value of quantitative, qualitative, and global assessments.

REFERENCES

Aaronson, N. K., Ahmedzai, S., Bergman, B., Bullinger, M., Cull, A., Duez, N. J., Filiberti, A., Flechtner, H., Fleishman, S. B., de Haes, J. C. J. M., Kaasa, S., Klee, M., Osoba, D., Razavi, D., Rofe, P. B., Schraub, S., Sneeuw, K., Sullivan, M., & Takeda, F. (1993). The European Organization for Research and Treatment of Cancer QLQ-C30: A quality of life instrument for use in international clinical trials in oncology. *Journal of the National Cancer Institute, 85*(5), 365–376.

Aaronson, N. K., Cull, A., Kaasa S., & Mirjam, A. & Sprangers, G. (1994). The EORTC modular approach to quality of life assessment in oncology. *International Journal of Mental Health, 23*(2), 75–96.

Allison, P. J., Locker D., & Feine, J. S. (1997). Quality of life: A dynamic construct. *Social Science and Medicine, 45*(2), 221–230.

Andrews, F. M. (1994). Social indicators of social quality of life. *Social Indicators Research, 1,* 279.

Axelsson, B., & Sjoden, J. (1999). Assessment of quality of life in palliative care-psychometric properties if a short questionnaire. *ACTA Oncology, 38*(2), 229–237.

Balducci, L. (1994). Perspectives on quality of life of older patients with cancer. *Drug & Aging, 4*(4), 313–324.

Bergner, M., Bobbitt, R. A., Kressel, S., Pollard, W. D., Gilson, B. S., & Morris, J. R. (1976). The sickness impact profile: conceptual formulation and methodology for the development of a health status measure. *Journal of Rheumatology, 9,* 780–799.

Bernhard, J., Hurny, C., Coates, A. S., Peterson, H. F., Castiglione-Gertsch, M., Gelber, R. D., Galligioni, E., Marini, G., Thurlimann, E., Forbes, J. F., Goldhirsch, A., Senn H. J., & Rudenstam, C. M. (1998). Factors affecting baseline quality of life in two international adjuvant breast cancer trials. *British Journal of Cancer, 78*(5), 686–693.

Bjoernsson, J. K., Tamasson, K., Ingimarsson, S., & Helgasson, T. (1997). Health-related quality of life psychiatric and other patients in Iceland: psychometric properties of the IQL. *Nordic Journal of Psychiatry, 51*(3), 1183–1191.

Bowling, A. (1995). What things are important in people's lives? A survey of the public's judgments to inform scales of health related quality of life. *Social Science and Medicine, 41*(10), 1447–1462.

Bowling, A., & Brazier, J. (1995). Quality of life in social science and medicine. *Social Science and Medicine, 41*(10), 1337–1338.

Buchholz, W. M. (1996). Assessment of quality of life. *The New England Journal of Medicine, 335*(7), 520.

Bulstein, D., & Mackowiak, J. (1997). Point of service outcomes data and its effect on asthema treatment: a salmeterol pilot investigation. *Medical Interface, 10*(2), 118–142.

Butler, R. (1994). Historical perspective on aging and quality of life. In R. Abeles, H. C. Gift, & M. G. Ory (Eds.), *Aging and Quality of Life.* (pp. 19–26). New York: Springer Publishing Company.

Cella, D. (1997). The functional assessment of cancer therapy-anemia (FACT-An) scale: a new tool for the assessment of outcomes in cancer anemia and fatigue. *Seminars in Hematology, 34*(3 Suppl 2), 13–19.

Cella, D., Hernnandez, L., Bonomi, A. E., Corona, M., Vaquero, M., Shiomoto, G., & Baez, L. (1998). Spanish language translation and initial validation of the functional assessment of cancer therapy quality of life instrument. *Medical Care, 36*(9), 1407–1418.

Cella, D., & Tulsky, D. S. (1990). Measuring quality of life today: methodological aspects. *Oncology, 4*(5), 29–37.

Cella, D. F., Tulsky, D. S., Sarafian, F., Linn, E., Bonomi, A. E., Silberman, M., Yellen, S. B., Winicour, P., Eckberg, K., Purl, S., Blenowski, C., Goodman, M., Barnicle, M., Stewart, I., McHale, M., Bonomi, P., Kaplan, E., Taylor, S., Thomas, C. R., & Harris, J. (1993). The functional assessment of cancer therapy scale: development and validation of the general measure. *Journal of Clinical Oncology, 11*(3), 570–579.

Coates, A., Gebski, V., Signorini, D., Murrary, P., McNeil, D., & Forbes, J. F. (1992). Prognostic value of quality-of-life scores during chemotherapy for advanced breast cancer. *Journal of Clinical Oncology, 10*(12), 1833–1838.

Cohen, R. S., Mount, B. F., Bruera, E., Provost, M., Rowe, J., & Tong, K. (1997). Validity of the McGill Quality of Life Questionnaire in the palliative care setting: a multi-centre Canadian study demonstrating the importance of the essential domain. *Palliative Medicine, 11*(1), 3–20.

Cummins, R.A., McCabe, M., Romeo, Y., & Gullone, E. (1994). The comprehensive quality of life scale (ComQol): instrument development and psychometric evaluation of college staff and students. *Educational and Psychological Management, 54*(2), 372–382.

Ebrahim, S. (1995). Clinical and public health perspectives and applications of health-related quality of life measurement. *Social Science and Medicine, 41*(10), 1383–1394.

Farquhar, M. (1995). Elderly people's definitions of quality of life. *Social Science and Medicine, 41*(10), 1439–1446.

Felce, D. (1997). Defining and applying the concept of quality of life. *Journal of Intellectual Disability Research, 41*(2), 126–135.

Fleishman, S. B., Kosty, M., Herndon, J., Kornblith, A. B., Duggan, D., Morris, J., Mortimer, J., Holland, J. C., & Green, M. R. (1994). Quality of life (QoL) predicts survival in advanced non-small lung cancer. *Proceedings of ASCO, 13*, 431.

Ganz, P. A., Bernhard, J., & Hurny, C. (1991). Quality-of-life and psychosocial oncology research in Europe: State of the art. *Journal of Psychosocial Oncology, 9*(1), 1–22.

Gill, T. M., & Feinstein, A. R. (1994). A critical appraisal of the quality-of-life measurements. *Journal of the American Medical Association, 272*(8), 619–624.

Gotay, C., Cook, C., & Wilson, M. (1998). Use of quality-of-life outcome assessments in current cancer clinical trials. *Evaluation & the Health Professionals, 21*(2), 157–178.

Guyatt, G. H., Eagle, D. J., Sackett, B., Willan, A., Griffith, L., McIroy, W., Patterson, C. J., & Turpie, I. (1993). Measuring quality of life in the frail elderly. *Journal of Clinical Epidemiology, 46*(12), 1433–1444.

Gwede, C., Friedland, J., Johnson, D., Casey, L., Cantor, A., Sauder, B., & Beres, K. L. (1996). Validation of the quality of life-radiation therapy instrument (QOL-RTI) in patients receiving definitive radiation therapy for locally advanced prostate cancer. *Proceedings of the 38ᵗʰ Annual ASTRO Meeting,* 1050.

Hjermstad, M. J., Sophie, J., Fossa, D., Bjordal, K., & Kaasa, S. (1995). Test/retest study of the European organization for research and treatment of cancer core quality-of-life questionnaire. *Journal of Clinical Oncology, 13*(5), 1249–1254.

Hurny, C., Berhard, J., Coates, A., Castigilone-Gertsch, M., Peterson, N F., Gelber, R. D., Forbes, J., Rudenstam, C., Simoncini, E., Crivellari, E., Goldhirsch, A., & Senn, H. (1996). Impact of adjuvant therapy on quality of life in women with node-positive operable breast cancer. *Lancet, 347,* 1279–1283.

Kiebert, G. M., de Hayes, J. C. J. M., & van de Velde, C. J. H. (1991). The impact of breast conserving treatment and mastectomy on the quality of life of early stage breast cancer patients: A review. *Journal of Clinical Oncology, 9*(6), 1059–1070.

Kuyken, W., Orley, J., Hudelson, P., & Sartorius, N. (1994). Quality of life assessment across cultures. *International Journal of Mental.Health, 23*(2), 5–27.

Lawton, P. M. (1991). A multidimensional view of quality of life in frail elders. In J. M. Birren, J. E. Lubben, J. C. Rowe, D. E. Deutchman (Eds.). *The Concept and Measurement of Quality of Life in the Frail Elderly* (pp. 4–23). San Diego, CA: Academic Press, Inc.

Leplege, A., & Hunt, S. (1997). The problem of quality of life in medicine. *Journal of the American Medical Association, 278*(1), 47–50.

Litwin, M. S., Hays, R. D., Fink, A., Ganz, P., Leake, B., Leach, G. E., & Brook, R. (1995). Quality-of-life outcomes in men treated for localized prostate cancer. *Journal of the American Medical Association, 273*(2), 129–135.

Marshall, P. A. (1990). Cultural influences on perceived quality of life. *Seminars in Oncology Nursing, 6*(4), 278–284.

Martin, A. J., & Stockler, M. (1998). Quality-of-life assessment in health care research and practice. *Evaluation & The Health Professions, 21*(2), 141–156.

Meran, J. G. (1996). Assessment of quality of life. *The New England Journal of Medicine, 335*(7), 521.

Moinpour, C., McMillen C., & Hayden, K. A. (1990). Quality of life assessment in southwest oncology group trials. *Oncology, 4*(5), 79–84.

Moore, K. D. (1999). Dissonance in the dining room: A study of social interaction in a special care unit. *Qualitative Health Research, 9*(1), 133–155.

Osoba, D. (1994). Lessons learned from measures health-related quality-of-life in oncology. *Journal of Clinical Oncology, 12*(3), 608–616.

Overcash, J., Extermann, M., Parr, J., Perry, J., & Balducci, L. (2001). Validity and reliability of the FCT-G scale for use in the older person with cancer. *American Journal of Clinical Oncology, 24,* 591–596.

Overcash, J., & Balducci, L. (2002a). General principles of cancer treatment in the older person with cancer. In J. Overcash & L. Balducci (Eds.), *Care, cure and healing in the older person with cancer: A guide for oncology nurses.* New York: Springer Publishing Company.

Overcash, J., & Balducci, L. (2002b). Epidemiology of cancer and aging. In J. Overcash & L. Balducci (Eds.), *Care, cure and healing in the older person with cancer: A guide for oncology nurses.* New York: Springer Publishing Company.

Payne, S. A. (1992). A study of quality of life in cancer patient receiving palliative chemotherapy. *Social Science and Medicine, 35*(12), 1505–1509.

Rogerson, R. (1994). Environmental and health-related quality of life: conceptual and methodological similarities. *Social Science and Medicine, 41*(10), 1373–1382.

Rosenberg, R. (1995). Health-related quality of life between naturalism and hermeneutics. *Social Science and Medicine, 41*(10), 1411–1415.

Sartorius, N. (1987). Cross-cultural comparisons of data about quality of life: a sample of issues. In N. K. Aaronson, & J. Beckman (Eds.), *The quality of life of cancer patients* (pp. 19–24). New York: Raven Press.

Scambler, G., & Hopkins, A. (1990). Generating a model noting epileptic stigma. *Social Science and Medicine, 30,* 1187–1196.

Schag, C. C., Coscarelli, A., & Heinrich, R. L. (1990). Development of a comprehensive Quality of life measurement tool: CARES. *Oncology, 4*(5), 135–138.

Schag, C. C., & Heinrich, R. L. (1984). Karnofsky performance status: reliability, validity and guide. *Journal of Clinical Oncology, 2,* 1870–1874.

Schipper, H., Clinch, J., McMurray, A., & Levitt, M. (1984). Measuring the quality of life of cancer patients: the functional living index-cancer: development and validation. *Journal of Clinical Oncology, 2*(5), 472–483.

Scitovsky, T. (1976). *The joyless economy.* New York: Oxford University Press.

Skevington, S. M. (1994). Social comparisons in cross-cultural quality of life assessment. *International Journal of Mental Health, 23*(2), 29–47.

Smart, C. R., & Yates, J. W. (1987). Quality of life. *Cancer, 60,* 620–622.

Sullivan, M., Karlsson, J., & Ware, J. E. (1995). The Swedish SF-36 health survey-I. evaluation of data quality, scaling assumptions, reliability and construct validity across general populations in Sweden. *Social Science and Medicine, 41*(10), 1349–1358.

Tannock, I., Gospodarowicz, M., Meakin, W., Panzarella, T., Stewart, L., & Rider, W. (1989). Treatment of metastatic prostatic cancer with low-dose prednisone: Evaluation of pain and quality of life as pragmatic indices of responses. *Journal of Clinical Oncology, 7*(5), 590–597.

Testa, M. A., & Lenderking, W. R. (1999). The impact of AIDS-associated wasting on quality of life. *The Journal of Nutrition, 129*(1), 282S–289S.

Testa, M. A., & Simonson, D. C. (1996). Assessment of quality-of-life outcomes. *The New England Journal of Medicine, 334*(13), 836–839.

The WHOQOL Group. (1995). The world health organization quality of life assessment (WHOQOL) position paper from the world health organization. *Social Science and Medicine, 41*(10), 1403–1409.

Uki, J., Mendoza, T., Cleeland, C. S., Nakamura, Y., & Takeda, F. (1998). A brief cancer pain assessment tool in Japanese: the utility of the Japanese brief pain inventory (BPI-J). *Journal of Pain & Symptom Management, 16*(6), 364–373.

Ware, J., & Sherbourne, C. D. (1992). The MOS 36–item short-form health survey (SF-36): conceptual framework and item selection. *Medical Care, 30*(6), 473–483.

Yamaoka, K., Ogooshi, K., Haruyama, K., Kobayyashi, K., Takeda, Y., Hayashi, F., Watanabe, M., & Hayashim, C. (1998). Validity of the Japanese version of the questionnaire for quality of life measurement (QOL20). *International Medical Journal, 5*(1), 23–29.

CHAPTER SIXTEEN

Strategies for the Enrollment of Older Patients into Clinical Trials of Cancer Treatment

Janine Overcash and Lodovico Balducci

I n the first chapter of this book we decried the lack of information related to the management of older cancer patients (Overcash & Balducci, 2002). In this chapter we examine the causes for the poor participation of older patients in clinical trials and we explore strategies to improve their enrollment.

THE STATE OF THE PROBLEM

In 1983, Beggs and Carbone examined the experience of the Eastern Co-operative Oncology Group, and found that only 10% of patients enrolled in the clinical trials of that group were aged 70 and older. This finding was disconcerting, because the enrollment did not reflect the prevalence of cancer, as 40% of neoplasms occur in the population over 70. Sixteen years later, in 1999, Hutchins et al. reviewed the experience of the South West Oncology Group (SWOG) and found a similar discrepancy between age of patients enrolled in clinical trials and prevalence of cancer. At the same time, the Cancer Acute Leukemia Group B (CALGB) explored differ-ent possibilities to account for the poor accrual of older patients. Ke-meny et al. (2000) found that women over 70 were as likely as younger women to consent to enter clinical trials, but the participation in clinical trials was offered to 51% of the younger and only 35% of the older eligible women. This study clearly revealed an age-related bias by the trial investigators. This important study has demonstrated what many of us already suspected, that is that older individuals are more often barred from clinical investigations for no other reason but the fact that they are old. At the meantime this study produced an unexpected and important finding—that older patients may be as accepting as the younger ones of clinical experimentation. Based on this finding, an extensive work of professional and public education appears necessary to promote access of older individuals to clinical research.

The willingness of older individuals to participate clinical trials emerged also by the large participation of these individuals in trials designed exclusively for the older aged person. These include trials for the management of non-Hodgkin's lymphoma (Bastion et al., 1997; Bertini et al., 1996; Bjorkholm et al., 1999; Coiffier et al., 2001; Gomez et al., 1998; Sonneveld et al., 1998; Tirelli et al., 1999; Zinzani et al., 1999), metastatic lung cancer (Gridelli et al., 2001), and breast cancer (Hainsworth et al., 2001).

Important clues for the planning of future clinical trials in older patients emerge from the review of this information. Older individuals are willing to participate in clinic trials, when the trials are appropriately explained and they perceive a potential benefit from their participation. A number of practitioners are uncomfortable about offering clinical trials of cancer treatment to older-aged persons. This discomfort may partly derive from lack of training in evaluating the older-aged person. Older individuals are more subject than younger individuals to some complications of cancer chemotherapy, including myelodepression and mucositis (Balducci et al., 2001), hence special provisions may be necessary for the management of these individuals. Functional status, rather than chronologic age, seems to predict the risk of myelotoxicity (Gomez et al., 1998). At the same time, it is important to recognize that a number of questions have been left unanswered by these clinical trials. These questions include: when is a clinical trial appropriate for the older-aged person? How should we classify the older person enrolled in clinical trials? Which clinical trials specific for the older-aged person are necessary? We'll explore these questions in the following section.

REMAINING QUESTIONS RELATED TO THE CLINICAL TRIALS FOR THE OLDER AGED PERSON

APPROPRIATENESS OF THE TRIAL

Ethical and medical principles coincide in stating that a clinical trial is appropriate when the potential benefits override the potential risk. Two characteristics of the elderly may influence this decision:

- Reduced life-expectancy;
- Reduced tolerance of cancer treatment.

The reduction of life expectancy for healthy elderly patients is mainly a consideration for enrollment into clinical trials of adjuvant chemotherapy or of management of chronic tumors with survival of several years (for example, stage D0 prostate cancer). This problem was afforded by Extermann et al., (2000), who calculated the threshold for risk of breast cancer recurrences at which adjuvant chemotherapy may be beneficial to healthy women aged 70 and older. Considering a 1% reduction in breast cancer mortality a desirable effect, adjuvant chemotherapy may be beneficial to a 70-year-old woman only if her risk of breast cancer death is 13% or higher; for an 80-year-old woman when the risk is 30% or higher. This study may be used as frame of reference to establish the suitability of clinical trials of adjuvant chemotherapy in general for individuals aged 70 and older. The calculation of risk of cancer death takes into account, in addition to the stage of cancer, the life expectancy of the patient, which in turns requires a comprehensive geriatric assessment involving comorbidity, functional status, and cognitive, emotional, and social resources (Balducci & Extermann, 2001).

The discussion of appropriateness of clinical trials cannot avoid the issue of high-dose chemotherapy with bone marrow transplant or autologous stem cell rescue. In the recent past, this treatment modality was considered prohibitive for older individuals. Recent experiences with non-myeloablative transplants in multiple myeloma has challenged this tenet (Badros et al., 2001). Older individuals in good general condition should not be excluded from clinical trials of this form of treatment, by reason of their age.

CLASSIFICATION OF OLDER CANCER PATIENTS INVOLVED IN CLINICAL TRIALS

As we already hinted, life expectancy and tolerance of treatment are important in the decision to enroll older cancer patients into clinical trials, and these parameters may best be evaluated by a Comprehensive Geriatric Assessment (CGA) (Balducci & Beghe', 2000; Naeim & Reuben, 2001). The information obtained from the CGA may be used also for other purposes, including stratification of the patients into clinical trials, according to the stage of their aging process, and correction of conditions that may interfere with participation in the clinical trials.

The staging system of aging proposed by Hamerman (1999) recognizes four stages of aging. The first stage is a primary stage. Persons in this stage are independent in all their instrumental activities of daily living (IADL) and have negligible comorbidity. This person should have no limitation in receiving any type of treatment. Persons in the intermediate stage are dependent in one or more IADLs, and may have some function-limiting comorbidity. The condition of these patients may be rehabilitated to some extent. The prevalence of this stage increases progressively between ages 75 and 95, and the majority of cancer patients aged 80 and older belong to this stage. These patients need special precautions when receiving aggressive treatment including cytotoxic chemotherapy. These special precautions may include reduction of the initial dose of treatment, provision of a "in-home" caregiver, etc. The third stage of aging is frailty. These are patients who have almost exhausted their functional reserve and have limited tolerance for even minimal stress. These patients are mainly candidates for palliative therapy. It is important to recognize that frail patients have an average life expectancy in excess of two years (Rockwood, 1999), thus effective and lasting palliation is desirable. For older women with painful bony metastases from breast cancer, or older men with painful metastases from prostate cancer, some form of low toxicity chemotherapy may be indicated. This includes taxanes at low doses, navelbine, gemcitabine, and capecitabine. There are currently two definitions of frailty. A classical definition (Balducci & Stanta, 2000), according to which the frail person has at least one of the following; dependence in one or more ADL, and/or three or more comorbid conditions, and/or one or more geriatric syndromes. A more modern definition, for which at least three of the following are necessary (Fried et al., 2001): weight loss of $\geq 10\%$ of the original body weight over one year; slow movements; difficulty in initiating movements; low grip strength; low energy level. Both definitions are helpful. The classical definition allows a more immediate diagnosis: if a person qualifies for frailty according to the classical definition, no further investigations of frailty are warranted. The new definition is more sensitive and should be employed when frailty is not obvious at the initial evaluation. In any case, frail patients are certainly not candidates for strenuous forms of cancer treatment. Near death is the final stage. This stage involves patients with a life expectancy of 6 months or less.

This staging system should be considered as a frame of reference, susceptible to evolution and fine-tuning with new understanding of aging. Two areas of development are particularly desirable: a more precise classification of the intermediate stage, which is of special concern to cancer patients, and currently encompasses patients of different function; and laboratory evaluation of aging. Recent studies have established the importance of certain laboratory determinations, including circulating concentrations of catabolic cytokines (Hamerman, 1999; Cohen, 2001) and D dimer (Cohen, 2001), in the diagnosis of frailty. It is reasonable that the laboratory may contribute to the staging of aging in the near future.

The obstacles that prevent enrollment of older individuals into clinical trials are of different nature and may involve comorbid conditions as well as social situations, including lack of transportation, or lack of care for a sick spouse or a sick relative, when the patient is the main caregiver for this person. In addition, the CGA allows identification of other areas that deserve attention, including nutritional risks, polypharmacy, and functional risk, which may be addressed before the enrollment into a clinical trial (Balducci & Yates, 2000).

SPECIAL CLINICAL TRIALS FOR OLDER INDIVIDUALS

Since old age by itself does not appear to be a contraindication to cancer treatment, the most desirable approach to the clinical research is inclusion of older individuals in general clinical trials, after proper screening for life expectancy and function. Yet, there are situations in which specific trials for older patients are desirable:

Before a number of specific trials were conducted in older patients with lymphoma (Bertini et al., Bjorkholson et al., Sonneveld et al., Tirelli et al., Zinzani et al), serious doubt lingered about the ability of older individuals to tolerate moderately toxic chemotherapy. The trials revealed that treatment of older individuals was feasible, but that support with colony-stimulating factors was indicated after age 70. Thus, trials focused on older individuals are essential to identify and correct specific problems. In the future this type of trial should include the use of non-ablative high dose chemotherapy with minitransplant, the prevention of mucositis in older individuals (Jacobson), and the clinical and functional consequences of chemotherapy induced anemia in the elderly (Balducci et al., 2001; Schijvers et al., 1999).

As previously mentioned, the majority of older cancer patients probably belong to the so-called "intermediate stage of aging" in the Hamermann classification (1999). Unfortunately, this stage is the least defined and includes patients who are near fully functional and patients who are near frail. Clearly, a more precise definition of the vulnerability of this group to the complications of treatment is desirable. The emerging concept of "vulnerable elderly" (Gill et al., 2001) may come "apropos" for this purpose. In addition, some basic biochemical evaluation prior to enrollment in clinical trials, including serum concentrations of Interleukin-6, tumor necrosis factor, and D dimer may provide useful prognostic information (Cohen et al., 2001; Hamerman et al., 1999). Management of special groups of older individuals, such as the frail elderly and the oldest old. We have already mentioned how the average life expectancy of the frail elderly is in excess of two years, and these patients deserve a palliative treatment beyond the use of opioids when experiencing symptoms of cancer. The oldest old is the population aged 85 and over, on which there is very little information. The majority of these persons may be frail because they may also have some undiscovered age-related conditions such as myelodysplasia, and acute myelogenous leukemia with MDR overexpression (Balducci & Extermann, 2001). Adoption of a common language, based on CGA, in the evaluation of the older aged person may also help to enhance care. This common language may prove invaluable in retrospective analysis of series of older individuals with cancer, to establish how function, comorbidity, social support, cognition, and depression affect the prognosis of cancer and cancer treatment.

Application of the National Cancer Center Network (NCCN) Guidelines for the management of older cancer patients is another positive step in providing better care. The NCCN issued these guidelines in 2000 (Balducci & Yates), but has provided no mechanisms for their implementation. The study of the implementation of guidelines in community practice is essential to establish the effectiveness of the guidelines, to establish Phase II trials of new forms of cancer treatment in older individuals, to hasten the detection of possible age-related complication, to establish the tolerability of these forms of treatment in older individuals, and to offer community based clinical trials capable to accommodate the majority of older individuals unable to travel to distant cancer centers.

CONCLUSIONS

The need for clinical trials in older patients with cancer may be summarized in four areas:

- Promotion of the enrollment of older individuals in existing clinical trials for the general cancer patient, as long as there is a reasonable chance that the trial may be beneficial to the older person. This goal requires an intensive work of public and professional education, to spread the word that age is not a contraindication to the best cancer treatment, that clinical trials represent the state of the art of cancer treatment, and that the benefits for older individuals may be enhanced by calculating their life ex-

pectancy and by proactively using antidotes to treatment-related toxicity.
- Studies of age-related problems, including special populations, special diseases, and special forms of treatment are needed at this time in health care.
- Understanding how various diagnoses affect the older person can enhance treatment options which will support a better plan of care.
- Lastly, studies of health care delivery, including implementation of guidelines, community based clinical trials, and standard evaluation of the older cancer patient.

The geriatric and the oncology nurses have a pivotal role in each area. They need to take the leadership in professional and public education to overcome ageism and to assure the proper flow of older individuals to clinical trials; this educational role should be espoused to an advocacy role for patients whom physicians or family wish to exclude from the best forms of cancer treatment. Nurses need to engage in the study of nursing policy and guidelines for the uniform evaluation of the older person, not unlike the evaluation of specific symptoms (pain, nausea and vomiting, quality of life, fatigue), today largely controlled by nursing practices. The promotion of clinical trials involving older individuals at local and national levels are other roles for the geriatric oncology nurse.

REFERENCES

Badros, A., Barlogie, B., Siegel, E., Morris, C., Desikan, R., Zangari, M. et al., (2001). Autologous Stem Cell transplantation in elderly multiple myeloma patients over the age of 70 years. *British Journal of Haematology, 114,* 600–607.

Balducci, L., & Beghe, C. (2000). The application of the principles of geriatric medicine to the older person with Cancer. *Critical Reviews in Oncology and Hematology, 35,* 147–154.

Balducci, L., & Extermann, M. (2001). A practical approach to the older patient with cancer. *Current Problems in Cancer, 25,* 1, 1–76.

Balducci, L., Hardy, C. H., Lyman, G. H. (2001). Hematopoietic growth factors in the older cancer patient. *Current Opinions in Hematology, 8,* 170–187.

Balducci, L., & Stanta, G. Cancer in the frail patient: A coming epidemic. *Hematology and Oncology Clinics of North America, 14,* 235–250.

Balducci, L., & Yates, G. (2000). Guidelines for the management of the older person with cancer. *Oncology, 14,* 11A, 221–227.

Bastion, Y., Blay, J. Y., Divine, M., Brice, P., Bordessoule, D., Sebban, C. et al. (1997). Elderly patients with aggressive non-Hodgkin's lymphoma: Disease presentation, response to treatment and survival. A Groupe d'Etude des Lymphomes de l'Adulte Study on 453 patients older than 69 years. *Journal of Clinical Oncology, 15,* 2945–2953.

Begg, C. B., & Carbone, P. (1983). Clinical trials and drug toxicity in the elderly. The experience of the Eastern Cooperative Oncology Group. *Cancer, 52,* 1986–1992.

Bertini, M., Freilone, R., Botto, B., Calvi, R., Gallamini, A., Gatti, A. M., et al. (1996). The treatment of elderly patients with aggressive non-Hodgkin's lymphomas: Feasibility and efficacy of an intensive multidrug regimen. *Leukemia Lymphoma, 22,* 483–493.

Bjorkholm, M., Osby, E., & Hagberg, H. (1999). Randomized trial of R-methu granulocyte Colony stimulating factors as adjunct to CHOP or CNOP treatment of elderly patients with aggressive non-Hodgkin's lymphoma. *Proceedings of the American Society of Hematology, 94,* 599a.

Coiffier, B., Ferme', C., & Hermine, O. (2000). Rituximab plus CHOP (R-CHOP) in the treatment of elderly patients with Diffuse Large B Cell Lymphoma: an update of the GELA study. *Blood, 11,* 725a.

Cohen, H. J., Pieper, C. F., & Harris, T. (2001). Markers of inflammation and coagulation predict decline in function and mortality in community-dwelling elderly. *Journal of the American Geriatrics Society, 49,* S1.

Extermann, M., Balducci, L., & Lyman, G. H. (2000). What threshold for adjuvant therapy in older breast cancer patients? *Journal of Clinical Oncology, 18,* 1709–1717.

Fried, L. P, Tangen, C. M., Walston, J., Newman, A. B., Hirsch, C., Gottdiener, J., et al. Cardiovascular Health Study Collaborative Research Group. (2001). Frailty in older adults. Evidence for a phenotype. *Journal of Gerontology, 56A,* M146–M156.

Gill, T. M., Desai, M. M., & Gahbauer, E. A. (2001). Restricted activity among community-living older persons: Incidence, precipitants, and health care utilization. *Annals of Internal Medicine, 135,* 313–321.

Gomez, H., Mas, L., Casanova, L., Pen, D. L., Santillana, S., Valdivia, S., et al. (1998). Elderly patients with aggressive non-Hodgkin's lymphoma treated with CHOP chemotherapy plus granulocyte-macrophage colony-stimulating factor: Identification of two age subgroups with differing hematologic toxicity. *Journal of Clinical Oncology, 16,* 2352–2358.

Gridelli, C., Cigolari, S., & Bilancia, D. (2000). Phase II study of gemcitabine and Gemcitabine-Vinorelbine in advanced NSCLC Elderly patients with the phase III miles (Multicenter Italian Lung cancer in the Elderly Study) Randomized Trial. *Proceedings of the American Society of Clinical Oncology, 19,* 532a.

Hainsworth, J. D., Burris, H. A., Yardley, D. A. et al (2001). Weekly docetaxel in the treatment of elderly patients with advanced breast cancer: a Minnie Pearl Cancer research Network Phase II trial. *Journal of Clinical Oncology, 19,* 3500–3505.

Hamerman, D. (1999). Toward an understanding of frailty. *Annals of Internal Medicine, 130,* 945–950.

Hamerman, D., Berman, J. W., Albers, G. W., Brown, D. L., & Silver, D. (1999). Emerging evidence for inflammation in conditions frequently affecting older adults: report of a symposium. *Journal of the American Geriatrics Society, 47,* 995–999.

Hutchins, L. F., Unger, J. M, Crowley, J. J., Coltman, C. A. Jr, & Albain, K. (1999). Underrepresentation of patients 65 years of age or older in cancer treatment Trials. *New England Journal of Medicine, 341,* 2061–2067.

Kemeny, M., Muss, H. B., Konblith, A. B. (2000). Barriers to participation of older women with breast cancer in clinical trials. *Proceedings of the American Society of Clinical Oncology, 19,* 602a.

Jacobson, S. D., Cha, S., & Sargent, D. J. (2001). Tolerability, dose intensity and benefit of 5FU based chemotherapy for advanced colorectal cancer (CRC) in the elderly. A North Central Cancer Treatment Group Study. *Proceedings of the American Society of Clinical Oncology, 20* (384a), 1534.

Naeim, A., & Reuben, D. (2001). Geriatric syndromes and assessment of the older cancer patient. *Oncology* (Huntington), *15,* 1567–1577.

Overcash, J., & Balducci, L. (2002). General principles of cancer treatment in the older person with cancer. In J. Overcash & L. Balducci (Eds.), *Care, cure and healing in the older person with cancer: A guide for oncology nurses.* New York: Springer.

Rockwood, K., Stadnyk, K., MacKnight, C., McDowell, I., Hebert, R., & Hogan, D. B. (1999). A brief clinical instrument to classify frailty in elderly people. *Lancet, 353,* 205–206.

Schrijvers, D., Highley, M., De Bruyn, E., Van Oosterom, A. T., & Vermorken, J. B. Role of red blood cell in pharmakinetics of chemotherapeutic agents. *Anticancer Drugs, 10,* 147–153.

Sonneveld, P., de Ridder M., van der Lelie, H., Nieuwenhuis, K., Schouten, H., Mulder, A., et al. (1995). Comparison of doxorubicin and mitoxantrone in the treatment of elderly patients with advanced diffuse non-Hodgkin's lymphoma using CHOP vs. CNOP chemotherapy. *Journal of Clinical Oncology, 13,* 2530–2539.

Tirelli, U., Errante, D., Van Glabbeke, M., Teodorovic, I., Kluin-Nelemans, J. C., Thomas, J., et al. (1998). CHOP is the standard regimen in patients ≥ 70 years of age with intermediate and high grade non-Hodgkin's lymphoma: results of a randomized study of the European Organization for the Research and Treatment of Cancer Lymphoma Cooperative Study. *Journal of Clinical Oncology, 16,* 27–34.

Zinzani, P. L., Storti, S., Zaccaria, A., Moretti, L., Magagnoli, M., Pavone, E., et al. (1999). Elderly aggressive histology non-Hodgkin's lymphoma: First line VNCOP-B regimen: experience on 350 patients. *Blood, 94,* 33–38.

CHAPTER SEVENTEEN

The Cost of Cancer Prevention and Treatment in the Older Person

Lodovico Balducci and Martine Extermann

U ndoubtedly, the progressive expansion of the older population (Yancik & Ries, 2000) will lead to a progressive increment in health care costs (Balducci, Hardy, & Lyman, 2001). Aging is associated with increased prevalence both of comorbidity and of functional dependence, which call for expensive in-home or institutional care (Balducci & Extermann, 2001; Balducci et al., 2001). It is a known fact that the 12% of the population over 65 accounts for more than 50% of hospital visits and hospitalizations. As the available resources to pay for health care are limited, it behooves both health care customers and providers to find ways to minimize the cost without compromising the outcome of care. In this chapter, we explore the cost of cancer prevention and cancer treatment in the older person and the potential roles of the nurse in cost management.

THE STUDY OF COST

DEFINITION

Though one commonly refers to the price of an object or of a service as "cost," it actually represents the charges a seller or a provider levy on the customer (Fenn et al., 1996). The cost is the minimal amount of money necessary to provide a certain object or service. Whereas charges are negotiable within the limits of profitability, the cost is not negotiable, or more simply stated, the object or service desired couldn't be obtained at a lower cost. For example, the real cost of a drug or of a hospital day is the cost below which a manufacturer or the hospital administration would undergo a loss. A corollary of this definition of cost is that cost is an absolute value, irrespective of who pays for it. For example, the cost of managing infusional chemotherapy at home may be cheaper than in-hospital administration, though the patient's bill may be higher if he/she needs to pay the fee for the infusion pump. Likewise, the prevention of anemia of cancer patients with erythropoietin (Balducci et al., 2001) may prevent functional dependence and thus decrease the global cost related to patient management, but from the insurance standpoint this approach is more expensive, because the insurance company has to pay for the medication, whereas the cost of home care is generally placed upon the patient or his or her family by the system. Any study of medical cost should try to distinguish the actual cost from the questions who is going to pay. The construct of cost we propose is real, but problematic to measure. In practice, customary charges are used in lieu of cost in most cost-analysis (Anonymous, 1998; Fenn, McGuire, Backhouse & Jones, 1996). This is a legitimate approach as long as one appreciates that in the cost so determined there is room for negotiation.

Different Types of Medical Costs

The costs involved in the management of a disease, including cancer, are generally subdivided into four subgroups (Anonymous, 1998):

(1) Direct Costs. These include the costs of the visit, of the medications, and of hospitalization, as well as the cost of supplies and reha-bilitative devices.

(2) Indirect Costs, Medically Related. These include the cost of trans-portation to and from the treatment center, of meals out of home, and of overnight staying in a hotel.

(3) Indirect Costs, Medically Unrelated. These include the days of work lost by the patient or a family member, and the cost of other aspects of the disease, such as babysitting children left home alone when the parent goes to a clinic visit.

(4) Intangible Costs. These include pain and suffering and long-term, unpredictable complications of the disease, such as the cost of di-vorce or psychiatric treatment for a person who has been the care-giver of a sick parent.

In a recent consensus conference held at the National Institutes of Health (Anonymous, 1998), the agreement was made to include in the computation only direct and indirect, medically related costs. This seems a fair approximation for the management of an acute illness, in which the indirect medically unrelated and the intangible costs are likely negligible and mostly absorbed by the employer or by disability insurance. The issue is more complex in the case of chronic illness and especially for older patients, when these costs are more substantial. For example, the fatigue coalition has recently explored the social consequences of fatigue, which is the most common chronic symptom among cancer patients, and found that approximately 50% of the patients and 25% of the caregivers were compelled to accept a less profitable job, or to become unemployed as a result of fatigue (Cleeland, Demetri, & Glaspy, 1999). The consequences of fatigue may be even more devastating for the older person, as fatigue may lead to functional dependence. Clearly, depending whether medically unrelated and intangible costs are or are not accounted for, the addition of erythropoietin to prevent anemia-related fatigue to the treatment plan may result in reduced or increased treatment cost (Heyman et al., 2001).

Cost Assessment

Four different approaches are commonly used for cost assessment (Table 17.1) (Laupacis et al., 1996). Cost minimization is the simplest and most intuitive analysis, when the outcome of different interventions is exactly the same. In the case of cancer treatment, Lyman et al. (1992) studied the cost of adding G-CSF for the prevention of neutropenic infections, in the course of cytotoxic chemotherapy, and concluded that the colony-stimulating factors reduced the cost of treatment when the risk of neutropenic infections was 40% and higher. Other investigators concluded that the use of colony-stimulating factors during the consolidation phase of the management of acute myeloid leukemia in patients over 60 reduced the cost of treatment (Bennett, Stinson, & Laver, 2000). In the same line, Hillner et al (2001) concluded that the addition of bisphosphonates to the management of women with breast cancer metastatic to the bones, though beneficial in terms of pain control, was associated with a significant cost increase in the USA (Hillner, 2001). Cost analyses are sensitive to the cost structure of the care in the country. For example, a Canadian analysis based on the same data found the treatment with biphosphonates to be much less costly in Canada (Deranitsaris & Hsu, 1999; Extermann, 2000).

Cost minimization is the analysis of choice when the outcome is exactly the same. The definition of outcome may be elusive, however. In the case of bisphosphonates, for example, though the survival is not improved by the addition of these agents to the treatment, the quality of life may be, due to a reduction in pain and risk of bone

TABLE 17.1 Common Approaches to Cost Assessment

Approach	Explanation
Cost-minimization	When two different approaches to the same condition yield the same outcome, choose the least expensive.
Cost-effectiveness	Cost for unity of outcome, example such as year of life gained. This approach is mainly used for public health policies. For example, accepted social costs of an intervention are around $60,000.00/year of life gained.
Cost-utility	Like cost-effectiveness, but in this case the outcome unit is the perceived benefit to the patient (utility), generally including an estimation of quality of life.
Cost-benefit	Like cost-effectiveness, but the unit of outcome in this case is economical, in other words this approach considers the cost of treatment as an investment and the outcome as the positive or negative profit from that investment. This is the most controversial and least used approach.

fractures. The cost-minimization approach should be complemented, then, by a cost/utility analysis, to establish how beneficial this approach has been to the patient quality of life.

At this point we wish to emphasize one more time, that the cost-minimization analysis is legitimate only when the outcome of two interventions is identical. A very common misinterpretation of cost minimization, which may disproportionately affect older cancer patients, is the deliverance of an inferior form of treatment to minimize cost.

Cost/effectiveness analysis is mostly employed to study the cost of population based interventions, such as cancer screening. The goal of this analysis is to establish whether a certain policy is affordable. Though the concept of affordability is not clearly explained, it is customary to consider any policy costing less than $60.000,00/year of life saved as affordable (Kerlikowske, Salzmann, Phillips, Crawley, & cummings, 1999). When different interventions produce similar results, the most cost-effective is of course the least costly. For example, a recent study compared the cost of screening individuals aged 50 and older for cancer of the large bowel with yearly hemoccult testing of the stools, yearly hemoccult testing and sigmoidoscopy every 5 years and colonoscopy every 10 years (Frazier, Colditz & Fuchs, 2000). Though all interventions were affordable, colonoscopy every 10 years appeared as the most cost effective.

Cost-utility analysis is very appealing, especially in older individuals, because it studies outcome in terms of personal benefits. The outcome unit in this case is called QALY (quality-adjusted life years) (Green, Brazier, & Deverill, 2000). In simple terms, the patient has to establish the fraction of a year of healthy life; he/she estimates worthy a year with the disease or with the complications of treatment. For example, a man with early PSA recurrence of prostate cancer may live 15 years with castration and 10 years without. However, if one year without sexual activity is worthy to that man 50% of a year of full health, the QALY of that man will be 10 without and 7.5 with castration, and avoidance of castration will be preferable in his case. The utility of an intervention may be assessed by visual analog scale (VAS), time trade-off, and standard bargaining techniques (Green et al., 2000). Taking again the example of a man with a PSA-only relapse of prostate cancer having to decide whether or not to undergo castration, the time-trade-off technique involves asking how much of his life expectancy he would be ready to give up in order to avoid castration. The standard bargaining technique consists in asking the patient how many chances of immediate death from prostate cancer he would take to avoid castration, whether 5, 10, 20, 50, 60%. The value at which the patient considers death and impotence as equivalent is the number used to adjust the patient life expectancy for the risk of impotence.

The use of cost-utility is fraught with several problems. The first is the assessment of utility based on a patient prediction of the effects of cancer and cancer treatment on quality of life. Not on actual quality of life assessment; of course this objection applies to any forms of medical intervention and by itself would not be sufficient to deny cost/utility analysis. Secondly, there is no clear consensus on which technique is preferable to assess utility, in the absence of an external golden standard of utility. Lastly, the assessment of utility is dependent on the patient comprehension of the question and of the mechanism of the technique, and this may be problematic especially in older individuals. With these obvious limitations, cost/utility is still a very valuable instrument that should complement in most cases cost minimization, to introduce the patient's perspective on disease and treatment.

Not unexpectedly, cost-benefits are the most controversial and least used form of cost/analysis. In its most brutal form, cost benefit analysis says that young and wealthy executives should be treated for their cancer, retired or unemployed individuals should not, and everybody in between should be treated only if they are willing to pitch in some resources. A gentler approach investigates the willingness to pay (WTP) of a patient for a certain outcome; for example, how worthy is for the patient an extra year of life; and decides that the intervention is cost/beneficial when the willingness to pay is higher than the cost of the intervention. The main limitations of this approach are the fact that the WTP cannot be validated by objective standards and it is not clear what this approach may add to the more commonly used QALY.

Irrespective of the form of cost-analysis selected, cost determination is subjected to a number of variables that may change over time or in different practice sets. An "in depth" analysis of cost-assessment is beyond the scope of this review, but the introduction of three concepts may be helpful to interpret cost-analysis. These concepts are: threshold, sensitivity analysis, and two-way sensitivity analysis. Threshold is the value of a certain variable at which two courses of action are identical. Lyman, Sanderson, & Balducci, (1993) established the threshold for risk of neutropenic infection at which the cost of using or not using growth factors was 40% (Table 17.1). Then it was concluded that when the risk of neutropenic infections was higher than 40%, the cost was minimized by colony-stimulating factors. Sensitivity analysis is the process necessary to find the threshold and shows how the estimate of cost would vary with the change of one variable. In the same case, the cost threshold would have been higher had the cost of G-CSF been higher, and lower had the cost been lower. Of special interest is the two way sensitivity analysis, in which the effects of the simultaneous changes of two variables are explored. Lyman, Kuderer, Greene, & Balducci, (1998)studied how the cost of treatment with and without G-CSF would vary for simultaneous changes in risk of neutropenic fever and cost of hospitalization. The line represents the various thresholds for the risk of neutropenic fever. The space above the line represents the conditions where the use of G-CSF leads to cost-minimization. Clearly, if the cost of hospitalization doubles, the threshold for the risk of neutropenic fever drops to almost 20%. Threshold and sensitivity analysis are important to assess the variation of cost of different interventions in different circumstances, to gain a cost panorama that reflects as closely as possible the variations of the real world. Enabled by these simple instructions, we will examine now the cost of preventative and therapeutic interventions in the elderly.

COST AND COST-EFFECTIVENESS OF CANCER MANAGEMENT IN THE ELDERLY

PREVENTATIVE INTERVENTIONS

We will examine the cost and cost-effectiveness of two generally accepted screening interventions: screening of older women for cancer of the breast and of the large bowel. Though there are not randomized controlled studies testifying the effectiveness of mammography after age 70, two retrospective studies suggest that this intervention may be beneficial to older women (Balducci & Beghe', 2002). The Nijmegen study suggests that biannual mammography reduces the risk of breast cancer–related deaths up to age 75; Mccarthy et al. (2000) reviewed the Surveillance Epidemiology and End Result (SEER) data and concluded that women who had obtained at least two mammographic exams after age 70 had their risk to die of breast cancer almost halved. Kerlikowske (2000) studied the cost-effectiveness of performing biennial mammography in all women aged 70 to 79 and found the cost-effectiveness of the procedure to be $112000.00/year of life saved. This is more than double the cost/year of life saved for women aged 50 to 70 and is clearly out of the range of the interventions considered affordable. The difference in cost is easy to explain as the life gain in older women is expected to be much lower due to reduced life expectancy and more indolent tumors (Holmes et al., 1994). A creative approach to reduce cost is to screen regularly only women at risk of breast cancer, such as those women at the upper quintile of their bone-density (Kerlikowske, 2000). As monitoring bone density is recommended for all postmenopausal women, this test should not be added to the cost of breast cancer screening. With this provision, 95% of cancers would still be detected at the cost of approximately $60,000.00 per year of life saved. This analysis represents an excellent example of how cost-effectiveness may be promoted in the management of older individuals, without substantial compromise of the outcome. This analysis may also serve as baseline for the evaluation of other approaches such as a yearly physical examination of the breast by a professional. In two studies, yearly breast examination yielded results comparable to those of mammography, with the exception of the diagnosis of ductal carcinoma "in situ" (DCIS), which was found exclusively at mammography (Miller, Baines, & Wall, 2000; Mitra, 1994). Given the long development time of DCIS, the diagnosis of this entity in older women with reduced life expectancy may be irrelevant. The study of triennial mammography may be reasonable, given the slower cancer growth in elderly patients (Balducci & Beghe, 2002). Finally, the value of new interventions, including digital mammography and breast MRI, may add substantial cost to screening despite being more precise than regular mammography.

Screening for cancer of the large bowel with biannual hemo-occult examination of the stools proved beneficial in persons aged 50 to 80. No data from randomized controlled studies are available for serial sigmoidoscopy and colonoscopy, though these tests are generally considered as effective (Balducci & Beghe', 2002). A recent decision analysis established that the most cost-effective approach involves colonoscopy every ten years (Frazier et al., 2000). This study represents an interesting example of cost minimization in screening and provides a useful baseline for studying different approaches, including the necessity of screening after age 80, for which there are no data.

THERAPEUTIC INTERVENTION

We will examine the cost and cost-effectiveness of two interventions that are gaining more and more acceptance in the geriatric population: prophylactic use of G-CSF and adjuvant chemotherapy of breast cancer.

The National Cancer Center Network (NCCN) recently issued some guidelines for the management of cancer in older individuals. These guidelines include the prophylactic use of colony-stimulating factor in persons aged 70 and older treated with combination chemotherapy of dose intensity similar to CHOP (cyclophosphamide, doxorubicin [hydroxydaunorubicin], oncovin, and prednisone) (Balducci & Yates, 2000). This recommendation was based on the following considerations:

The risk of neutropenic infections, and possibly death, increases with age after age 70 in patients treated with CHOP and CHOP-like chemotherapy (Balducci, hardy, & Lyman, 2001). In at least one study (Bjorkholm, Osby, & Hagberg, 2000), the risk of neutropenic infections was higher than 40% and G-CSF reduced this risk by 50%, fulfilling the requirements proposed by Lyman et al., (1993);

The duration of hospitalization in older individuals with neutropenic infections may be longer than 4.7 days, which was the duration reported in the study of Lyman et al., (1993), thus the cost of hospitalization may be higher in older individuals, and the threshold for the use of growth factors lower (Lyman et al., 1998) and probably encompassing the risk of neutropenic infections found in most studies (Balducci et al., 2001).

This example illustrates very well how cost analysis may be used to promote a certain form of intervention in the elderly: First, intervention may avoid treament-related death, in which case cost-consideration will be secondary. Second, even if the outcome is the same with and without growth factors, as suggested by at least one study (Zinzani et al., 1999), the risk of neutropenic infection is high enough to predict that the use of growth factors may not increase the cost of managing these patients. These analyses may serve as background to study other approaches, such as oral antibiotics in addition to or in lieu of growth factors, and shorter and more intense courses of chemotherapy.

ADJUVANT CHEMOTHERAPY OF BREAST CANCER

The benefits of adjuvant chemotherapy of breast cancer in women aged 70 and older are controversial. The Oxford meta-analysis failed to demonstrate any gain in survival and disease-free survival for this group of patients; however, women over 70 represented only 3% of the whole population and that number might have been too small to detect any meaningful trends in survival (early breast cancer trialists collaborative group, 1998). In general, it is reasonable to consider women aged 70 and older as any other group of postmenopausal women, for whom adjuvant chemotherapy has a smaller benefit than in premenopausal women, but still is effective in reducing recurrence rate and mortality, especially in those with hormone-receptor-poor disease (early breast cancer trialists collaborative group, 1998) and in those with hormone receptor-rich tumor and high expression of HER2/neu (Ravdin, Green, & Albain, 1998).

As one can expect, the cost-effectiveness of adjuvant treatment declines with age, due to more reduced benefits in survival and increased risk of complications. Desch, Hillner, & smith (1993) calculated that anthracycline-based chemotherapy would be associated with a cost of around $100,000.00/ year of life gained, which is considered outside the limits of affordability. A constructive approach to this issue involves identification of women for whom chemotherapy is likely to be beneficial. Extermann (2000) calculated that a 70-year-old woman in average health would gain at least 1% in absolute survival from chemotherapy if her risk of relapse at 10 years is 21% or more. An 80-year-old woman would need to have a 36% risk of relapse or more to achieve the same benefit. On the other hand, if one seeks primarily to prevent relapse, a decrease in 1% in relapse is achieved with chemotherapy for a 70-year-old patient with a 13% risk of relapse, and an 80-year-old with a 15% risk of relapse. Desch et al. (1993) used a cost effectiveness approach to analyze the economic implications of adjuvant chemotherapy. One may ask if this approach is reasonable given the small albeit real benefits of adjuvant chemotherapy. Though the point may be argued, the approach is reasonable; unlike the management of metastatic disease, the situation of adjuvant chemotherapy is more similar to the issue of screening and early diagnosis, in that the benefits are relatively small, and late in time. The main reason of similarity is the fact that it is necessary to intervene on a large number of patients, to prevent the death of very few, that cannot be identified "a priori." This societal rather than individual perspective makes it reasonable to study adjuvant chemotherapy like any other public health intervention.

Identification of the patients for whom adjuvant chemotherapy has a reasonable chance to be beneficial will both reduce the cost and at the same time improve the therapeutic index of adjuvant chemotherapy, demonstrating once more that good medicine is the most cost-effective. The combination of these two analysis models; assessment of cost effectiveness in the general population and in the population more likely to benefit from the intervention, may be used to study the cost of adjuvant therapy in other diseases, including cancer of the large bowel and of the bladder.

A number of therapeutic interventions in elderly cancer patients await proper cost/evaluation. Among the most urgent one should include evaluation of the use of erythropoietin to mitigate chemotherapy-related anemia (Balducci et al., 2001), the study of pain management using intrathecal infusion of opioids, in lieu of oral medications, and the benefits of palliative chemotherapy in the frail patient (Balducci & Stanta, 2000). This review was meant as an invitation to approach these issues.

THE NURSE ROLE IN COST ANALYSIS

Whereas the studies of cost analysis are generally performed by health economists, the practicing oncology nurse has a fundamental role in studying and applying cost management. In the context of clinical practice it behooves any health professional to promote cost-effectiveness. The nurse may have a pivotal role in the following areas: improving patient flow and patient satisfaction through appropriate communication; studying the practice pattern of different physicians and tailoring the patient flow to different practice styles; individuating patients with special needs (patients with multiple problems or those who are known for attention-seeking behavior) and accommodating them at a time when they least may disrupt the management of other patients; and coordinating management and education in a way of avoiding redundancies and time wasting.

In the context of cost-related research, the nurse may have a pivotal role in assessing patient's utility, by studying and utilizing innovative communication techniques, as one of the nurse's prerogatives is to translate science and technology into a personal language that may have a lasting impact on the patient. Likewise, the nurse is in the best position, by training and profession, to translate a personal language into the objective language of numbers.

In the present world, where advocacy and science are often at odds, the nurse may also have a role of intermediary between these opposite forces. A number of expensive interventions have made their way into daily practice despite little scientific support. Three examples responsible to increase the cost of medicine by more than a billion dollars a year, without any additional medical advantage include a yearly mammography in lieu of biennial examination that has been employed in the majority of randomized clinical trials (Kerlikowske, Grady, Rubin, Sandrock, & Ernster, 1995). The use of chemical castration in lieu of orchiectomy may increase by as much as $100,000.00 per patient the cost of managing metastatic prostate cancer (Hillner, 2000). The third example is breast preservation with partial mastectomy and radiation therapy that appears more costly than total mastectomy with or without breast reconstruction, despite no proven benefits in patient quality of life (Kiebert, de Haas, & van der Velde, 1991). These examples highlight the need for thorough cost evaluation of new and expensive procedures before they make roots as standard practice. Often the patient and well-intentioned advocacy groups ask for the implementation of these procedures, based on incomplete information from the lay press or the Web, with results that may be disastrous to both the patient health and the health care finances (that is what happened in the case of high-dose chemotherapy and autologous stem cell rescue for breast cancer). As the most trusted patient confidante the nurse may represent the most effective patient educator in these controversial areas.

CONCLUSIONS

Aging may be associated with increased cost in areas of both cancer prevention and cancer treatment. Given limited health care resources, cost management is an imperative of modern medicine. Cost management involves proper analysis of the cost of any planned intervention and study of method to limit the intervention to the patients who may most benefit from it. Often cost management parallels sound clinical judgment. In any case, it is not legitimate to withhold life-saving or quality of life–improving procedures from older individuals for the purpose of reducing health care costs.

REFERENCES

Anonymous. (1998). Integrating economic analysis into cancer clinical trials: the National Cancer Institute-American Society of Clinical Oncology workbook. *Journal of the National Cancer Institute Monographs, 24,* 1–28.

Balducci, L., & Beghe (2002). The application of the principles of geriatrics to the management of the older person with cancer. *Critical Reviews in Oncology and Hematology, 35*(3), 147–154.

Balducci, L., & Extermann, M. (2001) A practical approach to the older patient with cancer. *Current Problems in Cancer, 25,* 1–76.

Balducci, L., Hardy, C. L., & Lyman, G. H. (2001). Growth factors in the older cancer patients. *Current Opinions in Hematology, 23,* 106–120.

Balducci, L., Silliman, R. A., & Diaz, N. (In press). Breast cancer: An oncological perspective. In L. Balducci, G. H. Lyman, & W. B. Ershler (Eds.), *Comprehensive geriatric oncology.* Second edition. London: Harwood Academic Publishers.

Balducci, L., & Stanta, G. (2000). Cancer in the frail patient: a coming epidemic. *Hematology and Oncology Clinics of North America, 14,* 235–250.

Balducci, L., & Yates, G. (2000). General guidelines for the management of older patients with cancer. *Oncology, NCCN Proceedings, November 2000,* 221–227.

Bennett, C. E., Stinson, T. J., Laver, J. H. (2000). Cost analyses of adjunct colony stimulating factors for acute leukemia: Can they improve clinical decision making. *Leukemia/ Lymphoma, 37,* 65–70.

Bjorkholm, M., Osby, E., & Hagberg, H. (1999). Randomized trial of R-methu granulocyte Colony stimulating factors as adjunct to CHOP or CNOP treatment of elderly patients with aggressive non-Hodgkin's lymphoma. *Proceedings of the American Society Hemotology, 94,* Abstract 2665.

Cleeland, C. S., Demetri, G. D., & Glaspy, J. (1999). Identifying hemoglobin levels for optimal quality of life: results of an incremental analysis. *Proceedings of the American Society of Clinical Oncology, 16,* Astr 2215.

Desch, C. S., Hillner, B. E., & Smith, T. J. (1993). Should elderly receive chemotherapy for node-negative breast cancer? A cost-effectiveness analysis examining total and active life-expectancy outcome. *Journal of Clinical Oncology, 11,* 777–782.

Dranitsaris, G., & Hsu, T. (1999). Cost utility analysis of prophylactic pamidronate for the prevention of skeletal related events in patients with advanced breast cancer. *Support Care Cancer, 7,* 271–279.

Early Breast Cancer Trialists' Collaborative Group: Polychemotherapy for early breast cancer; an overview of the randomized trials. *Lancet, 352,* 930–942

Extermann, M. (2000).Pamidronate associated with high incremental costs per adverse event avoided in patients with metastatic breast cancer. Commentary. *Evidence-Based Oncology, 1,* 95–96.

Extermann, M., Balducci, L., & Lyman, G. H. (2000). What threshold for adjuvant therapy in older breast cancer patients? *Journal of Clinical Oncology, 18,* 1709–1717.

Fenn, P., McGuire, A., Backhouse, M., & Jones, M. (1996). Modeling programme cost in economic evaluation. *Journal of Health Economics, 15,* 115–125.

Frazier, A. L., Colditz, G. A., & Fuchs, C. S. (2000). Cost-effectiveness of screening for colorectal cancer in the general population. *Journal of the American Medical Association, 284,* 1954–1961.

Green, C., Brazier, J., & Deverill, M. (2000). Valuing health-related quality of life.

A review of health state evaluation technique. *Pharmacoeconomics, 17,* 151–165.

Hayman, J. A., Langa, K. M., Kabeto, M. U., Katz, S. J., DeMonner, S. M., Chernew, M. E., et al. (2001). Estimating the cost of informal caregiving for elderly patients with cancer. *Journal of Clinical Oncology, 19,* 3219–3225.

Hillner, B. E. (2000). Role of perspective and other uncertainties in cost-effectiveness assessments in advanced prostate cancer. *Journal of the National Cancer Institute, 92,* 1704–1706.

Hillner, B. E. (2001). Pharmacoeconomic issues in bisphosphonate treatment of metastatic bone disease. *Seminars in Oncology, 4* (suppl 11), 64–68.

Kerlikowske, K., Grady, D., Rubin, S. M., Sandrock, C., & Ernster, V. L. (1995). Efficacy of screening mammography. A meta-analysis. *Journal of the American Medical Association, 273,* 149–154.

Kerlikowske, K., Salzmann, P., Phillips, K. A., Crawely, J. A., & Cummings, S. R. (1999). Continuing screening mammography in women aged 70 to 79 years. *Journal of the American Medical Association, 282,* 2156–2163.

Kiebert, G. M., de Haes, J. C. J. M., & van der Velde, C. J. H. (1991). The impact of breast conserving treatment and mastectomy on the quality of life of early stage breast cancer patients: a review. *Journal of Clinical Oncology, 9,* 1059–1070.

Laupacis, A., Feeny, D., Detsky, A. S., & Tugwell, P. X. (1993). Tentative guidelines for using clinical and economic evaluation. *Canadian Medical Association Journal, 148,* 927–929.

Lyman, G. H., Lyman, C. G., Sanderson, R. A., & Balducci, L. (1993). Decision analysis of hematopoietic growth factor use in patients receiving cancer chemotherapy. *Journal of the National Cancer Institute, 85*(6), 488–493.

Lyman, G. H., Kuderer, N., Greene, J., & Balducci L. (1998). The economics of febrile neutropenia: implications for the use of colony-stimulating factors. *European Journal of Cancer, 34*(12), 1857–1864.

McCarthy, E. P., Burns, R. B., Freund, K. M., Ash, A. S., Shwartz, M., Marwill, S. L., et al. (2000). Mammography use, breast cancer stage at diagnosis, and survival among older women. *Journal of the American Geriatrics Society, 48,* 1226–1233.

Miller, A. B., To, T., Baines, C. J., & Wall, C. (2000). Canadian national breast screening study-2 13–year results of a randomized trial in women aged 50–59 years. *Journal of the National Cancer Institute, 92,* 1490–1499.

Mitra, I. (1994). Breast screening: the case for physical examination without mammography. *Lancet, 343,* 342–344.

Ravdin, P. M., Green, K. S., & Albain, V. Initial report of the SWOG correlative study of C-ERBB-2 expression as a predictor of outcome in a trial comparing adjuvant CAFT with tamoxifen (t) alone. *Proceedings of the American Society of Clinical Oncology, 97* a; A374.

Yancik, R., & Ries, L. A. G. (2000). Aging and cancer in America: demographic and epidemiologic perspectives. *Hematology/Oncology Clinics of North America, 14,* 17–24.

INDEX

Page numbers followed by *f* indicate figures. Page numbers followed by *t* indicate tables.

Exercise, 228

Facial changes, with aging, 74
FACT-G. *See* Functional Assessment
    in Cancer Therapy Scale
Failure to thrive, 33, 90
Falls, 33, 90
Family caregivers, CARE model,
    242–256
  case example, 252–253
Family members, elder, younger,
    proportions over time, 15*f*
Family of patient, during dying
    process, 202*t*
Farnesyl transferase inhibitors, 162
Fat intake, breast cancer, 48
Fatigue, 168–180
  with anemia, 189–190
  antineoplastic chemotherapy,
    172–173
  assessment of, 175–176
  cancer treatment and, 171–176
  fatigue diary, 172
  interventions for, 176
  measurement of, 173–175
    Cancer Related Fatigue Distress
      Scale, 175
    Functional Assessment of Can-
      cer Therapy-Anemia, 174
    Multidimensional Fatigue Symp-
      tom Inventory, 174–175
    Piper fatigue scale, 173–174
    Schwartz Cancer Fatigue Scale,
      174
  pathophysiology of, 170–171
  Piper fatigue scale, 173–174
  radiation therapy, 172–173
  biotherapy, 173
  surgery, 171–172
Fecal occult blood test, colon
    cancer, 57–58
Finasteride, 5 alpha reductase
    inhibitor, prostate cancer,
    53
Flexible sigmoidoscopy, 57
  colon cancer, 57
Fludarabine, 147, 153

Fluororacil, 147
Fluorouracil, 146
Folate deficiency, 182, 186
Folstein Minimental status, 33, 90
Fractures, bone, spontaneous, 33
Friends
  as domain of personhood, 194
  social support from, 225
Functional Assessment in Cancer
    Therapy Scale, 266
Functional Assessment of Cancer
    Therapy—Anemia, 174
Functional Living Index-Cancer, 266
Functional reserve, 93–97
Functional status, 33
Future, perceived, as domain of
    personhood, 194

Gastrointestinal system, changes in,
    with aging, 76
GDS. *See* Geriatric Depression Scale
Gender
  life expectancy, 10–14*t*
  probability of developing invasive
    cancers, by site, 16*t*
Generative imagination, 210
Gentuzumab ozogamicin, 161
Geriatric Depression Scale, 33, 90
Geriatric Quality of Life
    Questionnaire, 265
Glands, changes in, with aging, 77
Goals
  of health care decision, 120
  of prevention, treatment, 15
Guidance, as form of social support,
    227
Guilt, during dying process, 209
Gum, nicotine, smoking cessation,
    52

Habits preferences, as domain of
    personhood, 194
Hair, changes in, with aging, 77
Health care decision, 120–126
  measures of, 123–126
Health-care facility, limited access to,
    as barrier to screening, 27

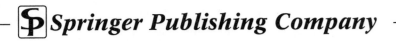
Springer Publishing Company

Persistent Pain in Older Adults

An Interdisciplinary Guide for Treatment

Debra K. Weiner, MD, Keela Herr, PhD, RN, and Thomas E. Rudy, PhD, Editors

Primary goals of this book are to increase awareness of the complexity involved when caring for older adults with persistent pain and to provide practitioners with the tools to approach complex management issues. Experts from many disciplines—including traditional and complementary medicine, nursing, psychology, and pharmacology provide evidence-based information and suggestions for treatment strategies.

The volume contains state-of-the-art clinically practical information and suggestions for treatment strategies aimed specifically at older adults. A valuable guidebook for geriatricians, nurses, psychologists, and advanced students.

PARTIAL CONTENTS:

- What is Unique About the Older Adults' Pain Experience? *S. W. Harkins*
- An Approach to Musculoskeletal Disorders, *M. Feletar, et al.*
- Functional Assessment and Outcomes, *J. C. Rogers and S. M. G. Gwinn*
- Pharmacologic Management: Noninvasive Modalities, *D. R. P. Guay, et al.*
- Invasive Pharmacologic and Non-Pharmacologic Modalities, *S. P. Lordon, et al.*
- Exercise Prescription, *M. J. Farrell, et al.*
- Complementary and Alternative Medicine Modalities, *L. A. Gerdner, et al.*
- Persistent Pain and Neuropsychological Function, *L. Morrow, et al.*
- The Ethics of Pain Management, *G. Kochersberger*
- An Approach to Reimbursement Issues, *R. McIlvried and P. Bonino*

2002   416pp   0-8261-3835-7   hard

536 Broadway, New York, NY 10012 • Fax (212) 941-7842
Order Toll-Free: (877) 687-7476 • Order on-line: www.springerpub.com